Encyclopedic Dictionary
of
YOGA

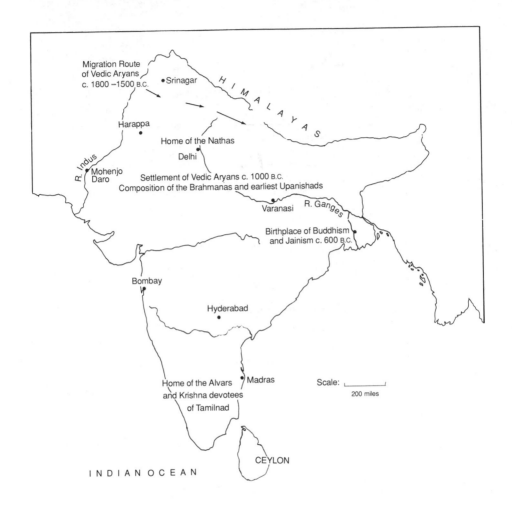

Migration Route
of Vedic Aryans
c. 1800 –1500 B.C.

• Srinagar

H I M A L A Y A S

Harappa
•

Home of the Nathas

Delhi
•

R. Indus

Mohenjo
Daro
•

Settlement of Vedic Aryans c. 1000 B.C.
Composition of the Brahmanas and earliest Upanishads

Varanasi
•

R. Ganges

Birthplace of Buddhism
and Jainism c. 600 B.C.
•

Bombay
•

Hyderabad
•

Home of the Alvars
and Krishna devotees
of Tamilnad

• Madras

Scale: └─────┘
      200 miles

CEYLON

I N D I A N   O C E A N

Map of India

THE PARAGON LIVING TRADITIONS SERIES, VOLUME ONE

Encyclopedic Dictionary

of

YOGA

GEORG FEUERSTEIN

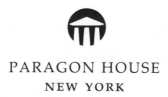

PARAGON HOUSE

NEW YORK

Ref.
181.45
F42e

First edition, 1990

Published in the United States by

Paragon House
90 Fifth Avenue
New York, NY 10011

Copyright © 1990 by Georg Feuerstein

Designed by Eve Kirch

Library of Congress Cataloging-in-Publication Data
Feuerstein, Georg.
Encyclopedic dictionary of Yoga / by Georg Feuerstein. — 1st ed.
    p.   cm. — (The Paragon living tradition series ; v. 1)
Includes bibliographical references.
ISBN 1-55778-244-X
1-55778-245-8 (pbk.)
1. Yoga—Dictionaries. I. Title. II. Series.
B132.Y6F46   1990   89-23068
181'.45'03—dc20   CIP

Manufactured in the United States of America

The paper used in this publication meets the minimum requirements of
American National Standard for Information Sciences—Permanence of Paper
for Printed Library Materials, ANSIZ39.48-1984.

The Paragon Living Traditions Series of Encyclopedic Dictionaries

We live in an age of spectacular contrasts. On the one hand, the scientific enterprise and its associated ideology of scientism (science as a quasi-religious tradition) has alienated countless people from their spiritual roots. On the other hand, never before in the history of humankind have so many religious and spiritual traditions coexisted relatively peacefully and with a growing awareness (except in the most fundamentalist quarters) that the Truth lies beyond doctrinal formulations. Cultural and religious pluralism is today offering people choices that did not exist before. At the same time, this bewildering range of possible life-styles and answers to life's big questions make such a choice difficult.

This series of encyclopedic dictionaries is intended to give the lay reader—and this is all of us outside our own narrow spheres of specialization—easily accessible and reliable information about major religious-philosophical-spiritual traditions. The purpose behind this series is not only to help those readers who are faced with a choice to choose more intelligently but also to encourage those who have made their choice to cultivate an attitude of tolerance, as well as to promote the ongoing dialogue between traditions. So long as we know only one tradition, we do not truly know any. Comparison helps to deepen our understanding and appreciation of our own tradition and another's way of life.

90–29491

ACKNOWLEDGMENTS

The author and the publishers would like to gratefully acknowledge the following sources for illustrations included in this volume. Every effort has been made to obtain permission for copyrighted material.

Illustrations #2, 11, 18, and 23: photographs reproduced by permission of Richard Lannoy, Bath, England;

Illustrations # 8, 10, 13, 16, 32, 41, 47, 62, 66, 74, 75, 76, and 82: photographs reproduced by permission of Reinhard Gammenthaler, Berne, Switzerland;

Illustrations #7 and 38: photographs from *Slaves of the Lord* by Vidya Dehejia. Reproduced by permission of Munshiram Manoharlal, New Delhi;

Illustration #19: photograph from *Patanjali & Yoga* by Mircea Eliade. French Edition copyright 1969 by Funk & Wagnals. Reproduced by permission of Schocken Books, published by Pantheon Books, a division of Random House, Inc.;

Illustrations #24 and 25: photographs from *India in Pictures* by Eugen Kusch. Reproduced by permission of Verlag Hans Carl, Nuremberg, West Germany;

Illustration #28: photograph reproduced by permission of G. Eleanore Murray, Calimesa, California

Illustrations #46, 57, 67, 70, and 72: photographs from *The Complete Illustrated Book of Yoga* by Swami Vishnudevananda. Copyright 1988 by Harmony Books. Reproduced by permission of Harmony Books, a division of Crown Publishers, Inc.;

Illustration #55: photograph of an illuminated manuscript page of the Ramayana. Reproduced by permission of Freer Gallery of Art, Washington, DC;

Photograph of Gopi Krishna. Reproduced by permission of Gene Kieffer, Kundalini Research Foundation, Darien, CT;

Photograph of Paramahansa Yogananda. Reproduced by permission of Self-Realization Fellowship, Los Angeles;

Photographs of Sri Ramakrishna and Swami Vivekananda. Reproduced by permission of Ramakrishna-Vivekananda Center, New York;

Illustrations #6, 30, 71, and 84: photographs from *Tantra* by Philip Rawson. Published by Thames and Hudson, London;

Illustration #44: photograph from *Yoga Art* by Ajit Mookerjee. Published by Thames and Hudson, London;

Illustration #58: drawing from *Kali* by Ajit Mookerjee. Published by Thames and Hudson, London;

Illustration #29: drawing from *Tools For Tantra* by Harish Johari. Published by Inner Traditions International, Rochester, Vermont;

Illustrations #15 and 20: photographs from *Indian Sculpture* by W. and B. Forman. Published by Spring Books, London;

Illustration #33: *Eine durch Miniaturen erlauterte Doctrina Mystica* by Fausta Nowotny. Published by Mouton & Co., The Hague, Netherlands;

Illustration #14: drawing from *Sri Caitanya* by Tridandi Svami. Published by Oxford & IBH Publishing Co., New Delhi;

Illustrations #26, 53, and 73: photographs from *Gheranda-Samhita* edited by Swami Digambarji and M. L. Gharote. Published by Kaivalyadhama S. M. Y. M. Samiti, Lonavla, India;

Illustration #52: photograph from *A Reappraisal of Yoga* by Georg Feuerstein and Jeanine Miller. Published by Rider & Co., London;

Illustration #77: photograph from *Introduction to the Bhagavad-Gita* by Georg Feuerstein. Published by Rider & Co., London.

CONTENTS

PREFACE

Yoga is an immensely rich and highly complex spiritual tradition. It comprises a great many approaches, schools, teachers, and technical vocabularies. In view of its sheer versatility and long history of nearly three thousand years, Yoga must be counted as the world's foremost tradition of psychospiritual transformation. Although there are numerous books available on Yoga, very few reflect that astounding richness. Over the years, I have endeavored to convey some of the subtleties of the different yogic paths in my various publications.

The present encyclopedic dictionary is another effort of mine to give an authentic portrayal of the Yoga tradition and to unlock its wealth for Western practitioners, historians of religion, and Indologists. There are several dictionaries of Yoga in existence, but these are either too obscure and not readily available or they are inadequate and unreliable. In the former category belongs the *Yoga Kośa* compiled by Swami Digambarji and Dr. Mahajot Sahai. It was published in 1972 by the Kaivalyadhama S. M. Y. M. Samiti in Lonavla, Poona, India. While this compilation contains many valuable and detailed references, its scope is limited, and its organization is such that only Sanskritists can benefit from it. Another noteworthy publication is Dr. Ram Kumar Rai's *Encyclopedia of Yoga*, which was first published in 1975 by Prachya Prakashan, Varanasi, India. Like the *Yoga Kośa*, this compilation lists the entries in Sanskrit alphabetical order and is therefore relatively inaccessible to the lay reader. Also, the selection of concepts is somewhat uneven and the descriptions are occasionally digressive. Neither dictionary contains English entries or cross-references. Among the popular dictionaries, mention must be made of Ernest Wood's *Yoga Wisdom*, published in 1970 by the Philosophical Library. This book has only some three hundred entries, which are not always accurate. Slightly bigger but suffering from the same shortcoming is Harvey Days's *Yoga Illustrated Dictionary*, published in 1971 by Kaye & Ward, London.

The idea of preparing a dictionary that would combine comprehensiveness with accessibility occurred to me almost ten years ago. I was then offered a contract by an English publishing house for a compilation of seven hundred pages, an ambitious project by any standards. Alas, the worsening economic situation in Britain forced my publisher into near bankruptcy and to cancel their contract with me. Manchester University was interested in taking on the project but failed to find an American copublisher to share the prohibitive costs. I was obliged to abandon the project. Then, in 1988, I decided to offer a much abbreviated version of the dictionary to Paragon House and was delighted when a contract for the book came through. As I was working on the dictionary, however, I realized that the agreed-on length of eighty thousand words was simply inadequate to do justice to the Yoga tradition. I ended up more than doubling the length of the manuscript. Fortunately, my intention to produce a more substantial dictionary was welcomed by my publisher, and I believe that their decision to allow me to go ahead with an expanded version will serve both lay readers and professional users of this work.

This dictionary is arranged and written in such a way that, despite the wealth of detail given, it will inform rather than overwhelm the lay reader, while at the same time providing valuable references for the professional Yoga researcher and historian of religion. This compilation can usefully be consulted in conjunction with the technical dictionaries mentioned above. Yet it has several unique features, which make it an encyclopedic dictionary rather than a mere word list. First, each entry is carefully cross-referenced (as indicated by asterisks), so that the reader can follow up on pertinent conceptual linkages. Second, there are a fair number of orientational entries that furnish the reader with an overview of a given aspect of the Yoga tradition, such as its history, psychology, or major branches. Third, the entries are all in English alphabetical order and, moreover, include key words in English, with references to their Sanskrit equivalents or other relevant Sanskrit concepts.

This is not a concordance. Therefore, scholars should not look for an exhaustive listing of occurrences of a given term. The idea behind this dictionary is to provide a selective range of concepts sufficient to give an authoritative coverage of the many aspects of Yoga theory and practice and to provide valuable guidelines for further research. I have inevitably covered some of the Yoga scriptures more thoroughly than others. This was dictated partly by their relative importance and partly by my own research interests. It remains for future generations of Indologists to compile a more comprehensive encyclopedia based on the minutiae of research. I believe that this dictionary will make such a task somewhat easier.

I have spent long days during the months of February to August 1989 converting my notes and ideas into a publishable manuscript. Computer technology, luckily, made this mountainous task somewhat more manageable.

I would like to express my heartfelt thanks to all those many friends, colleagues, and correspondents who over the years have furthered my interest in Yoga and spiritual life in general. I have already named some of them in my previous books. Here I specifically wish to thank the late Professor Mircea Eliade, one of the giants of Yoga research and comparative religion, for giving me encouragement when it was most needed; Dr. Tony Alston for his exemplary studies on Vedānta and various kindnesses during the past ten years; Dr. Lance Cousin, of Manchester University, England, for his academic feedback on part of the early manuscript; Ray Offord, of Manchester University Press, for continuing to express an interest in this dictionary over the years, which finally prompted me to resume work on it where I had left off ten years earlier; Reinhart Gammenthaler, a Swiss citizen who is an initiate of *hatha-yoga*, for supplying this volume with fine photographs of many of the more intriguing Yoga postures; Lydia de Pole for executing some of the drawings; Kenneth Stuart, editor-in-chief of Paragon House for adopting my idea of the Paragon Living Traditions series of dictionaries, launched by the present work; Don Fehr, my editor, for his patience and unfailing kindness; and not least my wife, Trisha, for lovingly cheerleading me through the final stages of this compilation, which at times seemed endless, and for relieving me of some of my other tasks.

Ever since my first encounter with the world of Yoga some twenty-five years ago, Yoga has claimed my attention again and again, both personally and professionally. I am greatly indebted to the masters of ancient and modern times, who have taught me much. I like to think of this dictionary as a small token of my appreciation and gratitude, and as my contribution to keep the tradition of authentic Yoga alive.

Georg Feuerstein
August 1989
Northern California

Note on the Transliteration and Pronunciation of Sanskrit

For the convenience of the lay reader, I have adopted a simplified form of transliterating Sanskrit words. Of the various diacritical marks used to indicate sounds that have no corresponding equivalents in the English alphabet, I have retained only macrons (the dash on top of the vowels *a*, *i*, and *u*). This sign indicates that a vowel is to be lengthened. Thus, the word *rāja* in *rāja-yoga*, for instance, is pronounced *rahja*.

Vowel sounds in Sanskrit have an open pronunciation. For example, *yoga* is not pronounced as if the *o* were followed by a *u*, but the *o* is similar to the *o*-sound in *jogurt*. Likewise, the long *ī* in the words *īshvara* ("lord") is pronounced *eeshvara*, not with an *i*-sound as in the name Isaac. The word *kundalinī*, which occurs frequently in this dictionary, is pronounced *koondaleenee*, with all vowels except for the final *ī* being short.

The Sanskrit language has no *th*-sound. Thus, the word *hatha-yoga* ("forceful Yoga") is pronounced as *hat-ha yoga*. The same is the case with all other syllables containing an *h*-sound, viz., *gha, kha, jha, cha, dha, bha*, and *pha*. In other words, to give one more example, the term *phala* ("fruit, result") is not pronounced *fala* but *p-hala*.

INTRODUCTION

Yoga is one of the most remarkable accomplishments of human ingenuity and surely one of the most fascinating products of spiritual aspiration. It is India's mature answer to the universal question "Who am I?"—a question that, sooner or later, will impinge on any self-inspecting individual. When our belly is full and when we have achieved our ambitions and are supposed to be happy and content, we may suddenly be overcome by a great restlessness and a feeling of emptiness. We begin to realize that we are strangers to ourselves. This crisis, which often strikes in the middle of life but which can also announce itself much sooner, either leads to resignation and an emotional landslide toward old age, or to a passionate quest for self-understanding through which we can discover and renew ourselves.

Our modern science-oriented civilization discourages spirituality and deeper existential questioning. The Christian religion has to a large extent become synonymous with morality; the mystical impulse within it has all but been forgotten. Hence, in our century, millions of sensitive Western men and women have turned to the East for spiritual nourishment and guidance. In their quest, many have discovered Yoga and have been greatly enriched by that encounter. For some, Yoga has strengthened their Christian faith. For others, it has led to a spirituality that transcends ideological leanings as far as this is possible. A few have taken the plunge into the doctrinal structure of Hinduism.

Yoga is an esoteric tradition within the versatile religious culture of Hinduism. It is one of the world's oldest branches of spiritual inquiry, and surely the longest and most intense experiment of the human spirit. The purpose of the yogic experiment has been to explore not the behavior of matter but the very limits of consciousness. For, the Indians realized early on that consciousness has primacy over matter—a notion that is gradually being resuscitated through the efforts of avant-garde quantum physics and parapsychology. What is more, that experiment is continuing even today; notwithstanding India's creeping secularization, Yoga adepts and schools have so far held their own. More importantly, Yoga has definitely arrived in the Occident and is undergoing a promising revival at the hand of creative Western teachers of this ancient discipline.

The Sanskrit word *yoga*, we are told in countless books, means "union." This is only half the truth. Its closest literal equivalent in the English language is "yoke." Yoga is the art of yoking the "lower" (or ego) personality to the "higher" Truth, of disciplining the body-mind so that it becomes fitted to Reality. The earliest and most popular Yoga book is the *Bhagavad-Gītā* ("Lord's Song"). This beautiful pre-Christian scripture, composed in melodious Sanskrit, defines Yoga as "balance" or "equanimity" (*samatva*). Such balance is the result of controlling the mind, or attention, which seems naturally disposed to flit hither and thither. Yoga is centering—the center being the transcendental Being, whether it be called God or higher Self. Thus, the word *yoga* signifies both the state of harmony and the means of realizing it. The underlying idea is that we can only truly be ourselves when we go beyond the ego-self, beyond what we normally believe ourselves to be: a man or a woman, a parent, a professional, owner of a car and a suburb home, happy or sad, witty or boring, chatty or reserved. Our essential nature is none of these things. It is pure Being-Consciousness. When our life is balanced and our mind enjoys equanimity, we feel closer to this truth.

Yoga is a whole way of life lived in the light of that pure Being-Consciousness that is our authentic identity. It is not simply a body of exercises or a set of ideas. It is the theory *and* practice of centering, of harnessing the body-mind so that it permits Being-Consciousness to manifest itself in and through us.

Yoga has a history of nearly 3,000 years, as compared to 2,000 years of Christianity and perhaps 250 years of "modern" secular civilization. Its taproot lies in archaic shamanism, and its long evolution is tied to the gradual unfolding of the plural cultures of India, notably Hinduism, Buddhism, and Jainism. As I have shown in my book *Yoga: The Technology of Ecstasy*, which traces the history of the various branches and schools of Yoga, the earliest faintly yogic ideas and practices are to be found in the sacred in canon of Hinduism—the Vedas. Mystical and psychocosmological speculations are present already in the *Rig-Veda*, a collection of Sanskrit hymns "seen" by the seers of yore. In its oldest portions, this hymnody may date back to about 1500 B.C. This date coincides with the final days of the great Indus civilization, whose archaeological remains also include some evidence suggestive of yoga-like notions. Other, more concrete speculations and practices of a proto-yogic type can be found in the *Atharva-Veda*, a collection that abounds in magical incantations, which is younger by a few hundred years.

Those early endeavors to explore the possibilities of the human spirit, remarkable as they are, can only barely be called Yoga. But they form the nucleus for the diversified psychotechnology that has come to be associated with the name of Yoga. Strictly speaking, they are still characteristic of the tradition of asceticism (*tapas*), which marks the dawn of religion and spirituality in India, as elsewhere. The ascetic, or *tapasvin*, aspires to gain control over the powers (or deities) animating the universe.

By contrast, the *yogin* is primarily (and ideally) concerned with the transcendence of the ego, the gods, and the world as a whole. His grand ideal is liberation, variously styled *moksha*, *mukti*, *kaivalya*, *apavarga*, and *nirvāna*, What is liberation? There is no unanimity among the different schools of esotericism. However, their answers are sufficiently similar to provide us with a workable definition: Liberation is the condition of radical freedom, in consciousness, from the bonds of the conditional personality with its ingrained habit patterns, relative unawareness, and fundamental lovelessness. It is, at the same time, the condition of pure Consciousness, unaffected by the fluctuations of the mind—one's ever-changing opinions and moods. Fundamental to liberation is the shift from the ego-identity to the Self-identity: The liberated adept (*mukta-siddha*) no longer experiences his or her body-mind as an impenetrable boundary of awareness. Rather, standing firmly in pure Consciousness (*cit*), he or she experiences the body-mind as arising in that Consciousness. Regardless of the different metaphysical positions that have been elaborated in the course of the long evolution of Yoga, this pure Consciousness—the transcendental Witness (*sākshin*)—is the common denominator. It is called *ātman* ("Self") in the Sanskrit scriptures. It is our innermost Essence, just as it is the deepest Foundation of the cosmos.

This Self cannot be experienced. It can, however, be realized. That is to say, a person can "awaken" as that Self. Self-realization is widely held to be utterly blissful. But this is only to say that it is the antithesis of the ordinary ego-identity, which, because of its inherent limitation (in space and time), is inevitably associated with the experience of pain and suffering. Self-realization is not pleasurable, for pleasure—like pain—is only something the ego-personality can experience. The Self does not get caught up in experiences. It simply notices ("witnesses") their occurrence in the body-mind, rather as the peak of a high mountain abides forever above the good and bad weather of the lower regions.

This does not mean, however, that the Self-realized sage is an unfeeling monstrosity. On the contrary, Patanjali, the founder of Classical Yoga, describes such a one as being acutely sensitive, "like an eyeball." The reason for this sensitivity is best summed up in the words of the Latin writer: *Homo sum, humani nihil a me alienum puto*, "I am human; I count nothing human as foreign to me."

The Yoga adept arrives at Self-realization only after a long struggle with the human condition. In the course of that personal ordeal, he or she has had to face all the numerous liabilities and weaknesses associated with being human. Having transcended them by transcending the ego, he or she can now look upon others with compassion. He or she understands that those who are still struggling with themselves and with existence at large are also on a journey of self-discovery—and Self-discovery. Though their pace may be slow and hesitant, and they may not even be aware of their journey, they, too, are already liberated, already free. Of course, the sage no longer exclaims: *Homo sum*, "I am human." Rather, his confession is: *Aham brahma asmi*, "I am the Absolute." I am the transcendental Self. Yet, his transcendence of the human condition peculiarly capacitates him to empathize with those who persist in identifying with the body-mind rather than the Self.

Observing their confusion, uncertainty, dis-ease, and actual physical and mental suffering, the sage feels compelled to communicate the gospel of humanity's essential freedom. Alas, the noise of our technological civilization has deafened our ears to the gentle but persuasive song of the bearers of wisdom of bygone ages and of our own time.

Notwithstanding its noblest discovery—the existence of the Self beyond the vicissitudes of the body-mind—the tradition of Yoga has retained many features of the antecedent tradition of asceticism. Thus, the *yogin* is typically celebrated as a possessor not only of wisdom but also of paranormal powers (*siddhi*). To the ordinary Indian, he is a knower and a miracle worker. This is in keeping with what we know of other spiritual traditions. Holiness and power go hand in hand. Even the mature *yogin* who has not yet realized the Self is thought to possess mysterious abilities that place him above ordinary persons.

But the practitioner of Yoga is frequently warned not to abuse that power, and sometimes even not to use it at all, lest it should distract him from the spiritual path. The exercise of power of any kind is fraught with danger, since it is apt to feed the ego and lure it away from the great ideal of liberation, which essentially consists in ego-transcendence. Once the Self is realized, powers of all kinds are said to become spontaneously available to the adept, and without endangering his or her hard-won freedom. The genuine *yogin* will always treat the paranormal powers and power in general with great circumspection. His prime motive is to constantly step beyond the self, until the Self is realized. And when the Self has been realized, self-transcendence continues as a spontaneous act.

In most schools of Yoga, Self-realization means the realization of the singular Self (*ātman*), the universal essence of Selfhood. This is a suprapersonal event, for, the Self exists beyond the particular configuration of one's personality. It is the same Self in all beings. This idea is fundamental to the various schools of Advaita-Vedānta, or Hindu nondualism. In its formative phase, Yoga was closely aligned with the ramifying metaphysical tradition of Vedānta, as expounded in the Upanishads. The oldest scriptures of this literary genre belong to the eighth century B.C. They teach a pantheism or, better, pan-en-theism: There is only one Reality, the *brahman*, which is experienced as the multiform cosmos by unenlightened beings. Through proper initiation, renunciation, and meditation, the spiritual aspirant can realize the prior singular Reality beyond the mind and the senses. For that Reality is not only the Ground of objective existence; it is also a person's true identity, the transcendental Self (*ātman*). The idealist doctrine of the identity of the *brahman* with the *ātman* is the quintessential notion common to all Upanishadic or Vedntic thought. The Yoga tradition evolved out of these metaphysical speculations and their attendant spiritual disciplines.

Yoga was originally also most intimately associated with the Sāmkhya tradition, which is marked by a realist philosophy with a strong cosmological bent. Sāmkhya is concerned with defining the categories of existence, as they emerge in hierarchic order out of the perennial World-Ground called *prakriti* ("procreatrix"). Beyond the World-Ground and its psychomaterial evolutes stands the primal Person, the *purusha*, or pure Consciousness. Vedānta, Yoga, and Sāmkhya together formed the intellectual milieu of Upanishadic times—the milieu into which Gautama the Buddha was born.

His teaching, which has sometimes been looked upon as a pragmatic version of Yoga, is founded in a rejection of metaphysical speculation, especially the notion of an eternal Self (*ātman*). Instead, the Buddha emphasized practical discipline—his noble eightfold path to liberation—to countermand the ever-present tendency to theorize about spiritual life rather than to engage it. A similar discipline-oriented approach characterizes the teaching of Vārdhamana Mahāvīra, the founder of historical Jainism, who was an older contemporary of the Buddha. Both Buddhism and Jainism, the other two great religious cultures spawned on Indian soil next to Hinduism, had a strong influence on the further evolution of Yoga. Particularly Mahāyāna Buddhism influenced the philosophical formulation of Yoga under Patanjali, who seems to have lived in the second century A.D.

Yoga is first clearly spoken of in the *Katha-Upanishad*, which was probably composed in the fifth or sixth century B.C. This work propounds what is called *adhyātma-yoga*, the "Yoga of the inmost self," by which the sage may come to know the great God hidden in the cave of the heart. Then, in the third century B.C., the anonymous composer of the *Bhagavad-Gītā*—the New Testament of Hinduism—made a unique attempt at integrating the various yogic approaches then current. Most importantly, the *Gītā* introduced the ideal of devotion (*bhakti*) to the Divine as a "super-person" (*purusha-uttama*), thus instituting the path of *bhakti-yoga*, which quickly gained great popularity.

However, it was Patanjali's *Yoga-Sūtra* ("Aphorisms of Yoga") that gave Yoga its classical form as one of the six philosophical "viewpoints" (*darshana*) of Hinduism. Although Patanjali's work was very influential, since it proffered valuable definitions of the fundamental concepts of the yogic path, his metaphysical dualism was never looked upon favorably within mainstream Hinduism. Notwithstanding the fact that Patanjali's school came to be regarded as *the* philosophy of Yoga, many other yogic schools continued to exist and flourish alongside of it.

These non-Classical schools of Yoga retained their Vedntic (nondualist) foundations and in the course of time led to the fascinating developments of Post-Classical Yoga. The schools of Post-Classical Yoga show a marked Tantric influence. Tantrism, which originated in the early post-Christian era and gathered momentum in the sixth century A.D., is a pan-Indian syncretic movement that greatly transformed Hinduism and Buddhism and to a lesser extent also Jainism. Because of its enormous breadth, Tantrism is very difficult to define. It is more a cultural style than a philosophy, and from the outset purported to be *the* teaching for the present "dark age" (*kāli-yuga*), which commenced with the death of the God-man Krishna, supposedly in 3006 B.C.

In simplified terms, Tantrism translated the ancient panentheistic intuition that the world arises in the all-encompassing Being into ritual action and a deep philosophical understanding. It elevated the age-old popular belief in the Divine as Female, or *shakti*, to a metaphysical principle of the first order. This resulted in a certain reevaluation of the female gender, but primarily it led to a reappraisal of the body as a manifestation of the Divine and thus as a positive instrument for attaining liberation.

An important tradition within Tantrism is the Siddha movement, dating back to the sixth century A.D. A *siddha* is a spiritual adept who has attained perfection (*siddhi*) through a transubstantiated body endowed with all kinds of paranormal powers (*siddhi*). Out of this tradition of "body cultivation" (*kāya-sādhana*) grew the different schools of the "forceful Yoga" (*hatha-yoga*). The origins of *hatha-yoga* are quite obscure but are traditionally connected to the name of Gorakshanātha, a tenth-century master.

The teachers of *hatha-yoga* have created important manuals, some of which are still extant and in use today. These show an astonishing variety of techniques for manipulating the life force (*prāna*) of the human body, primarily by means of breath control and mental concentration. The idea behind these practices is that a strong and healthy body is needed to gain liberation, or enlightenment, and to manifest its paranormal effects. In the course of time, many *hatha-yogins* lost sight of the spiritual goal of this tradition and focused more on its therapeutic and prophylactic aspects, or exploited it as a means for cultivating paranormal abilities. Hence *hatha-yoga* fell into disrepute, especially among the more educated classes of Hindu and Buddhist society, who favored a more meditative and intellectual approach.

There are today several million people who practice one or the other form of Yoga—from the physical exercises of *hatha-yoga* to the mental disciplines of *rāja-yoga*; to the mysterious *kundalinī-yoga*, which seeks to control the vast psychophysical powerhouse of the body; to the seemingly glamorous but difficult orientation of *tantra-yoga*, with its manipulation of the sexual drive; to the approach of the heart favored in *bhakti-yoga*; to the conscious execution of actions, which is the essence of *karma-yoga*.

Many Western practitioners are simply in search of health, beauty, longevity, and a more meaningful life. Medical research on *hatha-yoga* has shown that many of its techniques are remarkably potent therapeutic instruments. They can restore health to an ailing body; they can, to some extent, slow the aging process; they can even reverse some of its effects. Meditation is demonstrably a wonderful tool for cultivating equanimity. Perhaps the best known approach is that of "Transcendental Meditation," introduced to the West by Maharshi Mahesh Yogi in the late 1960s. Behind this designation lies an ancient method—the meditative recitation of sacred syllables known as *mantra-yoga*. Research on TM practitioners has shown that they derive all kinds of physical and mental benefits from this method. Some of the findings and conclusions have possibly been somewhat exaggerated, from an understandable enthusiasm. But, in substance, they confirmed what *yogins* have claimed for many centuries, namely that Yoga is a powerful transformative approach. Modern research on Yoga has also brought home the fact that the *yogins* were first-class experimenters with a keen understanding of the interaction between consciousness and the body. Very many aspects of Yoga practice still await open-minded scientific exploration.

In the meantime, Yoga has become part of the cultural kaleidoscope of the Western world. This has prompted C. G. Jung, among others, to caution against any simplistic imitation of Eastern traditions. His warning is valid. However, what we encounter as Yoga in the West are mostly adopted and adapted forms, unfortunate popularizations that distort the intention behind Yoga and hence no doubt also diminish the effectiveness of the original methods and approaches. But there are also genuine approaches that combine ancient yogic wisdom with modern medical and psychological knowledge.

The neophyte is advised to make every effort to inform himself or herself about the tradition of Yoga before embarking on any approach or before choosing a teacher or instructor. My book *Yoga: The Technology of Ecstasy* and the present work contain ample material for this kind of preliminary study. In fact, I venture to suggest, both books can serve as trustworthy companions for even more seasoned travelers on the yogic path.

An important question for the serious student of Eastern traditions is whether the initiatory nature of authentic Yoga is a possibility for Westerners. Traditional Yoga is typically transmitted by a qualified teacher (*guru*). Can Westerners benefit from a pupilage involving a *guru*? There is no way of answering this question briefly, without running the risk of inviting misunderstanding or reinforcing existing prejudices, whether they be for or against the figure of the *guru*. I have addressed this question in some depth—from a historical, a psychological, and an experiential point of view—in my book *Crazy Wisdom: The Outer Limits of Religion and Morality*, also published by Paragon House. The only advice worth giving in this context is to use good common sense and to trust one's bodily felt wisdom, and to continue to do so after one has reached a decision.

What remains to be said is that Yoga has survived for over two thousand years, mainly through being skillfully adapted to different historical and cultural contexts. There is every indication that it will continue to be with us. It seems desirable to try to understand it so that we can benefit from the cumulative wisdom of its practitioners in our modern quest for self-definition. This encyclopedic dictionary is an attempt to make such an understanding possible—both for practitioners of Yoga and others who care to comprehend this tradition as part of the complexity of our pluralistic society.

Orientation for the Lay Reader

This encyclopedic dictionary covers a considerable amount of information about the Yoga tradition. There are a number of entries that furnish valuable overviews, containing references to specific subcategories. Thus, the reader unacquainted with Yoga may profitably first consult the following entries: *Hinduism, Yoga, Classical Yoga, History, Psychology, Parapsychology, Divine, Freedom, Guru*. These entries contain sufficient references to guide the reader to the next conceptual level in understanding this rather complex tradition. For instance, he or she may next want to look up the descriptions given of the different major branches of Yoga, such as *rāja-yoga* ("royal Yoga"), *hatha-yoga* ("forceful Yoga"), *bhakti-yoga* ("Yoga of love"), *karma-yoga* ("Yoga of action") and *mantra-yoga* ("yoga of sound").

Encyclopedic
Dictionary
of
YOGA

Abandonment. In ancient India, there was a prominent trend toward leaving the conventional world and living an ascetic life in the seclusion of forests and caves. This movement of world renunciation (called *tyāga* or *samnyāsa*) started about 800 B.C., and the *Upanishads are an early reflection of this emerging ideal. That movement soon had grown strong enough to become a social problem. In response, the Hindu lawgivers invented the ideal of the stages of life (*āshrama*). According to this social model, a person had to complete the student and

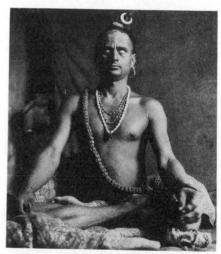

2. *Hindu renouncer (samnyāsin).*

householder (*grihastha*) stage before he or she could retire from the world. See also *vairāgya*.

abhāva-yoga ("Yoga of nonbeing") is a compound found in some of the *Purānas. The *Kūrma-Purāna (II.11.6), for instance, understands it thus: "[That method] in which one contemplates [one's] essence as void and [yet] all-illuminating, and by which one beholds the Self is called the 'Yoga of nonbeing.' " A similar definition is given in the *Linga-Purāna (II.55.14), where it is said to effect the *mind's extinction (*citta-nirvāna*). The *Shiva-Purāna* (VII.2.37.10), again, explains it as that in which the *world is contemplated without any perception of *objects. This appears to be the equivalent of supraconscious enstasy (*asamprajnāta-samādhi*). Cf. *bhāva-yoga*.

abhaya ("fearlessness"). Fear is integral to individuated human existence. As the ancient *Brihadāranyaka-Upanishad* (I.4.2) puts it: "Fear arises when there is an other." Fearlessness is the fruit of perfect *Self-realization, or *enlightenment (*bodha*), that is, the recovery of non-duality. Cf. *bhaya*.

abhaya-mudrā ("seal of fearlessness"). This is one of the classical hand gestures found in Mahāyāna *Buddhist and *Tantric iconography. It is used by *adepts to dispel fear (*bhaya*) in others. All fear is groundless, for our true nature is unalloyed bliss (*ānanda*). See also *mudrā*.

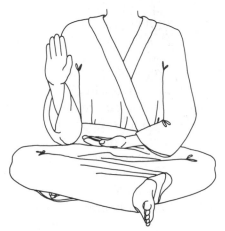

abhimāna ("pride") a function of the "inner organ" (*antahkarana*), or psyche. It must be overcome through insight into the fact that one is not identical with the ego-personality. See also *darpa*.

3. *Abhaya-mudrā, hand gesture bestowing fearlessness.*

Abhinava Gupta was born in the middle of the tenth century A.D., was regarded as an *incarnation of *Shesha and widely hailed as a miracle worker. He is the most renowned scholar and *adept of Kashmiri *Shaivism, demonstrating that intellect and spiritual virtuosity are not necessarily in conflict. Legend has it that he went into a remote cave with twelve hundred of his disciples, never to be seen again. Abhinava Gupta has left behind numerous writings, and his most famous work is the voluminous *Tantra-Āloka* ("Luster of *Tantra"), which is a systematic presentation of the teachings of the *Kaula sect and *Tantrism.

abhinivesha ("will to live"). According to *Classical Yoga, the will to live, or thirst for life, is one of the five causes of suffering (*klesha*). *Patanjali, the author of the *Yoga-Sūtra* (II.9) observes: "The thirst for life flowing on by its own nature is rooted even in the sage." Ultimately, *abhinivesha* springs from spiritual ignorance (*avidyā*), whereby a person wrongly identifies with the body and becomes subject to the survival instinct. See also *trishnā*.

abhisheka, or the "sprinkling" of water, is often used in yogic ceremonial contexts, particularly in *Tantrism. It is a ritual of empowerment, a form of initiatory baptism, by which the aspirant's spiritual endeavors are blessed. The term is also used to denote initiation in general. See also *dīkshā*.

abhyāsa. "Practice," or practical application (*exercitium*), is one of two essential aspects of spiritual life; the other is dispassion (*vairāgya*), or renunciation. The *Yoga-Bhāshya* (I.12), the oldest extant commentary on the *Yoga-Sūtra*, compares the *mind, or psyche, to a stream that can flow in two directions. One starts with spiritual ignorance and ends in evil (i.e., *rebirth), the other starts with discrimination and ends in what is good (i.e., *liberation). The latter is governed by renunciation, which checks the outflow of *attention toward worldly objects, and the practice of discrimination (*viveka*), which opens higher evolutionary possibilities. The *Shiva-Samhitā* (IV.9), a late *hatha-yoga text, declares: "Through practice comes perfection; through practice one will attain liberation."

abhyāsin ("practitioner") is a synonym for *yogin or *sādhaka. The feminine form is *abhyāsinī*.

Absolute. All spiritual traditions of India recognize the existence of an ultimate, transcendental *Reality, though different schools propose different conceptions of it. Most are agreed that the Absolute is without qualities and is supramaterial, supraconscious, and suprapersonal. All these traditions insist that the Absolute is identical to the very essence of the human being, the *Self, and is realizable as such by transcending the *mind. However, they offer different speculations about the relationship between the Absolute and that innermost essence. The most radical solution is that of *Advaita-Vedānta, which sees no distinction whatsoever between the Absolute (*brahman*) and the essential aspect of the psyche, the transcendental *Self (*ātman*). In *Classical Yoga, however, many such essential Selves (*purusha*) are supposed to exist, and one of them is unique in that It has never been, nor ever will be, subject to the illusion of *embodiment. That special Self is called the "Lord" (*īshvara*), the equivalent of *God in *Patanjali's Yoga.

Absorption. The ability to allow *attention to become absorbed in the object of contemplation is fundamental to all schools of *Yoga. Meditative absorption (*dhyāna) is a more advanced stage of concentration (*dhāranā), because of the degree of sensory inhibition that is involved. See also *laya*.

Abstinence. The voluntary disciplining of the sexual drive is a very important practice in most traditional schools of spirituality, including *Yoga and *Tantra. It is considered a primary means of accumulating psychospiritual energy in the *body, which is then employed to focus the *mind on spiritual goals. See also *brahmacarya*, Sexuality.

abuddha ("unawakened"). In some schools of *Preclassical Yoga, this term denotes the transcendental *Self, which is called *budhyamāna. See also *apratibuddha*.

ācāra ("conduct"). Apart from having the general meaning of "behavior," this word is also a technical term standing for a particular approach to *Self-realization. Thus, in *Tantrism a distinction is made between a "right-hand approach" (*dakshina-ācāra) and a "left-hand approach" (*vāma-ācāra). Whereas the former orientation employs mainstream methods, the latter is unconventional insofar as it makes use of *sexuality, alcohol, and other similar means that are controversial in the context of spiritual practice.

In the *Kula-Arnava-Tantra (II), seven ways of life are distinguished in ascending order: (1) the *veda-ācāra* (the Vedic way of rituals); (2) the *vaishnava-ācāra* (the way of the *Vishnu worshippers); (3) the *shaiva-ācāra* (the way of the *Shiva worshippers); (4) the *dakshina-ācāra* (the right-hand way); (5) the *vāma-ācāra* (the left-hand way); (6) the *siddhānta-ācāra* (the doctrinal way); and (7) the *kula-ācāra* (the way of *kula, which is the feminine principle, or *shakti). The *kula-ācāra* is hailed as the most excellent and most secret of all approaches to *Self-realization. See also Kaula sect.

ācārya ("preceptor"). *Yoga is traditionally an initiatory teaching, handed down from *teacher to *pupil by word of mouth. The preceptor is a teacher who may or may not have the function of a *guru, or spiritual guide proper. Sometimes the two terms are used interchangeably. The *Brahma-Vidyā-Upanishad (51–52), which is one of the *Yoga-Upanishads, distinguishes three kinds of preceptors: the "prompter" (*codaka*), the "awakener" (*bodhaka*), and the "bestower of *liberation" (*moksha-da*). The *Mahābhārata* epic (XII.313.23) likens the preceptor to a ferryman, and his knowledge to a ferry. See also *upādhyāya*.

ācārya-sevana ("service to the preceptor") is sometimes considered among the practices of self-discipline (*niyama*). See also *guru-sevā, sevā*.

ācārya-upāsana ("veneration of the preceptor"). Because of the central importance given to the *teacher in the yogic tradition, all schools emphasize that the pupil (*shishya*) must assume a reverential attitude toward the teacher, without which spiritual *transmission cannot occur. The person of the teacher serves as a means of self-transcendence for the disciple. This must not be confused with adulation, though at times *guru-yoga* has suffered from this kind of excess. According to the *Bhagavad-Gītā* (XIII.7), an ancient *Yoga scripture, veneration of the preceptor is a manifestation of wisdom (*jnāna*). See also *guru-bhakti, guru-sevā, sevā*.

Action. The spiritual practitioner (*yogin*, *sādhaka*), is expected to know how to act in the world in accordance with the higher principles of the *cosmos. For him or her, right action is action that is not only morally sound (i.e., virtuous) but also conducive to spiritual growth, or *progress. Otherwise, action is karmically binding, that is, it reinforces spiritual blindness (*avidyā*) and thus leads to reincarnation. In Sanskrit, the word for action and the *fate created by action is the same, namely *karman* (or *karma*).

Action became a subject of keen philosophical inquiry in India with the *Upanishads (about 800 B.C.), but notably with the *Bhagavad-Gītā* several centuries later. The fundamental existential question "What must I do?" is closely connected to the question "Who am I?" For the Upanishadic sages and later also for the *yogins*, human action is played out in the finite realms of conditional reality, and it cannot touch the transcendental *Self, or *Reality. The sense that "I" act is an illusion, and so are, in the final analysis, the consequences of "my" actions. Upon *enlightenment, actions are experienced as simply arising, without there being an ego-identity. See also *karma-yoga*.

Actor or **agent.** The conditional ego-personality (*jīva*, *ahamkāra*), presumes itself to be the performer of *actions, which, according to *Classical Yoga and *Vedānta, is an illusion. In the view of Classical *Sāmkhya, however, the transcendental Self (*purusha*) is the doer of all deeds. This is also the view of Kashmiri *Shaivism. By contrast, Classical Yoga subscribes to the opinion that the *Self is the passive enjoyer (*bhoktri*) of the experiences of the finite human personality. The Self apperceives the contents of *consciousness but, by virtue of its inherent *purity, also acts as an attractive force in the evolutionary play, which accounts for the gradual upliftment of individuals and whole world cycles (*yuga*). See also *kartri*.

Adept. The accomplished spiritual practitioner, who has climbed to the top of the ladder of spiritual life, is not only a master of the discipline but, above all, a master (*svāmin*) of his or her own self-body-mind. An adept is generally considered to be an *enlightened being, or one who has awakened from the "dream" of conventional life and has realized the Self (*ātman*). Such a being is known as a *siddha* or *mahāsiddha*. See also Crazy adept, *sādhaka*.

ādhāra ("support," "prop"). This term refers to different places in the *body on which the *yogin* focuses his *attention not only to discipline the *mind but also to harness the body's psychosomatic energy (*prāna*). Sometimes six, nine, and even sixteen such supports are distinguished. The set of sixteen is frequently presented as comprising the following body parts: thumbs, ankles, knees, thighs, prepuce, genitals, *navel, *heart, neck, throat, *palate, *nose, spot between the eyebrows, forehead, *head, and the *brahma-randhra* ("brahmic fissure") at the crown of the head.

    The word *ādhāra* is also used specifically to indicate the lowest of the bodily centers (i.e., the *mūlādhāra-cakra*). See also *desha*, *cakra*.

adharma. The word *dharma* has a great many different meanings, and so does *adharma*. Generally speaking, the latter word stands for "lawlessness" or "anomy," indicating a lack of virtue or righteousness, as well as moral and spiritual chaos. In the *Bhagavad-Gītā* (IV.7), the God-man *Krishna declares that he incarnates in every age (*yuga*) to stamp out lawlessness and reestablish the spiritual order on earth.

ādhibhūta. This adjective means "pertaining to the elements." In the *Bhagavad-Gītā*, this term is used to refer to the perishable (*kshara*) manifestation of the Imperishable (*akshara*). Cf. *ādhidaiva*, *ādhyātman*.

ādhidaiva. This adjective means "pertaining to the deities (*deva*)," that is, to one's *destiny, which is thought to be governed by higher powers. In some contexts, this word refers to the transcendental *Self. Cf. *ādhibhūta*, *ādhyātman*.

adhikāra ("qualification"). In the setting of *guru-yoga, the *transmission of spiritual knowledge and *power, requires that the *student is truly qualified to receive what is given. The unqualified person was traditionally supposed to be excluded from such transmission, since it could damage him or her, as well as the *teacher.

adhikārin ("qualified [person]"). The various traditions of *Yoga resort to all kinds of criteria for determining who is a qualified practitioner (*sādhaka), that is, the competent person who is worthy of being initiated and instructed in the great esoteric lore of *liberation. Thus, in the *Shiva-Samhitā (III.16–19), a positive frame of mind, or *vishvāsa, is said to be the primary qualification. This is followed by faithful application, *veneration of the *teacher, impartiality, sense restraint, and a moderate *diet.

According to this *hatha-yoga work (V.10ff.), the weak (mridu) aspirant is unenthusiastic, foolish, fickle, timid, ill, dependent, rude, ill-mannered, and unenergetic. He is considered fit only for *mantra-yoga, or the recitation of empowered sounds (*mantra). The mediocre (madhya) aspirant, on the other hand, is endowed with even-mindedness, patience, a desire for virtue, kind speech, and the tendency to practice moderation in all things. He is considered capable of practicing *laya-yoga, or the dissolution of the *mind through meditative *absorption.

The exceptional (adhimātra) aspirant shows such qualities as firm understanding, an aptitude for meditative absorption (*laya), self-reliance, liberal-mindedness, bravery, vigor, faithfulness, the willingness to worship the *teacher's "lotus feet" (both literally and figuratively), and delight in the practice of *Yoga. The extraordinary (adhimātratama) aspirant, who may practice any type of Yoga, demonstrates the following thirty-one virtues: great energy, *enthusiasm, charm, heroism, scriptural knowledge, the inclination to practice, freedom from *delusion, orderliness, youthfulness, moderate eating habits, control over the *senses, *fearlessness, *purity, skillfulness, *liberality, the ability to be a refuge for all people, capability, stability, thoughtfulness, the willingness to do whatever is desired by the teacher, *patience, good manners, observance of the moral and spiritual law, the ability to keep his struggle to himself, kind speech, *faith in the *scriptures, the readiness of the Divine), knowledge of the vows pertaining to his level of practice, and, lastly, the active pursuit of all forms of Yoga.

ādhyātman. This adjective means "pertaining to the self." When used as a noun, it often refers to the innermost *Self, or one's essential nature. Cf. *ādhibhūta, ādhidaiva.*

Ādinātha ("Primal Lord"). This appellation applies to the original teacher of the *Kaula or *Nātha tradition, who is identified with God *Shiva himself. He is held to be the first great adept (*mahā-siddha*) in the long line of master *teachers.

Adoration. See *ārādhana.*

advaita ("nonduality") signifies the interconnectedness of everything, which is founded in the singularity of the transcendental *Reality. Cf. *dvaita.*

Advaita-Vedānta means literally the "nondual end of the *Vedas" and refers to the metaphysics expounded in the *Upanishads and all those scriptures that base themselves on the Upanishads in one way or another. Nondualism (*advaita*) is the dominant philosophical tradition within *Hinduism. It comprises many different schools. Some are radically pantheistic, others monotheistic, and yet others panentheistic, or even qualifiedly nondualistic (see, e.g., *Rāmānuja).

*Yoga was originally panentheistic: The world emerged from and is contained in the *Divine but is not merely identical with it. The spiritual *path is a movement in *consciousness through progressive levels of the hierarchy of existence, until the original Consciousness (*cit*), or transcendental *Self, is realized. That Self experiences itself as an integral part (*amsha*) of the ultimate *Reality.

*Patanjali, who consolidated *Yoga as a philosophical system (*darshana*), appears to have favored a dualistic (*dvaita*) metaphysics presuming an eternal chasm between *Consciousness (or Spirit) and matter. Reversing the position of the *Upanishads, he contrasted the transcendental Self (*purusha*) with the transcendental ground of Nature (*prakriti*). See also Shankara, Vedānta; cf. Vishishta-Advaita.

Avaya-Tāraka-Upanishad ("Upanishad of the Nondual Deliverer"). This is one of the *Yoga-Upanishads and belongs to the post-Christian era. In nineteen short passages, this work propounds *tāraka-yoga, in which internally or externally perceived *light phenomena (known as photisms) play an important role. The "nondual deliverer" is the transcendental *Consciousness, which reveals itself to the *yogin in a "multitude of fires." See also *tāraka.*

āgama ("tradition"). In the narrower sense, this is one of the three means of valid knowledge (*pramāna*) admitted in *Classical Yoga. It stands for testimonial or authoritative *knowledge, that is, knowledge acquired through sensory perception or inferred by a trustworthy person. See also *smriti*, *shruti*.

Āgama refers to a work within a particular genre of sacred *Hindu literature belonging to *Shaivism. Some two hundred such scriptures are known, though they have barely been studied. They are presented as revelations (*shruti*) of God *Shiva. Their counterparts in *Vaishnavism are known as *Samhitās, and in *Shaktism as *Tantras.

Traditionally, twenty-eight Āgamas are recognized as forming the revealed canon of the *Shiva community of South India. These scriptures are equivalent to the four *Vedas of North Indian *Brāhmanism and are sometimes collectively referred to as the "fifth Veda." Like the *Tantras, they purport to be for the spiritual aspirant of the present "dark age" (*kāli-yuga*) who lacks the moral and mental capacity to follow more conventional *paths to *liberation. Regrettably, few of these texts have so far been published in book form, and fewer still have been translated into English.

āgāmi-karma ("present karma"). See *karma*.

Agastya (Tamil: Akattiyar), or Agasti, is the name of several individuals. Thus, a seer (*rishi*), Agastya composed several of the hymns of the ancient *Rig-Veda*. He was married to Lohāmudrā, the daughter of the ruler of the Videha tribe. The *Rig-Veda* (I.179.4) has preserved a conversation between them. The name Agastya is also associated with works on grammar, medicine, gemology, and other sciences. Agastya is remembered to have been of small stature, and in iconography is generally depicted as a dwarf. He is mentioned in a number of *Brāhmanas, the *Mahābhārata* and *Rāmāyana* epics, as well as several *Purānas. His hermitage is said to have been in the extreme south of the Indian peninsula. Agastya was a great adept (*siddha*) who is to South India what *Matsyendra is to the North. His fame spread as far as Indonesia.

Aghora ("Nonterrible"). This is an epithet of God *Shiva, paradoxically referring to his terrifying aspect, which presumably is not so for the initiate worshipper of that deity (*deva*).

Aghorī sect. This is a *Tantra-based cult that evolved from the more widespread *Kāpālika ascetic order some time in the fourteenth century A.D. Its followers, known as Aghorī Panthīs, have always been held in low esteem because of their many eccentric practices, such as the use of human skulls as vessels, the frequenting of cemeteries, the eating of refuse, and not least cannibalism (until the end of the nineteenth century).

āgneyī-dhāranā-mudrā ("fiery concentration seal") is one of the five *concentration techniques described in the *Gheranda-Samhitā (III.75f.). The practitioner is asked to focus his *attention and *life force on the (digestive) "fire" (*agni) in the abdominal region for 150 minutes, which stimulates the psychosomatic energy there. Accomplishment in this practice is said to make one immune against the heat of flames. See also dhāranā, mudrā, panca-dhāranā.

agni ("fire") is one of the five material elements (*bhūta) that compose the manifest *cosmos in its grossest dimension. It can also stand for digestive and psychosomatic heat. See also tattva, vahni.

Agni, the God of Fire, figured as a central deity of the ancient *Vedic religion. He was closely associated with the Vedic sacrificial fire ritual. The symbolism of Agni is open to many interpretations, including his tentative equation with the "serpent power" (*kundalinī-shakti) in some contexts. See also deva.

agni-sāra-dhauti ("cleansing by means of fire") is a synonym for vahni-sāra-dhauti.

agni-yoga ("fire Yoga"). This is the process whereby the "serpent power" (*kundalinī-shakti) is awakened through the joint action of *breath (or controlled psychosomatic energy) and *mind. There is also a modern spiritual school by that name, which was founded by Russell Paul Schofield. Here visualization is used in combination with the *body's psychosomatic energy (*prāna) in order to dissolve undigested perceptual and emotional experiences that have created a blockage in the body-mind. This approach is also known as Actualization.

aham ("I"). Normally, this personal pronoun refers to the conditional *ego, the *ahamkāra. But in Kashmiri *Shaivism, it designates the transcendental *Self, and is also known as ahamtā, or "I-ness."

aham brahma asmi ("I am the Absolute"). This is one of the famous dicta of *Advaita-Vedānta, which was introduced in the early *Upanishads, and which is also reiterated in medieval *Yoga scriptures that avow nondualism. It is more an ecstatic exclamation than a philosophical proclamation. In the condition of *enlightenment, the "I" is no longer the ego-personality (*ahamkāra) but the transcendental Self (*ātman).

ahamkāra means literally "I-maker." This is the *ego, or principle of individuation. In *Sāmkhya philosophy, it is regarded as one of the eight primary evolutes of *Nature and thus stands for a whole evolutionary category (*tattva). However, often it simply denotes the ego-illusion, that is, the sense of being a particular body-mind, of having certain properties ("my feelings," "my ideas," "my children," etc.), and of being an *actor originating *actions.

All spiritual traditions are agreed that the ego-sense must be transcended. Sometimes this is wrongly interpreted as a demand to be altruistic. Something much more profound is intended, namely a radical shift in our sense of who we are: From self-identity, we are asked to move to Self-Identity—from ahamkāra to *ātman. See also asmitā, jīva.

āhāra ("food" or "diet"). Dietary rules have formed a very important part of *Yoga practice from the earliest times. Thus the *Chāndogya-Upanishad (VII.26.2), which belongs to the eighth century B.C., speaks of the close link between dietary *purity and purity of being. A favorite saying of modern *yogins is "You are what you eat."

The *Bhagavad-Gītā (XVII.8f.), a pre-Christian work on nondualist *Yoga, distinguishes foods according to the predominance of the qualities *sattva, *rajas, and *tamas in them.

Foods that promote life, lucidity (*sattva), strength, *health, *happiness, and *satisfaction, and that are savory, rich in oil, firm, and heart [gladdening] are agreeable to the sattva-natured [person].

Foods that are pungent, sour, salty, spicy, sharp, harsh, and burning are coveted by the rajas-natured [person]. They cause *pain, *grief, and *disease.

And [food] that is spoiled, tasteless, putrid, stale, left over, and unclean, is food agreeable to the tamas-natured [person].

Not all yogic authorities—both ancient and modern—are in agreement over what constitutes a good diet. But, without exception, they emphasize the importance of exercising restraint over the intake of food. This rule is known as *mita-āhāra. See also anna-yoga, laghv-āhāra, upavāsa.

āhāra-jaya ("mastery over food"), that is, disciplined eating, is sometimes listed among the moral observances (*yama), which shows the great importance of this discipline. See also anna-yoga.

ahimsā ("nonharming"). This word is often translated as "nonviolence," but something more fundamental is intended by it. *Patanjali, the originator of *Classical Yoga, regards it as one of the five moral observances (*yama), which make up what he calls the "great vow" (mahā-vrāta), which must be kept under all circumstances. Other authorities list ahimsā under the five restraints (*niyama). It is generally defined as the practice of abstaining from harming others physically, mentally, and vocally at all times. In our time it was "Mahatma" Gandhi who advocated ahimsā as a viable moral and political practice. In doing so, he articulated an age-old tradition within *Hinduism. However, his radical approach is not characteristic of all *Hindu schools of thought. For instance, *Brāhmanism permits the slaughter of animals for sacrificial purposes. Also, the teachings of the *Bhagavad-Gītā, the oldest work on *Yoga, are set against the historical background of one of ancient India's fiercest wars. Here the God-man *Krishna admonishes Prince *Arjuna to participate in the *war rather than feel dejected about having to kill kinsmen and former teachers among the enemy. Because of the militaristic tenor of these teachings, the *Bhagavad-Gītā has often been interpreted as an allegory about our inner struggle. Cf. himsā.

aishvarya ("lordship"). This is one of the great magical attainments (*siddhi) by which the *yogin is said to gain mastery over the manifest and unmanifest aspects of the *cosmos, similar to the supremacy of the "Lord" (*īshvara). Some *Yoga authorities take such powers literally; others understand them metaphorically, which is perhaps more in keeping with contemporary sensibilities. See also vibhūti.

ajapa-mantra, also known as ajapa-gāyatrī. This is the "unpronounced *mantra," the sound hamsa that is continually produced by the *body as a result of the breathing process. The syllable ham is connected with inhalation, and sa with exhalation. According to the *Gheranda-Samhitā

(V.84–85) and other medieval texts, this sound is automatically "recited" in the human body 21,600 times during each twenty-four-hour cycle. The same work (V.90) instructs that one should recite this potent sound (*mantra*) consciously and even double its *recitation in order to effect the state of exaltation (*unmanī*). This idea is embedded in an esoteric teaching according to which the continuous sound *hamsa-hamsa-hamsa* can also be heard as *so'ham-so'ham-so'ham*, which means "I am He . . ." See also *gāyatrī, japa, mantra-yoga.*

ājnā-cakra means literally "command wheel." This is one of the seven major psychosomatic energy centers (*cakra) of the human *body. It is located in the middle of the head at the level of the eyebrows. This center is also known as the "third eye." It derives its name from the fact that it is the receiver for the *guru's telepathic communications to the *student. Hence it is also called *guru-cakra.* The *ājnā-cakra* is graphically depicted as a gray or white two-petaled lotus. It contains a symbolic representation of the phallus (*linga)—as a symbol of masculine creativity, or *shiva—

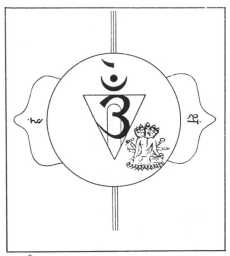

4. *Ājnā-cakra, the psychoenergetic center situated in the middle of the head.*

placed within a downward-pointing triangle, a symbol of the feminine principle, or *shakti. This center is connected with the sense of individuality (*ahamkāra*), the lower mind (*manas*), and the sacred syllable *om. Its presiding deities are Parama-Shiva ("supreme *Shiva") and the Goddess Hākinī. It is the penultimate station in the ascent of the "serpent power" (*kundalinī-shakti*) along the spinal axis. Its activation is said to lead to all kinds of psychic powers (*siddhi*), notably *clairvoyance and the ability to communicate telepathically.

ajnāna ("ignorance") is a synonym for *avidyā* ("nescience"). It signifies spiritual blindness as a result of which we experience ourselves as individuated body-minds that know physical *pain and psychic torment and that are doomed to age and die. It is the opposite of spiritual wisdom (*jnāna, vidyā*), which is conducive to genuine self-knowledge and, ultimately, *Self-realization.

akarman ("inaction"). According to the *Bhagavad-Gītā* (III.8), inactivity is impossible in the manifest world, because the very constituents of *Nature, the *gunas, are forever in motion. Hence life cannot be maintained without a minimum of *action. Instead of abstention from action, this work proposes the ideal of action transcendence (*naish-karmya-karman). Cf. *karman, karma-yoga*.

ākāsha. This old Sanskrit word means literally "radiance." Early on, it acquired the meaning of "space" or "ether," and served as a frequent comparison for the transcendental *Self, which is described as being brighter than a myriad of suns. Thus, in the ancient *Brihad-Āranyaka-Upanishad* (II.1.17), the *ākāsha* is said to be located in the *heart, the secret seat of the *Self. In medieval works such as the *Advaya-Tāraka-Upanishad*, the term has the specific meaning of "luminous [inner] space," which describes a set of mystical experiences in which *light phenomena play an important role. Five types of *ākāsha* are differentiated: (1) the *guna-rahita-ākāsha* ("ether/space devoid of qualities"); (2) the *parama-ākāsha* ("supreme ether/space"), which resembles palpable darkness lit up by the resplendent "deliverer" (*tāraka); (3) the *mahā-ākāsha* ("great ether/space"), which is bright like the conflagration at the end of time; (4) the *tattva-ākāsha* ("ether/space of verity"), which is effulgent beyond compare; and (5) the *sūrya-ākāsha* ("solar ether/space"), which is brilliant like 100,000 suns. The *yogin is said to merge with these luminous realities, which are stepping-stones to the transmental (*amanaska) state.

In later times, *ākāsha* came to be regarded as the finest of the five material elements (*bhūta) of the manifest *cosmos. In this sense, the concept is similar to Aristotle's "quintessence" and the "luminiferous ether" of nineteenth-century physics—a notion that was abandoned at the beginning of our century. See also *kha, madhya-lakshya, tāraka-yoga, tattva, vyoman*.

ākāsha-cakra ("ether wheel"). According to the *Siddha-Siddhānta-Paddhati* (II.9), an old work on *hatha-yoga, this is the ninth psycho-energetic center in the human *body. It has sixteen petals facing upward. The middle of the pericarp is shaped like three peaks. See also *vyoma-cakra*.

ākāsha-gamana ("walking in the ether"). This is a yogic power (*siddhi) that corresponds, if understood physically, to *levitation or, if understood psychologically, to visualization involving the *mind's journey through "other dimensions." In the latter sense, it is a precondition for the magical technique of entering the body of another being (*para-deha-pravesha*), mentioned for instance in the *Yoga-Sūtra* (III.38). See also *khecaratva, mano-gati*.

ākāshī-dhāranā-mudrā ("ethereal concentration seal") is one of the five *concentration techniques described in the *Gheranda-Samhitā* (III.80f.). This practice consists in focusing one's *attention and *life force, through breath control, on the *ether element for 150 minutes, which stimulates the psychosomatic energy. This is also known as *nabho-dhāranā*, and is said to be capable of "breaking open the door to *liberation." See also *dhāranā, mudrā, panca-dhāranā*.

Akattiyar. See Agastya.

aklishta ("nonafflicted"). According to the *Yoga-Sūtra* (I.5), the textbook of *Classical Yoga, this term applies to one of two basic categories of mental activity (*vritti*), and it is thought to be conducive to *liberation. See also *klesha, klishta*.

akshara can mean "immobile," "imperishable," and "lettered." It refers to both the *Absolute and its symbol *om. Cf. *kshara*.

Akshy-Upanishad ("Eye Upanishad") counts among the general Vedānta *Upanishads. The text has two parts, of which the latter part deals with the seven stages (*sapta-bhūmi*) of Yoga defined as the "supraconscious, nonartificial obliteration of "consciousness."

Akula, meaning "nonflock," is one of *Shiva's many epithets. See also Kaula sect; cf. *kula*.

Akula-Āgama-Tantra is a scripture belonging to the *Kaula tradition of *Matsyendra. Its first section deals with the sixfold path of *hatha-yoga*. In the third section the five "ingredients" of *Tantrism, the *makaras*, are explained as being a part of yogic practice, but their literal enactment is condemned.

Akula-Vīra-Tantra, of which there appear to be two versions, is a short work belonging to the *Kaula sect. The *akula-vīra*, or "akula hero," is the supreme *Reality. See also *Vīra*.

ālambana ("foundation") is the *object or stimulus of *consciousness acting as a prop for concentration (*dhāranā*). See also *bīja*.

ālambusā- or **ālambushā-nādī** ("plenteously misty channel") is one of the principal conduits (*nādī*), or pathways of life energy, of the *body. It is generally thought to originate in the "bulb" (*kanda*), in the lower abdomen, but its termination point is variously described as being in the eyes, the ears, or the mouth.

ālasya ("sloth"). This is one of the obstacles (*antarāya*) of *Yoga and is explained in the *Yoga-Bhāshya* (I.30) as inactivity resulting from bodily and mental heaviness. The *Shiva-Purāna* (V.26.35) calls this one of the great enemies that must be conquered. Already in the pre-Christian *Mahābhārata* epic (XII.263.46), it is said to be one of the factors that prevent one from reaching *heaven. It can effectively be combatted by *sīt-karī-prānāyāma*, which is one of the chief types of *breath control employed in *hatha-yoga. See also *styāna, tandrā.*

al-Bīrūnī. This famous Persian traveler visited India in the first half of the eleventh century. He composed a rather free Arabic rendering of the *Yoga-Sūtra*, the textbook of *Classical Yoga, together with a lengthy commentary that could have been the *Tattva-Vaishāradī*. His translation, entitled *Kitāb Patanjal*, adds little to our knowledge of *Patanjali's Yoga, and in fact al-Bīrūnī seems to have misunderstood many of the more intricate technical matters.

Alchemy is the prescientific craft of using natural elements to produce seemingly supernatural results, notably physical *immortality. Whether in China, India, or Europe, the alchemists sought after the elixir of life, the philosopher's stone, that would outwit Nature's law of entropy. From the reports of such seasoned travelers as *al-Bīrūnī and Marco Polo, we learn that Indian *yogins have also practiced alchemy. Indeed, *Yoga is a form of alchemy, since it aims at the transmutation of human *consciousness and—in *Tantrism and *hatha-yoga—even at the transubstantiation of the *body. At the center of the medieval *Siddha tradition lies the quest for a "divine body" (*divya-sharīra*) endowed with a variety of paranormal abilities (*siddhi*) and thoroughly enlightened. The word *siddha means "perfected" and refers to a spiritual *adept whose *enlightenment has permanently changed his body's chemistry. See also Magic, Occultism.

alinga ("signless"). In *Classical Yoga this is the highest (or deepest) level of the hierarchy of Nature (*prakriti*). It is the state of undifferentiated existence. In the *Tattva-Vaishāradī* (I.45), a principal commentary on the *Yoga-Sūtra*, it is defined as the equipoise of the three primary constituents (*guna*) of Nature. By contrast, in *Pre-Classical Yoga, the term is sometimes used synonymously with *purusha*, the transcendental *Self. See also Cosmos, *linga*, *tattva*.

Allāma Prabhudeva, a twelfth-century *adept, is remembered as the head of an order of more than three hundred enlightened beings, including about sixty women. He is mentioned in the *Hatha-Yoga-Pradīpikā* (I.8) as one of the *teachers of *hatha-yoga*.

aloluptva ("nonwavering"). According to the *Shvetāshvatara-Upanishad* (II.12), this is one of the characteristics of the first stage of yogic accomplishment where the practitioner is firmly committed to the spiritual process.

Altered states of consciousness. This term, as defined by psychologist Charles Tart, who wrote a definitive work on the subject, means a state of *consciousness that the experiencer feels to be qualitatively different from his or her ordinary mental functioning. The high value placed on the routine state of consciousness in our culture is a noteworthy historical oddity. Most premodern cultures valued such altered states as dreams, visions, trances, ecstasies. By contrast, we tend to regard these states with perplexity and unease, seeing in them "abnormal" (i.e., deficient) manifestations of the psyche. The counterculture of the 1960s, mainly through the widespread exposure to "mind-altering" drugs like LSD, has led to a softening of our attitude toward nonordinary states of awareness. This is most apparent in the growing New Age movement. However, altered states of consciousness are still only imperfectly understood. Most importantly, the condition of *enlightenment must be carefully distinguished from altered states, for it implies a transcendence of the *mind itself, even though this widely made claim is rejected by many psychologists. See also *dhāranā*, *dhyāna*, *samādhi*.

Ālvārs. Southern *Vaishnavism remembers twelve *ālvārs*, who inspired the people with their devotional hymns expressing their burning love for the *Divine in the form of *Vishnu. These propagators of *bhakti-yoga* lived in the seventh and eighth centuries A.D. Their hymns were gathered in the Tamil compendium known as the *Nalayirap-Pirapantam* (Sanskrit: *Nalayira-Prabandha*). Most of the approximately four thousand hymns are by Tirumankaiy and *Namm. The only woman saint in this group is *Āndāl, of whom 107 hymns have survived.

amanaskatā ("transmindedness") or **amanaska** (the "transmental") is the sublime condition of *enlightenment in which the mind (*manas*), is transcended. It is also called "exaltation" (*unmanī*).

Amanaska-Yoga is a work on *hatha-yoga* ascribed to Īshvara Vāmadeva. It consists of two chapters with a total of 208 stanzas and expounds what it calls *tāraka-yoga*. However, this teaching is not identical with the photistic *Yoga of the *Advaya-Tāraka-Upanishad*. Rather, it is a technique for the simultaneous stabilization of one's *gaze, *breathing, and *attention, founded in the *renunciation of everything.

amānitva ("humility"). According to the *Bhagavad-Gītā* (XIII.7), this virtue is a manifestation of wisdom (*jñāna*). Cf. *abhimāna, darpa*.

Amaranātha-Samvāda ("Dialogue With the Immortal Lord") is a twelfth-century Marathi text ascribed to *Goraksha, the great preceptor of *hatha-yoga*.

Amaraugha-Prabhodha ("Immortal Flood of Illumination") is a work of seventy-four stanzas ascribed to *Goraksha. Many of its verses correspond to those of the *Hatha-Yoga-Pradīpikā*, one of the classic manuals of *hatha-yoga* still used today.

amarolī-mudrā (*"amarolī* seal"). The word *amarolī* is difficult to translate; it means the "immortal (*amara*) nectar." This "seal" (*mudrā*) is one of the techniques that have brought *hatha-yoga* into disrepute with pollution-conscious brahmins. The *Yoga-Tattva-Upanishad* (128) describes it as the daily drinking of the *amarī*, or urine. The *Hatha-Yoga-Pradīpikā* (III.96ff.) contains a more detailed description of this practice: One should enjoy the middle flow of one's urine, discarding the first flow since it increases bile (*pitta*) and the last flow because it lacks essence. This is regarded as a variety of *vajrolī-mudrā*. See also *sahajolī-mudrā*.

āmbhasī-dhāranā-mudrā ("aqueous concentration seal"). This is one of the five *concentration techniques described in the *Gheranda-Samhitā* (III.72ff.) as follows:

> The [*water] element is said to be like a conch, the moon, or white like the *kunda* flower, and auspicious. Its seed [syllable] is the letter *va*, [which is] its ambrosia, and *Vishnu is connected with it. One should concentrate the *mind and *breath for five *ghatikās* [about 150

minutes] thereon. This is the aqueous concentration that destroys all *evil, affliction, and *sorrow. Whoever know this seal will never meet with *death even in the deepest water. It should carefully be kept secret. By disclosing it, success is forfeited.

See also *panca-dhāranā*.

amrita ("immortal), **amritatva** ("immortality"). *Enlightment is frequently equated with *immortality, for the transcendental *Self is deathless. In the literature of *hatha-yoga*, however, the word *amrita* has a technical meaning. It refers to the nectar of immortality that trickles down from an esoteric center in the *head and is wasted by ordinary mortals because they do not know its secrets. The intrinsic connection between this nectar and immortality is succinctly captured in the *Kaula-Jnāna-Nirnaya* (XIV.94), which poses this question: "How can there be immortality (*amaratva*) without [the flowing of] the nectar?"

The nectar is variously called *soma, sudhā, amara-vārunī*, and *pīyūsha*. It is of brilliant white-reddish color and is exquisitely bliss inducing. According to the *Shiva-Samhitā* (II.7f.), a late work on *hatha-yoga*, the nectar of immortality has two forms; one flows through the left conduit (the *idā-nādī*) and nourishes the *body; the other flows along the central pathway (the *sushumnā-nādī*) and creates the "moon" (*candra*). The nectar's flow increases when the "serpent power" (*kundalinī-shakti*) has ascended from the base center to the psychoenergetic center at the throat.

The *Hatha-Yoga-Pradīpikā* (IV.53) states that the whole *body should be flooded with this ambrosia, which produces a superior body endowed with enormous strength and vigor and which is free from *disease. This practice also prevents aging and bestows immortality as well as the eight magical powers (*ashta-siddhi*). See also *khecarī-mudrā*.

Amrita-Bindu-Upanishad ("Upanishad of the Immortal Drop"), consisting of only twenty-two stanzas, is one of the *Yoga Upanishads. Based on *Vedānta metaphysics, it teaches a form of Yoga that combines renunciation with recitation (*japa*) of the sacred syllable *om*.

Amrita-Nāda-Upanishad ("Upanishad of the Immortal Sound"), consisting of thirty-eight verses, is one of the *Yoga-Upanishads. It expounds a *Vedānta-based sixfold *Yoga (*shad-anga-yoga*). The text is prefixed with four verses dealing with a method for the recitation of the *pranava* (i.e., *om*) coupled with the adoration of God *Rudra.

amrita-nādī ("conduit of immortality"). According to the modern Indian sage Ramana Maharshi and the contemporary American adept Da Free John, the *amrita-nādī* is the esoteric structure that extends from the *head to the *heart to infinity. It is said to complete the circuit formed by the axial pathway (*sushumnā-nādī*), which runs from the base of the spine to the crown of the head. See also *nādī*.

amsha ("part," "fragment"). In the panentheistic teaching of the *Bhagavad-Gītā* and the *Bhāgavata tradition in general, the *cosmos and the embodied selves are merely a fragment of the immeasurable body of the *Divine. Individual beings are the cells of the infinite organism that is the "Lord" (*bhāgavat*).

anāhata-cakra ("wheel of the unstruck [sound]"). This esoteric center, which is also known as the "lotus of the heart" (*hrit-padma*), has been recognized as a special locus of the sacred within the human *body since the time of the *Vedas. The heart has anciently been celebrated as the seat of the *Divine and as the location where the immortal sound *om, which is not produced by anything, can be heard.

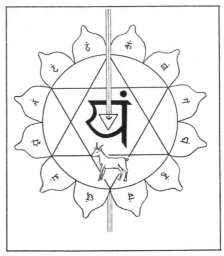

This psychoenergetic center is generally held to have twelve petals of deep red color. Its "seed syllable" (*bīja-mantra*) is *yam*, which pertains to the *wind ele-

5. *Anāhata-cakra, the psychoenergetic center located at the heart, considered to be the seat of the transcendental Self.*

ment. The center's presiding adept is Pinākin, the presiding *Goddess is the yellow-colored, three-eyed Kākinī. The heart center is likened to the legendary wish-fulfilling tree. It is the abode of the "swan" (*hamsa*), that is, the life force (*prāna*). Regular *contemplation of this esoteric structure yields a variety of paranormal abilities (*siddhi*), including immeasurable knowledge, *clairaudience, and *clairvoyance. See also *dahara*.

ānanda ("bliss") can connote both joy and transcendental *bliss. The *Hatha-Yoga-Pradīpikā* (IV.75), a classic work on *hatha-yoga, distinguishes between bliss as a mental state (*citta-ānanda*) and as the unqualified innate delight (*sahaja-ānanda*) pertaining to the *Absolute. In *Classical Yoga, the term denotes one of the accompanying phenomena of conscious enstasy (*samprajnāta-samādhi*). See also *sukha*.

Ānanda Bhairava. In the *Hatha-Yoga-Pradipika (I.5), he is mentioned as a great *teacher of *hatha-yoga. Nothing is known about him, however. See also Bhairava.

ānanda-maya-kosha ("sheath composed of bliss"). The highest or most subtle of the five "envelopes" (*kosha*) covering the transcendental *Self. Its substance is bliss (*ānanda*).

ānanda-samāpatti ("blissful coinciding [with the object of contemplation]"). According to the *Yoga-Bhāshya (I.17) and other commentaries on the *Yoga-Sūtra, this is a high-level conscious enstasy (*samprajnāta-samādhi*) consisting of the experience of pure *bliss. However, the bliss experienced in *ānanda-samāpatti*, or *ānanda-samādhi*, is conditional and temporary. In his *Tattva-Vaishāradī (I.17), the scholar *Vācaspati Mishra explains that the experience of bliss is generated when the *yogin's introverted *attention rests on one of the sense organs (*indriya*), which contain a preponderance of the *sattva (luminosity) constituent of *Nature. This experience is thus different from the "formless enstasy" (*nirvikalpa-samādhi*) of *Vedānta, which reveals the transcendental Being-Consciousness-Bliss (*sac-cid-ānanda*). Here bliss is considered an essential aspect of the ultimate *Reality.

Ānanda-Samuccaya is a rare thirteenth-century work on *hatha-yoga consisting of eight chapters totaling 277 stanzas. Among other things, the text deals with the psychoenergetic centers (*cakra*) and "channels" (*nādī*) as well as the other esoteric structures of the *body.

Ananta ("Infinite") is an epithet of God *Vishnu who is said in the *Mahābhārata epic (XII.175.19) to be "difficult to be known even by *adepts owing to his infinity." Ananta, or Shesha, is the "thousand-headed" cosmic serpent of *Hindu mythology who serves as God *Vishnu's couch. The name Shesha ("Remainer") is explained by the fact that Shesha remains after the destruction of the *cosmos. He is invoked by *Vyāsa at the beginning of his *Yoga-Bhāshya as the "Giver of *Yoga who is himself yoked in Yoga."

Ananta is also the name of the author of a late work entitled *Yoga-Sūtra-Artha-Candrikā ("Moonshine on the Meaning of the Yoga Aphorisms").

ananta-samāpatti ("coinciding with the infinite"). According to the *Yoga-Sūtra* (II.47), this is a precondition of the proper performance of posture (**āsana*) and presumably refers to the subjective experience of one's "widening out" in the state of deep relaxation (**shaithilya*). Some of the Sanskrit commentators think that this is a reference to the serpent-king *Ananta. See also *samāpatti*.

anātman ("non-Self"). This technical term denotes everything that is experienced as being different from the transcendental *Self (**ātman*), that is, the phenomenal world and the ego-personality. In *Buddhism, *anātman* refers to the fact that nothing in Nature has an eternal essence.

Anatomy. Conventional medical anatomy based, as the word suggests, on dissection is concerned with the material structures of the physical *body. Yogic anatomy, by contrast, is primarily concerned with the esoteric structures of the human body-mind, as it is experienced in such *altered states of consciousness as *meditation and *ecstasy or *enstasy. These esoteric structures include the distribution channels (**nādī*) and the vortices (**cakra*) of the life force (**prāna*). It also deals with the shock wave that rocks the body when its hidden psychospiritual power is tapped—the **kundalinī-shakti*. Earlier generations of *Yoga researchers typically regarded the *cakras* and *nādīs* as fanciful representations of the nervous system. But the *yogins were well aware of the difference between their models of the body and the medical model of India's indigenous naturopathic system of health care, the **Āyur-Veda*.

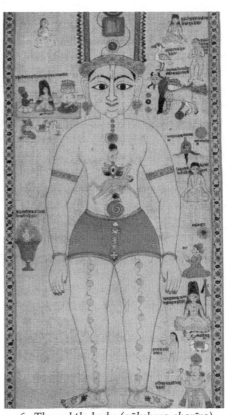

6. *The subtle body (sūkshma-sharīra) with its various psychoenergetic foci.*

The plurality of yogic models is an indication of the fact that the *cakras and *nādīs are not altogether objective structures. Neither are they purely fictitious. A convenient way of looking at the different *cakra* models is that they are intended to be maps for the **yogin* on his inward odyssey, during which he discovers the psychosomatic structures of his being, only to transcend them in the unqualified radiance of original Being (**sat*), or transcendental Consciousness (**cit*). The purpose of yogic anatomy is thus to guide the *yogin* through and beyond the wonderland of the inner world of the psyche, which is interlinked with the physical vehicle.

anavasthitatva ("instability"). This is one of the obstacles (**antarāya*) of **Yoga, and is occasionally also referred to as "mental unsteadiness" (*citta-anavasthiti*).

ānava-upāya ("atomic means"). In Kashmiri **Shaivism, this is a technical term referring to the approach to **Self-realization, or **enlightenment, through individual effort. The adjective "atomic" (*ānava*) is derived from the word **anu* signifying here the individuated psyche, which is a "fragment" (**amsha*) of the Whole. Cf. *anupāya, upāya*.

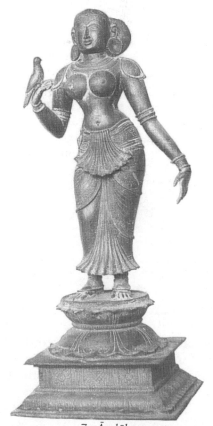

Āndāl is still venerated as one of the great female poet-saints of South India. She was a worshipper of God **Vishnu and lived in the early ninth century A.D. Andal's poetry is reminiscent of the bridal mysticism of medieval Europe, though she tended to use far more explicit erotic imagery to express her adoration of the **Divine. See also Ālvārs, Vaishnavism.

anga ("limb"). In addition to referring to the **body or, more specifically, to the male genitals, this term also denotes the constituent practice categories of the yogic **path. The **Yoga-Rāja-Upanishad (2), a late work, speaks of four

7. *Āndāl.*

basic categories that are common to all paths: posture (*āsana*), breath restriction (*prāna-samrodha*), meditation (*dhyāna*), and enstasy (*samādhi*). The best known tradition is the eightfold path, or *ashta-anga-yoga*, taught by *Patanjali. Another prominent approach is the sixfold path (*shad-anga-yoga*) taught for instance in the *Maitrāyanīya-Upanishad (VI.18). Also known are a "sevenfold discipline" (*sapta-sādhana*) and a fifteenfold path (*panca-dasha-anga-yoga*). In *Classical Yoga, a distinction is made between "outer limbs" (*bahir-anga*) and "inner limbs" (*antar-anga*), whereby the latter comprise the higher mental practices.

Anger. See *krodha*.

animan ("atomization"). This is one of the great paranormal powers (*siddhi*) resulting, according to the *Yoga-Sūtra (III.44f.), from the mastery over the *elements. It is the *adept's capacity to make himself infinitely small.

anīshvara ("lordless). This term, which appears in a few passages of the *Mahābhārata epic (notably XII.238.7 and 289.3), has given rise to scholarly debate. Some authorities have interpreted it in the sense of "atheist" but it is more likely to stand for the unliberated self, that is, the individuated psyche (*jīva*) who is not the "Lord" (*īshvara*).

anna ("food"). See *āhāra*.

anna-maya-kosha ("sheath composed of food"). According to an ancient *Vedānta doctrine, this is the lowest or coarsest of the five "envelopes" (*kosha*) covering the transcendental *Self, i.e., the physical body.

anna-yoga ("Yoga of food"). This contemporary term describes *Yoga as a spiritual discipline focusing on our relationship to food—its cultivation and consumption. See also *āhāra*.

antahkarana ("inner instrument"). This *Sāmkhya term, which is also met with in *Yoga and *Vedānta texts, signifies the psyche. According to the *Sāmkhya-Kārikā (32), the textbook of Classical Sāmkhya, it comprises the higher mind (called *buddhi*), the "I-maker" (*ahamkāra*), and the lower mind (called *manas*). In *Classical Yoga, the term *citta is used instead.

anta-kāla ("end time"). This refers to the time of a person's *death, one's final hour, which holds a particular obligation for the spiritual practitioner. From a materialistic point of view, death is simply the final and irrevocable cessation of the individual body-mind, which is followed by eternal oblivion. This view is denied by all spiritual traditions. Thus, already in the ancient *Bhagavad-Gītā (VIII.5f.), we find a passage that emphasizes the importance of dying well, and how one's last thoughts or intentions determine one's postmortem existence. The God-man *Krishna admonishes:

> And he who in the last hour, abandoning the *body, remembers Me alone, goes hence—he arrives at My state; there is no doubt of this.

> Also, whatever state [a man] remembers when he abandons the body in the end, even to that [state] does he go, o Kaunteya [*Arjuna], forever forced to become that state.

Such esoteric knowledge dates back to the earliest *Upanishads. The *Bhāgavata-Purāna (V.8.1ff.), a ninth-century work, contains the popular story of Bharata that illustrates this age-old *ars moriendi*. Bharata was so intent on the young deer he had saved from the lion's clutches that he forgot to pursue his *Yoga practice and consequently was promptly reborn as a deer.

Expressing a classic yogic teaching, the *Shat-Cakra-Nirūpana (38), a medieval *Tantric work, advises the *yogin to focus his *attention on the *ājnā-cakra (the brain core) at the moment of death. See also *kāla*, *prayāna-kāla*.

antar-anga ("inner limb"). In the *Yoga-Sūtra (III.7), this is the technical term for the last three constituents of the eightfold *path, namely concentration (*dhāranā), meditation (*dhyāna), and enstasy (*samādhi). See also *ashta-anga-yoga*; cf. *bahir-anga*.

antarāya ("obstacle"). The *Yoga-Sūtra (I.30), the textbook of *Classical Yoga, lists the following impediments on the yogic *path: illness (*vyādhi), languor (*styāna), doubt (*samshaya), heedlessness (*pramāda), sloth (*ālasya), dissipation (*avirati), false vision (*bhrānti-darshana), nonattainment of the higher levels (*alabdha-bhūmikatva*) of the spiritual path, and instability (*anavasthitva*) in a given level of attainment. These are also called "distractions" (*vikshepa) of *consciousness, and the *Yoga-Sūtra (I.29) prescribes the practice of recitation (*japa) and contemplation (*bhāvanā) of the sacred syllable *om for their swift removal.

The *Linga-Purāna (I.9.1ff.) offers a slightly different list, which includes lack of *faith (ashraddhā), suffering (*duhkha), and depression (*daurmanasya). This work states that such obstacles can be removed through constant practice and devotion to one's *teacher. The *Vedāntic *Uddhāva-Gītā (X.33), which is an imitation of the *Bhagavad-Gītā inserted into the voluminous *Bhāgavata-Purāna (XI), additionally regards the paranormal powers (*siddhi) as obstacles for the person who seeks union with the Lord, calling them "time wasters." See also upasarga, vighna.

antar-dhauti ("inner cleansing"). According to the *Gheranda-Samhitā (I.12ff.), a classical manual of *hatha-yoga, this practice comprises the following four techniques: swallowing air and expelling it through the anus at will; completely filling the stomach with water (a risky practice); stimulating the "*fire" in the abdomen by repeatedly pushing the navel back toward the spine, and washing one's prolapsed intestines (a dangerous practice if done without proper supervision).

antar-lakshya ("inner sign"). This technical term belongs to the discipline of *tāraka-yoga. It refers to one of three kinds of inner luminous experiences (*lakshya). The *Advaya-Tāraka-Upanishad (13) describes it as the photistic experience of the *Absolute as the *light of awareness hidden in the cave of the higher mind (*buddhi). For the anonymous author of the *Mandala-Brāhmana-Upanishad (I.2.6), the object of this experience is the "serpent power" (*kundalinī-shakti), which is resplendent like myriads of lightning streaks; or it is the blue radiance that can be experienced into the middle of the eyes or in the *heart when one fixes the *mind thereon. Reference to this practice is also made in the *Siddha-Siddhānta-Paddhati (II.27). Cf. bahir-lakshya, madhya-lakshya.

anu ("atom"). The idea that the physical objects are composed of minute indivisible parts is not a twentieth-century discovery. Ancient Greek cosmologists like Democritus speculated about this well over two thousand years ago. The notion was also current in India at that time, though it is difficult to say whether it was arrived at independently.

In Kashmiri *Shaivism, anu is a technical term referring to the individuated, "atomic" being (*jīva), as opposed to the universal transcendental *Self. See also parama-anu.

Anugītā ("Secondary Song") is closely modeled after the *Bhagavad-Gītā* and, like the *Gītā*, forms part of the great Indian national epic, the *Mahābhārata* (XIV.16–51). The *Anugītā* purports to be a recapitulation of the teachings communicated by the God-man *Krishna to Prince *Arjuna at the eve of the Bharata *war. This second instruction occurs after the battles have been fought and the moral order (*dharma) has been restored.

anugraha ("favor"). Divine *grace is frequently cited as the principal means of *Self-realization. In *Classical Yoga, the "Lord" (*īshvara) is said to incline toward the *yogin who strives for *perfection. See also *kripā, prasāda*; cf. Effort.

anumāna ("inference") is widely considered in *Hindu metaphysics as a valid means of knowledge (*pramāna). The *Yoga-Bhāshya* (I.7) defines it as "the [mental] activity referring to that relation which is present in things pertaining to the same class as the thing to be inferred (*anumeya), which is absent from things pertaining to different classes, and which is chiefly [concerned with] the ascertainment of the genus." This is further developed in the *Tattva-Vaishāradī*, where the logical structure of inference is examined.

anupāya ("without means"). This is a technical term of Kashmiri *Shaivism, which refers to the spontaneous realization of the *Self without any effort. Cf. *ānava-upāya, upāya*.

anvaya ("nexus"). This is a technical expression of *Classical Yoga. The *Yoga-Bhāshya* (III.44) explains it as referring to the primary constituents (*guna) of *Nature which inhere in everything.

anyatā-khyāti ("vision of otherness"). In *Classical Yoga, this denotes the enstatic "vision" of the distinction between the transcendental *Self and the *sattva, which is the highest aspect of (insentient) *Nature. It is synonymous with *viveka-khyāti*.

ap ("waters") is a feminine plural word derived from the verbal root *ap* ("to be active"). The water element is one of the five material elements (*bhūta) thought to compose the physical realm of *Nature, including the human *body. It is specifically connected with the five bodily liquids, namely saliva, urine, semen, blood, and *perspiration. The water element is sometimes said to govern the bodily region from the anus down to the knees. Its symbol is the crescent moon (*ardha-

candra), and its color is white, with *vam* being its "seed syllable" (*bīja-mantra*). See also *jala, tattva*.

apāna ("down-breath"). This is one of the principal currents of the life force (*prāna*), of which the *breath is its external manifestation. Together with the "forth-breath" (*prāna*), *apāna* is the great piston that powers the *body. According to various *Yoga-Upanishads, it resides in the lower half of the body—from the genitals down to the knees or, alternatively, from the belly down to the shanks or even the feet. This aspect of the universal life energy is responsible for the evacuation of waste matter and is connected with exhalation. When it is "mingled" with the *prāna and the "*fire" at the *navel, it is instrumental in arousing the "serpent power" (*kundalinī-shakti*).

aparānta-jnāna ("knowledge of one's end"). Foreknowledge of one's *death through omens (*arishta*) and dreams is one of the yogic powers (*siddhi*). It is important for the *yogin to die well, that is, to die consciously so that he can guide the death process and possibly effect *liberation during his last moments of bodily existence. There are numerous legends and anecdotes of contemporary *yogins* who correctly predicted the time of their death, in some cases years before it actually occurred. See also *jnāna*.

aparigraha ("greedlessness") is one of the five practices of moral restraint (*yama*) in *Classical Yoga. When practiced to the point of perfection, it yields knowledge of the "wherefore" of one's birth, as the *Yoga-Sūtra* (II.39) states. Already the *Bhagavad-Gītā* (IV.21), composed in the pre-Christian era, calls for the *abandonment of all possessions. This has given rise to schools of thought favoring radical world *renunciation. But other scriptural authorities, like the *Bhāgavata-Purāna* (III.28.4), espoused a minimalist interpretation of greedlessness, understanding it as "possessing as much as is necessary."

apas ("water") is the singular form of *ap*.

apavāda ("refutation") is a key term of *Vedānta that is also found in some works of *Post-Classical Yoga. It denotes the intellectual procedure whereby the erroneous predications (*adhyāropa*) about the nature of reality can effectively be exposed as such. Thus, it is a systematic attack on the consensus point of view of ordinary *consciousness, which, it is argued, fails to realize that *Reality is not finite and painful but infinite and blissful (*ānanda*).

apavarga ("turn-off") is a synonym for *moksha*, *mukti*, *kaivalya*.

apratibuddha ("not fully awakened") is a synonym for *abuddha* in *Pre-Classical Yoga. Cf. *budhyamāna*.

apunya ("demerit" or "demeritorious"). Many *Hindu schools look upon demerit almost as a material substance that is accumulated in the body-mind, determining its *destiny. It is a part of the doctrine of *karma*. Cf. *punya*.

ārādhana ("adoration") is sometimes listed among the practices of self-restraint (*niyama*). It is synonymous with *īshvara-pūjana*.

ārambha-avasthā ("initial state"). This is the first of the four states (*avasthā*) of yogic accomplishment. According to the *Yoga-Tattva-Upanishad* (64), a medieval scripture, it consists in the recitation of the sacred syllable *om*, whereas the *Varāha-Upanishad* (V.72) explains it as the giving up of external *actions and functioning inwardly instead. The *Hatha-Yoga-Pradīpikā* (IV.70f.), however, interprets it as that stage in which the "brahmic knot" (*brahma-granthi*) is pierced and *bliss arises out of the void (in the *heart) and various mystical *sounds can be heard. For the anonymous author of the *Shiva-Samhitā* (III.28), this stage is entered upon the *purification of the network of currents (*nādī*) in the *body.

Āranyaka ("[Treatise] Pertaining to the Forest") is a type of ancient ritual work composed by and for forest anchorites. This genre of scriptures preceded the *Upanishads and ideologically stood midway between their esotericism and the sacrificial ritualism of the *Vedas and *Brāhmanas.

arcanā ("worship") is often counted among the elements of self-discipline (*niyama*) and is also one of the aspects of the *Yoga of devotion (*bhakti-yoga*).

ardha-mātra ("half-measure") This is the symbol ⌣ placed above the syllable *om*. It is sometimes likened to a flame flickering above a candle.

arishta ("omen"). Omens play an important role in *Yoga. The *yogin invests even seemingly irrelevant and arbitrary events with deeper significance. Nothing is thought to be due to chance. According to the

Yoga-Bhāshya (III.22), an old commentary on the *Yoga-Sūtra*, there are three kinds of omens: those generated by oneself; those involving others; and omens involving deities (*deva*). Many scriptures furnish lists of omens relating to the death of a *yogin*, since this is an important spiritual transition and must be passed through with full awareness. See also *anta-kāla*.

ārjava ("rectitude") is sometimes counted as one of the practices of moral observance (*yama*). According to the *Bhagavad-Gītā* (XIII.7), uprightness is a manifestation of knowledge or gnosis (*jñāna*) and forms part of physical austerity (*tapas*).

Arjuna ("White" or "Bright") is the hero of the *Bhagavad-Gītā*, which is essentially a dialogue between Arjuna and the God-man *Krishna. Like Hamlet, Prince Arjuna typifies the indecisive individual, suffering from *doubt.

ārogya ("health"). According to the *Shvetāshvatara-Upanishad* (II.13), *health is one of the initial signs of spiritual *progress. That this is a more comprehensive concept than our Western notion of health is evident, for instance, from the *Hatha-Yoga-Pradīpikā* (II.2). This four-teenth-century work considers the following as manifestations of health: the ability to hold one's *breath as desired, increased activity of the gastric "*fire," and perception of the inner sound (*nāda*). Cf. *roga*, *vyādhi*.

Arrogance. See *abhimāna, darpa*; cf. *amānitva*.

Art. In India, the artist (*shilpin*) traditionally employed yogic *medi-tation for assisting the creative process. Any flaws in the artistic end product were attributed to laxity in *concentration and meditation. The textbooks not infrequently refer to the craftsman or artist as a *yogin* or *sādhaka*. Also, as a rule, these technical treatises contain prescrip-tions for the practice of *Yoga. Contemplation (*dhyāna*) is thought to produce "vision" or "audition" (as in the case of Vālmīki who inwardly heard the entire *Rāmāyana* epic). Traditional (religious) Indian art was never concerned with the pursuit of beauty for its own sake. Rather, the artist aspired to communicate the infinite through his creative work and to uplift the person "participating" in his art. See also Dance.

artha ("object, thing"). In certain technical contexts, this word means "intended object" or "content of *consciousness." It also has the meaning of "purpose." A further meaning is "material welfare," as the lowest of the four human concerns (*purusha-artha) recognized in *Hindu ethics. See also *vishaya*.

ārūdha ("ascended") designates the *adept who has risen to the top of the spiritual *path. According to the *Bhagavad-Gītā (VI.3), this term applies to the *yogin whose means is quiescence (*shama). The same scripture (VI.4) states that the condition of *yoga-ārūdha* is realized by that practitioner who has renounced all purpose (*samkalpa). Cf. *ārurukshu*.

ārurukshu ("desirous of ascending") designates the spiritual aspirant whose discipline consists, according to the *Bhagavad-Gītā (VI.3), in the performance of action (*karman) rather than the *renunciation of all activity. Cf. *ārūdha, siddha*.

asamprajnāta-samādhi ("supraconscious enstasy"). This is the technique leading to, and the experience of, the state of unified *consciousness beyond all cognitive content. In this superlative condition, subject and *object become one. In Vedānta, this is known as "formless enstasy" (*nirvikalpa-samādhi).

This realization presupposes the temporary deconstruction of the ordinary consciousness (*citta). All that is left is a residuum of subconscious tendencies (called *samskāra). If the state of supraconscious *enstasy is maintained over a prolonged period of time, these subconscious tendencies begin to neutralize one another, leading to ultimate and irreversible *liberation, or *enlightenment. At first, however, the supraconscious enstasy can be maintained only for brief intervals because the powerful subconscious "activators" (samskāra) causing the ordinary *waking state tend to reassert themselves. However, the periods of restriction (*nirodha) of the contents of consciousness become increasingly longer until the subconscious deposits (*āshaya) are completely eliminated. At this point, the ultraconscious enstasy is called "seedless" (*nirbīja). See also *dharma-megha-samādhi, samādhi*; cf. *samprajnāta-samādhi*.

āsana ("seat"). Originally, this term denoted the surface on which the *yogin is seated. That surface is supposed to be firm, neither too high nor too low, sufficiently big, level, clean, and generally pleasant. The

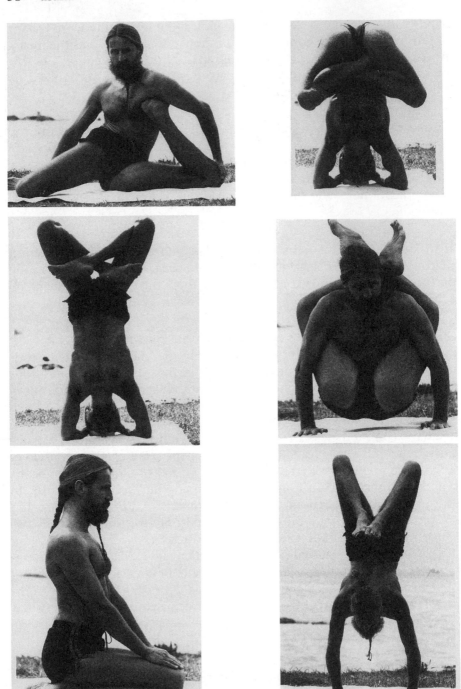

8. Select postures (āsana) of hatha-yoga.

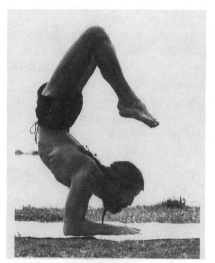
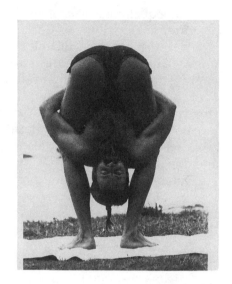
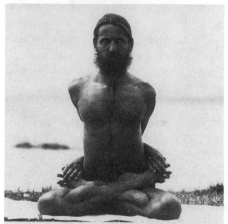
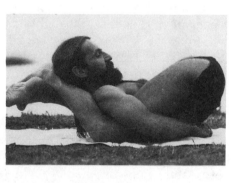
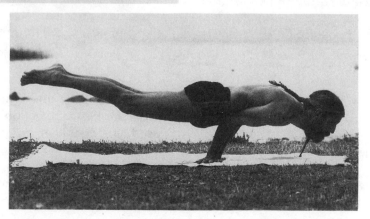

word is equally applied to the cover of the seat, which can be made of grass, wood, cloth, or different types of animal skin.

The most common technical significance of the term *āsana* is "posture." This is considered as one of the regular "limbs" (*anga) of the yogic *path and is usually listed first. The *Yoga-Sūtra (II.46), the textbook of *Classical Yoga, simply stipulates that the posture should be steady and comfortable. The latter qualification implies that it should be practiced in a state of relaxation (*shaithilya). A common piece of advice is that one should also sit up straight, with the trunk, neck, and head aligned.

Different postures are known and described in the scriptures of *Yoga. Originally, they served as stable poses for prolonged *meditation. Later, they were greatly elaborated and acquired a variety of therapeutic functions leading to the sophisticated *āsana* technology of *hatha-yoga. The scriptures of *Post-Classical Yoga declare that God *Shiva propounded 840,000 different postures. This figure is thought to represent the total number of classes of living beings. Of this wide variety, only a limited number of "seats" (*pītha) are said to have been recommended by *Shiva for spiritual practitioners. Thus, the *Goraksha-Paddhati (I.9) states that eighty-four postures are particularly suited, whereas the *Gheranda-Samhitā (II.2) claims that thirty-two are useful to human beings. Modern textbooks on *hatha-yoga describe as many as two hundred such postures.

According to the *Yoga-Sūtra (II.48), *āsana* desensitizes the *yogin to the impact of the "pairs of opposites" (*dvandva), such as heat and cold. Many scriptures of *Post-Classical Yoga extol posture as a means of conquering the worlds and as a preventive and curative panacea. Thus, the *Hatha-Yoga-Pradīpikā (I.17) claims that the regular practice of posture induces *stability, *health, and bodily *lightness. Probably in reaction to the hypertrophy of this aspect of yogic practice in later times, the *Garuda-Purāna (227.44) makes this criticism: "The techniques of posture or 'seat' (*sthāna) do not promote Yoga. Though called essentials, they all [merely] retard [one's *progress]." See also *nishadana*; cf. *bandha*, *mudrā*.

asat ("nonbeing"). According to the traditions of *Yoga and *Sāmkhya, *being can only arise from being, which implies a rejection of the doctrine of creation *ex nihilo*, as espoused, for instance, in Christian theology. See also *sat-kārya-vāda*; cf. *sat*.

Asceticism. *Yoga as we know it today emerged with the *Upanishads. Prior to that, a psychotechnology was prominent in India that is rooted in a more archaic mentality. This is the tradition of *tapas* or asceticism. It contributed to Yoga but also continued to flourish alongside it, and nowadays is mostly evident in the form of fakirism. The practitioner of this ascetic tradition relies on sheer will power rather than grace (*prasāda*), coercion and self-discipline rather than submission and *self-transcendence. The *tapasvin* seeks to win the support of the hidden forces of the universe—the *deities and spirits—in his struggle for power, notably magical abilities (*siddhi). See also *samnyāsa*.

āshaya ("resting place"). In *Classical Yoga, this term refers to the subconscious "deposit," often called "action deposit" (*karma-āshaya*), which is the network of subliminal activators (*samskāra) forming the structure of the subconscious or depth memory (*smriti). It is this *action residuum that is responsible for an individual's birth, span of life, and life experience. It must be transcended for *enlightenment to occur. See also *vāsanā*.

āshrama is derived from the Sanskrit word *shrama* meaning "effort." It refers, first of all, to a hermitage where an *adept instructs *disciples who exert themselves in a sacred way of life. Secondly, the word designates a stage of life, of which the *Hindu social model distinguishes the following four: the stage of the student (*brahmacārin*), which is called *brahmacarya*; the stage of the householder (*grihastha*), which is known as *gārhasthya*; the stage of the forest dweller (*vāna-prastha*), which is referred to as *vānaprāsthya*, and the stage of the renouncer (*samnyāsin*), which is called *samnyāsa*. See also *kutīra*.

ashta-anga-yoga ("Yoga of eight limbs"). This is the *path of yogic maturation proposed by *Patanjali, the founder of *Classical Yoga. It consists of the following eight practices: moral observance (*yama*), self-discipline (*niyama*), posture (*āsana*), breath control (*prānāyāma*), sensory inhibition (*pratyāhāra*), concentration (*dhāranā*), meditation (*dhyāna*), and enstasy (*samādhi*). See also *anga*; cf. *panca-dasha-anga-yoga, sapta-sādhana, shad-anga-yoga*.

ashta-siddhi ("eight powers"). This term applies to the classic set of eight paranormal powers (*siddhi), ascribed to yogic *adepts. According to the *Yoga-Bhāshya* (III.45), a work on *Classical Yoga, these comprise the following abilities: miniaturization (*animan*), levitation (*laghiman*), expansion (*mahiman*), extension at will (*prāpti*), freedom of will (*prākāmya*), universal mastery (*vashitva*), lordship (*īshitritva*), and perfect wish fulfillment (*kāma-avasāyitva*). See also *vibhūti*.

ashvinī—mudrā ("dawn horse seal") is one of the twenty-five "seals" (*mudrā) described in the *Gheranda-Samhitā (III). It is performed by repeatedly contracting the anal sphincter muscle. This is said to invigorate the *body, cure *diseases of the rectum, and awaken the "serpent power" (*kundalinī-shakti). Cf. yoni-mudrā.

asmitā ("I-am-ness") is the awareness of oneself as a discrete being. The *Yoga-Sūtra (II.6) lists "I-am-ness" as one of the five causes of affliction (*klesha) and defines it as the identification of the power of vision (i.e., the *mind) with the power of the visioner (i.e., the *Self). Furthermore, according to the *Yoga-Sūtra (I.17), this is one of the basic phenomena present in the state of conscious enstasy (*samprajnāta-samādhi). Some authorities state that there is an enstatic state that is exclusively composed of the feeling of "I-am-ness," which they call *asmitā-samāpatti. See also ahamkāra.

asmitā—mātra ("mere I-am-ness"). In *Classical Yoga, this is the principle of primary individuation, which represents a distinct level in the hierarchy of being. It is the generic pool of all individualized consciousnesses (*nirmāna-citta).

asmitā-samāpatti ("coincidence with 'I-am-ness' "). In *Classical Yoga, this is an advanced form of conscious enstasy (*samprajnāta-samādhi), which is based on the mere feeling of being present as an entity. See also sa-asmitā-samāpatti, samādhi.

asparsha-yoga ("intangible Yoga"). This is an apophatic *Yoga based on the metaphysics of nondualism and was first announced by *Gaudapāda, a renowned teacher of *Advaita-Vedānta. *Shankara, the great interpreter of that tradition, explains the term asparsha as that which is free from contact (sparsha) with everything and which is coessential with the *Absolute. Thus, this Yoga is not so much a *path as the practice of living from the *enlightened condition of nonduality. Cf. sparsha-yoga.

asteya ("nonstealing") is one of the practices of moral observance (*yama). According to the *Yoga-Sūtra (II.37), when this virtue is practiced to perfection, it yields all sorts of "gems," which is best understood symbolically. The *Yoga-Bhāshya (II.30) defines it as one's abstention from unauthorized appropriation of things belonging to another. In the *Shāndilya-Upanishad (I.1.7), a medieval *Yoga scripture, it is explained as the noncoveting of another's property physically, mentally, and vocally.

āstikya ("it-is-ness") is often regarded as one of the constituent practices of moral observance (*yama*) and also of self-discipline (*niyama*). the *Shāndilya-Upanishad* (I.2.4) explains as *faith in the knowledge of revelation (*shruti*) and tradition (*smriti*).

āsvāda ("taste"). In *Classical Yoga, this is the paranormal ability to taste "divine" delicacies. *Patanjali regards this as one of the flashes of illumination (*pratibhā*), a kind of supersense, which is considered to be an obstacle (*upasarga*) to *enstasy.

Atharva-Veda ("Knowledge of Atharvan") is one of the four *Vedic hymnodies. Belonging to the era of about 1000 B.C., this work consists of some six thousand magical incantations (in 730 hymns), though there are also a number of fascinating philosophical riddles and illuminating metaphysical passages that anticipate later *Sāmkhya and *Yoga ideas and practices, notably breath control (*prānāyāma*). See also Veda, Vrātya.

atikrānta-bhāvanīya ("he who is intent on transcendence"). The *Yoga-Bhāshya* (III.51) explains this high-level spiritual attainment as consisting in the intention to cause the "involution" (*pratiprasava*) of the constituents (*guna*) of consciousness, or *Nature. The *adept who has reached this level of the spiritual process enjoys the sevenfold wisdom (*saptadha-prajnā*). Cf. *mādhu-bhūmika, prajnā-jyotis, prathama-kalpika*.

atithya ("hospitality") is sometimes regarded as one of the constituents of yogic self-discipline (*niyama*).

ātivāhika-deha ("superconductive body"), or simply **ātivāhika**, is the migratory *body of the after-death state. According to the *Agni-Purāna* (369.9), this body receives its nourishment from the funeral oblations. It is an intermediate vehicle for the ceased identity prior to the acquisition of the body peculiar to a deceased spirit (*preta-deha*) and, subsequently, an "enjoyment body" (*bhoga-deha*) in which the deceased reaps the auspicious or inauspicious fruits of his earthly deeds either in *heaven or in *hell.

A different interpretation of the *ātivāhika* is found in the *Yoga-Vāsishtha* (III.57.29 et al.). Here it is equated with the universal, omnipresent "body" of the singular *Reality. This is glorified as the true body of human beings, the physical body being considered a mere illusion. See also Death, *deha*, *pitri-yāna*.

ātma-darshana ("Self-vision") is often used synonymously with *Self-realization, or *enlightenment. In the *Yoga-Sūtra* (II.41), this signifies the appearance of the transcendental *Self on the horizon of *consciousness in the highest mode of enstasy (*samādhi*). See also *purusha-khyāti*.

ātma-jnāna ("Self-knowledge") is not mere self-understanding in the Socratic sense but the *enstatic realization of the transcendental *Reality.

ātman ("self" or "Self"). Since Sanskrit does not have capital letters, the context alone determines whether the empirical self, or ego-personality (*jīva*), or the transcendental *Self is intended. It is not always easy to make this distinction, however, as is clear from the following passage in the *Bhagavad-Gītā* (VI.5–6):

> One should raise the *ātman* by the *ātman*; one should not let the *ātman* sink; for the *ātman* is indeed the *ātman's* friend, and the *ātman* is also the *ātman's* enemy.

> The *ātman* is the friend of the *ātman* of him whose *ātman* is subdued by the *ātman*; but for [him who is] bereft of the *ātman*, the *ātman* is like an enemy in enmity.

The word *ātman* is primarily a reflexive pronoun but since the time of the ancient *Upanishads it has been used to denote the transcendental *Self. As such, it is a key concept of *Hindu metaphysics, notably *Vedānta and Vedānta-based schools of *Yoga. The Hindu sages and philosophers have mustered considerable ingenuity in determining and communicating the nature of the *ātman*. The problem is that the *Self is by definition not within reach of the *mind and the *senses. "The form of the Self cannot be seen by the eye," states the *Mahābhārata* epic (XII.196.4), reiterating a point made already in the earliest *Upanishads. As the archaic *Brihad-Āranyaka-Upanishad* (III.7.23) declares in a well-known passage, the *Self cannot be grasped since it is the grasper, the seer, of everything. In other words, the *Self reveals itself only to itself. No finite act of cognition is involved. Hence the *Shiva-Samhitā* (I.62), a work on *hatha-yoga*, states: "Having abandoned the perception of false states [of *consciousness], the renouncer of all volition (*samkalpa*) certainly beholds the Self in the Self by the Self."

ātma-nivedana ("self-offering") is one of the aspects of the *Yoga of devotion (*bhakti-yoga*). It means total surrender of the *ego and the unconditional worship of the *Divine as it is possible only in the state of enstasy (*samādhi*).

Attachment. See *rāga, sanga, sneha.*

Attention is an intrapsychic process that is fundamental to all *Yoga. It is the focusing of the *mind, or *consciousness, upon a select object. As the scriptures of *hatha-yoga* point out again and again, it is closely associated with the flow of psychosomatic energy (*prāna*) in the *body. In other words, attention and *breath are interconnected—a fact that is exploited by the *yogin*. Attention permits consciousness to rest on ever more "subtle" (*sūkshma*) aspects of existence, until it is totally transcended in the condition of supraconscious enstasy (*asamprajnāta-samādhi*).

atyāhāra ("overeating"). According to the *Hatha-Yoga-Pradīpikā* (I.15), this is one of the six factors by which *Yoga is foiled. See also *āhāra*; cf. *mita-āhāra.*

aum. See *om.*

Aurobindo Ghose (A.D. 1872–1950) is remembered as one of modern India's most famous sages. Born into a wealthy Bengali family, Aurobindo Ghose was educated in England and later entered the service of the Maharaja of Baroda. During Curzon's viceroyalty, he became a leading figure in the Bengali nationalist movement. It was during his one-year imprisonment for political agitation that his spiritual transformation occurred. Upon his release, he renounced the world and settled in the town of Pondicherry

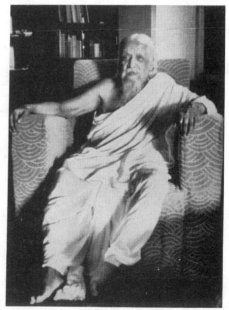

9. *Aurobindo Ghose.*

in South India. He was a prolific writer and published numerous books on philosophy, art, education, and, not least, *Yoga. Among his major publications are *The Life Divine*, *The Synthesis of Yoga*, and *Essays on the Gita*. His work has been continued by the French woman Mira Richard, better known as "The Mother," in whom Sri Aurobindo saw the embodiment of the divine *shakti*.

Sri Aurobindo described his spiritual approach as "Integral Yoga" (*pūrna-yoga*). It has been hailed as the only new philosophical system to emerge from contemporary India that is firmly founded in spiritual experience. Integral Yoga seeks to combine the quest for individual *liberation with the evolutionary destiny of humanity. This *Yoga purports to offer a viable spiritual *path for the present global crisis, which Sri Aurobindo understood as a transition from the mental to the supramental consciousness.

aushadhi ("herb" or "herbal concoction"). Certain drugs derived from plants are occasionally used by *yogins to procure *altered states of consciousness as well as paranormal powers (*siddhi*). Herbs play an important role in Indian *alchemy.

Auspicious posture. See *bhadra-āsana*.

avadhūta ("cast off") is the spiritual *adept who has "shaken off" all worldly things and concerns. According to the *Mandala-Brāhmana-Upanishad* (V.9), a medieval work, such a practitioner of radical *renunciation is accomplished in the practice of the highest type of supraconscious, supracognitive enstasy (*nirvikalpa-samādhi*). He is also known as a "supreme swan" (*parama-hamsa*), and is said to bring about the *liberation of 101 generations in his family. The *Mahānirvāna-Tantra* (XIV.149) distinguishes two types of *avadhūta*: the perfect one who is called "supreme swan" and the still imperfect one who is know as "wanderer" (*parivrāj*). See also Baul sect, Crazy adept, *samnyāsin*.

Avadhūta-Gītā is a late *Vedānta work that describes and extols the life-style of the *avadhūta* who, in his blissful state of *Self-realization, bows to no social convention but utterly renounces everything.

avasthā ("state"). *Yoga authorities distinguish several states or stages of maturity on the spiritual *path. Thus, the *Hatha-Yoga-Pradīpikā (IV.69) speaks of the initial state (*ārambha-avasthā), the active or "pot state" (*ghata-avasthā), the "accumulation state" (*paricāya-avasthā), and the "state of maturity" (nishpatty-avasthā). These are more often styled "levels" (*bhūmi).

The word avasthā is also used to describe the four or five states of *consciousness according to the Vedānta tradition. These are waking (*jāgrat), dreaming (*svapna), sleep (*sushupti), and the "fourth" (*turīya), which is the condition of *Self-realization. To these is sometimes added the state that transcends the "fourth" (*turīya-atīta), or radical *enlightenment.

Lastly, avasthā designates different states or stages of breath control (*prānāyāma).

avatāra ("descent"). This word is derived from the verbal root tri meaning "to cross over." It denotes a manifestation, or incarnation, of the *Divine on earth—particularly of God *Vishnu. Generally, ten such descents, or incarnations, are mentioned of him. However, the *Bhāgavata-Purāna also knows of sixteen, twenty-two, or twenty-three avatāras. The best known avatāra of these series are the God-men *Rāma and *Krishna. The divine incarnation for the present eon—the *kāli-yuga ("dark age")—is Kalki, or Kalkin, who is yet to come. Prophecy has it that he will appear riding a white horse and holding a blazing sword.

Aversion. See dvesha.

avidyā ("nescience") is a synonym for *ajnāna and generally denotes spiritual ignorance. In *Classical Yoga, avidyā is the principal among the five causes of affliction (*samsāra) of birth and *rebirth. The *Yoga-Sūtra (II.5) defines it as seeing that which is eternal, pure, joyous, and of the *Self as that which is transient, impure, sorrowful, and not of the *Self. Nescience is not merely the absence of *knowledge but a positive misconception about reality, just as a foe is not merely an absent friend but an enemy. Cf. jnāna, vidyā.

avirati ("dissipation"), or the squandering of one's energies on unworthy pursuits, is one of the nine obstacles (*antarāya) mentioned by *Patanjali.

avishesha ("unparticularized") is a technical term of *Classical Yoga, designating a distinct hierarchic level of Nature (*prakriti*). According to the *Yoga-Bhāshya* (II.19), it is composed of six ontic categories (*tattva*), namely the five potentials (*tanmātra*) and the principle of individuation (*asmitā-mātra*). See also Cosmos, *parvan*: cf. *vishesha*.

avyakta ("unmanifest") is a term that belongs to the ancient vocabulary of the *Yoga and *Sāmkhya traditions. It generally refers to the matrix of Nature (*prakriti*), the source of the manifest forms, corresponding to the Greek notion of *archē*. *Patanjali, the originator of *Classical Yoga, employs the synonyms *alinga* and *pradhāna* instead. See also Cosmos, *parvan*; cf. *vyakta*.

Awakening. The idealist traditions of the world, including some schools of *Yoga, compare our ordinary *waking state to a dream or hallucination: The reality we experience is not what there actually is but a conjured image, a projection, that is based on the mistaken assumption that reality is external to our experiencing *consciousness. The split into an experiencing subject (the ego-consciousness) and an experienced objective world is part of this dreamlike condition. Upon spiritual awakening, or *enlightenment, we understand that the duality (*dvaita*) between seer and seen is purely imaginary and that *Reality is singular. In this view, our ordinary state of awareness is one of diminished consciousness; it is a semiconscious condition governed by habit patterns (*vāsanā*).

This dream metaphor is, however, not used by *Patanjali, who believes that there is an ultimate, irrevocable chasm between the Self (*purusha*), and Nature (*prakrti*). See also *bodha*.

Awareness. See *caitanya*, *cit*, *citi*, Consciousness.

Āyur-Veda ("life science") is the native Indian system of *medicine. It is traditionally considered to be an appendix to the *Atharva-Veda*. Although the original scripture by this title is no longer extant, some of its medical lore has been preserved in the *Caraka-Samhitā* and other similar compilations.

B

baddha-padma-āsana ("bound lotus posture"), which is mentioned already in the *Goraksha-Paddhati* (I.96), is performed by clasping the big toes with one's hands, while being seated in the lotus posture (*padma-āsana) with one's arms crossed behind one's back. It is often recommended especially for the *purification of the psychoenergetic pathways (*nādī-shodhana). See also āsana.

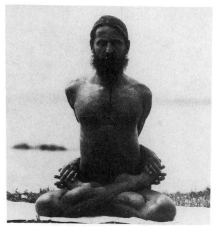

10. Baddha-padma-āsana.

bahir-anga ("outer limb"). In *Classical Yoga, this term applies to the first five "limbs" (*anga) of the eightfold *path, which are contrasted with the three "inner limbs" (*antar-anga). See also ashta-anga-yoga.

bahir-lakshya ("external sign") is one of the three kinds of photistic experience in *tāraka-yoga. The *Advaya-Tāraka-Upanishad (6) describes it as the perception of luminous "ether-space" (*vyoman) of blue, dark blue, red, and yellow color, at a distance of four, six, eight, ten, or twelve "breadth of thumb" in front of one's nose. This is preceded by the manifestation of rays of golden *light that, as one becomes accomplished, are seen at the rim of the eyes or on the ground.

bahish-krita-dhauti ("expelled cleansing") is one of the four types of internal cleansing (*antar-dhauti) used in *hatha-yoga. In the *Gheranda-Samhitā* (I.22), a medieval manual, we find the following description: One should perform the "crow seal" (*kākī-mudrā), then fill the abdomen with air, hold it there for ninety minutes and then force it down into the intestines. Next, one should stand in navel-deep water, draw out the intestines, and wash them until they are completely clean; then one should pull them back up again. This procedure, which should not be done without supervision, is said to yield a "shining body" (deva-deha). See also dhauti.

bala ("power," "strength"). Since ancient times, the practice of *Yoga has been said to lead to *power—both physical and psychic. This bears out the close historical association between Yoga and asceticism (*tapas). In the *Yoga-Sūtra* (III.46) of *Patanjali, bala is listed as one of the marks of bodily perfection (*kāya-sampad). However, the *Bhagavad-Gītā* (XVI.18) warns against the lust for power, which merely leads to repeated *rebirth. The word bala also signifies "strength" or "energy" as a positive requirement for *yogins. According to the *Mahābhārata* epic (XII.289.16), those who lack energy are bound to go astray. See also siddhi, vibhūti, vīrya.

Balance. See samatva.

bali ("offering") is one of the "limbs" (*anga) of the *Yoga of sacred sound (*mantra-yoga). This practice, which is an aspect of most forms of ritual Yoga, consists in the offering of fruit and flowers to one's chosen deity (*ishta-devatā).

bandha ("bond," "bondage") has a wide range of meanings in the Sanskrit literature and can stand for "tying" or "bridging" as well as "pledge" and "tendon." In *Yoga, it first and foremost signifies the human condition of finite existence, that is, the state of unenlightenment: Our spiritual ignorance (*avidyā) is our bondage. It keeps us tied to the cycle of existence (*samsāra)—from birth to *death to *rebirth to repeated death. In *Classical Yoga, bandha denotes the "correlation" (*samyoga) between the transcendental *Self or *purusha and the finite ego-personality, or *consciousness. This relation is sometimes described as that between fire and wood. Moreover, according to the

Yoga-Sūtra (III.1), the term refers to the "binding" of consciousness to a particular *object, or locus (*desha*), which is the very essence of *concentration.

Finally, *bandha* stands for a particular class of techniques in *hatha-yoga* that involve local stoppages of the flow of psychosomatic energy (*prāna*). In this sense, the word is often translated as "lock" or "constriction." Three such locks are generally distinguished: the *mūla-bandha* ("root lock"), the *uddīyāna-bandha* ("upward lock"), and the *jālandhara-bandha* ("water pipe lock"). According to the *Yoga-Kundaly-Upanishad* (I.40), a medieval work, these should be practiced when *breath control is mastered properly. See also *āsana, mudrā*.

Bath, bathing. See *snāna*.

Baul sect. The Bengali word *baul* (Hindi: *baur*) can be derived either from the Sanskrit term *vātula* meaning "mad" or from *vyākula* meaning "intent" or "perplexed." Both make reference to the ecstatic intoxication and religious fervor for which the Bauls are renowned. This loosely organized sect originated in Bengal during the Indian Middle Ages. Its members are chiefly recruited from the lower strata of society. The Bauls are noted for their unconventional manners and customs. As *yogin*-bards they are famous for their songs that more often than not revolve around the "man in the *heart," that is, the transcendental *Self immanent in the human *body. See also *avadhūta*, Sahajiyā.

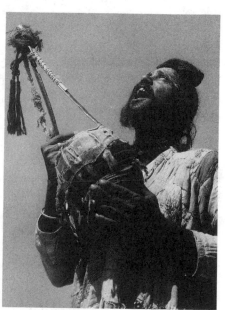

11. *Nabani Das, a modern Baul.*

Bellows breathing. See *bhastrikā*.

bhadra-āsana ("auspicious posture"). This yogic posture (*āsana*) is already mentioned in the fourth-century *Yoga-Bhāshya* (II.46), and is described in the *Tattva-Vaishāradī* (II.46) as follows: Bringing the soles of both feet near to each other at the scrotum, one should hollow the hands and place them above the feet in the shape of a tortoise. The *Gheranda-Samhitā* (II.9f.) states that one should place the heels cross-wise under the scrotum, cross one's hands behind the back, and catch hold of the toes. While performing the "water pipe lock" (*jālandhara-bandha*), one should fix one's gaze on the tip of the nose. This, it is said, cures all kinds of diseases. According to the *Hatha-Yoga-Pradīpikā* (I.53), this is also known as "Goraksha's posture" (*goraksha-āsana*). However, modern manuals of *Hatha-yoga* tend to distinguish between the *bhadra-āsana* and the *goraksha-āsana*. See also *āsana*.

Bhagavad-Gītā ("Lord's Song") is the most famous of all *Yoga scriptures. It is an episode in the vast national epic of India, the *Mahābhārata* (VI.13–40), into which it appears to have been neatly inserted prior to the Christian era. Like the epic as a whole, the *Gītā* belongs to what is called the "tradition" (*smriti*) literature of *Hinduism, but has for centuries in effect been treated as a part of the *Vedic canonical or *shruti* ("revelation") literature. According to its colophon, it wants to be understood as a secret teaching—an *upanishad*. It was probably composed in the third or fourth century B.C., but earlier and also later dates have been suggested. It is probable that the *Gītā* as we know it, consisting of seven hundred stanzas, is not all of a piece, though scholarship has so far failed to reconstruct a satisfactory *urtext*, or original version.

The teachings of the *Gītā* stem from the *Pāncarātra tradition of the ancient *Bhāgavata sect. They bear a unique stamp, and especially the *Gītā's* emphatic theism sets it off from other works of the same period. Its approach is markedly integrative, attempting to synthesize such diverse views as *Vedānta, *Sāmkhya, *Yoga, and orthodox *Brāhmanism, as well as the personal worship of God *Krishna. Purporting to be both a moral (*dharma*) teaching and mystical lore (*yoga-shāstra*), the *Gītā* advocates a three-pronged *path to *liberation, namely *karma-yoga, *jnāna-yoga, and *bhakti-yoga. The first two approaches are ex-pounded mainly in chapters I to XII, whereas the last six chapters are traditionally held to treat of the ideal and excellences of devotion (*bhakti*). Though not rejecting the kind of world-negating *asceticism that characterizes many *Upanishads, the *Gītā* nevertheless places the ideal of disinterested action (*naishkarmya-karman*) above that of the *renunciation of all *action. Yet, devotion (*bhakti*) is put forward as especially worthy of pursuit since it leads to a state of realization that is higher than mere "extinction in the world-ground" (*brahma-nirvāna*) insofar as it involves one's awakening in the divine person of *Krishna,

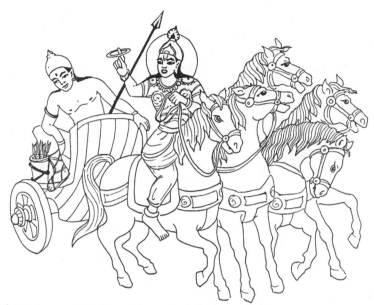

12. *Lord Krishna and Prince Arjuna in the war chariot where the teachings of the Bhagavad-Gītā were imparted.*

who is the all-encompassing suprapersonal (rather than impersonal) *Reality. See also *Anugītā, Avadhūta-Gītā, Ganesha-Gītā, Īshvara-Gītā, Uddhāva-Gītā.*

bhagavat ("blessed one"). This word generally refers to God *Krishna but is also applied to other personal *deities of the *Hindu pantheon. It suggests that the ultimate *Reality is not an abstract condition but living Being. See also *īshvara.*

Bhāgavata-Purāna or *Shrīmad-Bhāgavata.* This major *Purāna was probably composed about A.D. 750. It is the most important scripture of the *Bhāgavata sect. Its philosophical foundations are those of *Advaita-Vedānta, mellowed by the conception and *worship of the *Divine in personal form, as *Krishna. However, cultic rituals do not play as significant a role in this work as they do in the *Samhitā literature of the *Pāncarātra tradition. The *Bhāgavata-Purāna* is replete with *Yoga and *Sāmkhya teachings. All the elements of the eightfold *path (*ashta-anga-yoga*) are present, yet the overall focus is on *service and *devotion to the personal *God. Thus, the path propounded in this *Purāna is *bhakti-yoga.* This is contrasted with "Yoga," which presumably refers to the dualist approach of *Classical Yoga. Much space is given to instructions about visualizing the personal deity in *meditation.

Of particular interest is section XI.6–29, known as the *Uddhāva-Gītā ("Uddhava's Song"). In imitation of the *Bhagavad-Gītā ("Lord's Song"), this work expounds three types of *Yoga, namely *karma-yoga, *jnāna-yoga, and *bhakti-yoga. In one passage (IX.20), God *Vishnu declares that he is of nothing more fond than *devotion. Elsewhere *XXIII.41), the Uddhāva-Gītā speaks out against the kind of body-oriented Yoga that merely aims at the acquisition of paranormal powers (*siddhi), since, it is argued, the *body is after all mortal.

Bhāgavata sect. This sect has grown up around the *worship of the "blessed one" (*bhagavat), that is, God *Vasudeva, who is *Vishnu and *Krishna. The antiquity of Bhāgavatism is well established, but its history is still rather obscure. The earliest available sources of this sect are the *Bhagavad-Gītā and the Nārāyanīya section of the *Mahābhārata epic (XII.334–351). According to *Shankara's learned commentary on the Brahma-Sūtra (II.2.42f.), a classic summary of *Vedānta metaphysics, the word bhāgavata applies to the followers of the religious tradition known as *Pāncarātra, though this distinction is not always so clear-cut. See also Vaishnavism.

Bhairava is one of the terrifying forms of God *Shiva. This is also the name of an *adept of *hatha-yoga, who is mentioned in the *Hatha-Yoga-Pradīpikā (I.6). See also Ānanda Bhairava.

bhakta ("devotee," "worshipper"). Worship or devotion (*bhakti) is a spiritual practice by which the aspirant seeks to acknowledge his or her dependence on a higher power. The *Bhāgavata-Purāna (III.29.7ff.) distinguishes four types of devotee. The qualities of the first three are in consonance with the three primary qualities (*guna) of *Nature, whereas the fourth type is said to be nirguna, or beyond *Nature's primary constituents. According to the *Bhagavad-Gītā (IX.23), even those who are completely dedicated to the worship of a deity (*deva) other than God *Krishna in reality worship Krishna, because he is the recipient of all *sacrifices. However, because such worshippers do not know *Krishna to be the supreme *Being, they also do not attain final *liberation. There is always an exclusive element to such devotionalism, which is founded in theism, but the ultimate virtue of the worshipper is to discover the *Divine in all beings and forms.

bhakti ("devotion," "love"). This word is derived from the verbal root *bhaj* meaning "to participate in." It denotes "loving attachment" or "devotion." From the beginning, the term was intimately connected with the theistic traditions of *Hinduism. It made its first appearance in the *Shvetāshvatara-Upanishad* (IV.23), an early *Shaiva text, which demands devotion to the *Divine and one's *teacher.

However, originally the ideal of *bhakti* was mainly promoted among the worshippers of God *Vishnu who favored a strongly theistic philosophy. This orientation is best represented in the *Bhagavad-Gītā* (XVI.30) where the God-man *Krishna declares: "He who sees Me everywhere and who sees Me as all: to him I am not lost nor is he lost to Me."

The *Bhagavad-Gītā* (XVIII.54f.) distinguishes two degrees of *liberation—one without devotion, the other with devotion:

Having become [identical with] the world-ground (*brahman*) and being tranquil, he neither grieves nor craves. [Beholding] the same [*Reality] in all beings, he gains supreme love for Me.

Through love (*bhakti*) he really knows Me; how great I am and who. Then, having really known Me, he forthwith enters into that [supreme state of My Being].

These stanzas speak of what elsewhere is called the "higher love" (*para-bhakti*) of the person who, upon attaining *liberation, discovers that the ultimate *Reality is not impersonal but suprapersonal.

For the Marathi saint *Jnānadeva, whose *Jnāneshvarī* is hailed as the finest commentary on the *Bhagavad-Gītā*, devotion constitutes the fifth goal of humanity (*purusha-artha*). the *Bhāgavata-Purāna* (VI.9.47), again, insists that love and *knowledge are interdependent and that the one can be reached by means of the other. See also *bhakti-mārga*, *bhakti-yoga*, *guru-bhakti*.

bhakti-mārga ("road of devotion") refers to the devotional religious movement that swept across the south of India in the seventh to ninth centuries and across the north in the fourteenth to seventeenth centuries A.D. The modern Krishna Consciousness sect is a revival of those teachings. See also Bhaktivedanta Swami.

Bhakti-Sūtra of *Nārada is a medieval *Vaishnava work that was probably composed after *Rāmānuja's time. In eighty-four aphorisms, the sage Nārada explains in simple terms the essence of the devotional approach (*bhakti-yoga*) to the *Divine. He recommends contact (*sanga*) with the great *adepts and constant worship (*bhajana*) of *God, expressed in selfless *action, songs of praise, and listening to the scriptural expressions of his glory. *Liberation is gained through grace (*kripā*) alone. In aphorism eighty-three, he mentions *Shāndilya among other teachers of *bhakti.

Bhakti-Sūtra of *Shāndilya. In contrast to *Nārada's *Bhakti-Sūtra*, the work of the sage Shāndilya is more academic and polemical and has been more influential in philosophical circles. It consists of one hundred aphorisms distributed over three chapters, and it probably precedes the *Bhāgavata-Purāna*, which can be placed in the eighth century A.D. The earliest extant commentary on Shāndilya's compilation is the *Bhāshya* ("Speech") of Svapneshvara, a Bengali *Vaishnava who may have lived between A.D. 1300 and 1400. Another commentary is by the seventeenth-century scholar and spiritual practitioner *Nārāyana Tīrtha.

Bhaktivedanta Swami Prabhupada (A.D. 1896–1977) was the founder and spiritual head of the International Society for Krishna Consciousness, an offshoot of the ancient tradition of *Vaishnavism as taught in the first half of the sixteenth century by the ecstatic *Caitanya. Founded in 1966, the ISKC has published new translations of many ancient *Vaishnava scriptures, notably the *Bhagavad-Gītā* and the *Bhāgavata-Purāna*, and its renunciates made the "Hare Krishna" *mantra famous in the Western hemisphere. Bhaktivedanta Swami's teaching is a form of *bhakti-yoga.

bhakti-yoga ("Yoga of devotion"). This is one of the principal branches of the *Yoga tradition of *Hinduism. It is often presented as complementing the approaches of *jnāna-yoga and *karma-yoga. Later *Vaishnava authorities of this type of Yoga mention the following nine "limbs" (*anga): *shravana, or "listening" to the sacred scriptures; *kīrtana, or the "singing" of devotional songs in praise of *God; *smarana, or "remembering" the *Divine by meditating upon its form; *pāda-sevana, or "service at the feet" of the Lord; *arcanā, or ritual worship; *vandana, or "prostration" before the image of God; *dāsya, or "slavish" devotion to the Lord; *sākhya, or "friendship" through which the Divine raises the humble *devotee to the status of a friend, and *ātma-nivedana, or "self-offering," through which the worshipper enters into the immortal body of God. These aspects, or stages, of *bhakti-yoga* are most lucidly expounded by Rūpa Gosvāmin in his work

Bhakti-Rasa-Amrita-Sindhu ("Ocean of the Immortal Essence of Devotion").

According to the *Bhāgavata-Purāna* (III.28.7), there are many *paths of *bhakti-yoga*, depending on the different inner constitution (*svabhāva*) of practitioners. This scripture (III.29.14) also speaks of an *ātyantika* ("extreme") *bhakti-yoga* consisting in pure *devotion to the *Divine on the part of those who have resigned their will to the point where they do not even *desire to be uplifted to God *Vishnu's paradise but have become utterly devoid of personal motivation apart from the desire to be *God's instrument. This is also known as "unqualified devotion" (*nirguna-bhakti*). See also *prapatti*.

Bhanukin is an adept of *hatha-yoga* mentioned in the *Hatha-Yoga-Pradīpikā* (I.8). No further information is available on him.

Bhartrihari, the seventh-century poet and grammarian, is best known for his *Vairāgya-Shataka* ("Century of Dispassion") and *Shānti-Shataka* ("Century of Peace"). The former composition celebrates the ideal of *dispassion and depicts its author as still engaged in the struggle for *renunciation. The latter work, on the other hand, portrays him as having gained a certain spiritual vantage point. In this didactic poem (IV.10), the author condemns false *yogins* who, through painful self-castigation, acquire *powers but lack genuine inner *peace. Bhartrihari was the first to propound the *Advaita-Vedānta doctrine of *vivarta*, or illusory world emanation.

Bhartrihari, the eleventh-century king of Ujjain (western India), was, according to local tradition, converted to *Nāthism by the great teacher *Goraksha himself. According to other traditions, it was *Jālandhari who initiated him. One of the subsects of the *Kānphata sect is named after him.

bhāshya ("Speech," "Discussion"). See *Yoga-Bhāshya*.

bhastrikā or **bhastrā** ("bellows") is one of the eight types of breath control (*prānāyāma*) described in the *Gheranda-Samhitā* (V.74f.) and other scriptures of *hatha-yoga*. It is explained as follows: As the bellows of the black smith move the air to and fro, so should the breath be slowly moved through both nostrils. After twenty repetitions of this, the *yogin* should perform the "pot" (*kumbhaka*), that is, retention of the *breath. It is clear from the description found in the *Hatha-Yoga-Pradīpikā* (II.59ff.) that inhalation should be done through the right nostril and exhalation through the left. However, in the *Yoga-Kundaly-Upanishad* (I.32ff.) a reverse procedure is stipulated. The principal purpose of *bhastrikā* is to awaken the "serpent power" (*kundalinī-shakti*). See also *shakti-cālana*.

Bhāsvatī of *Harihrānanda Āranya. This is a twentieth-century Sanskrit commentary on the *Yoga-Sūtra*, offering many illuminating definitions.

bhava, which is derived from the verbal root *bhū* ("to be"), can mean such diverse things as "birth," "source," and "prosperity." In many contexts, however, the word denotes "existence" in the sense of *samsāra*.

bhāva, which is a derivative of *bhū*, means "being," "condition," "nature," "disposition," and "feeling." The last-mentioned connotation is found primarily in works on *bhakti-yoga*, which distinguish five principal feelings, or moods: *shānta-bhāva*, or the "tranquil mood" (of awe or humility); *dāsya-bhāva*, or the "slavish mood" (of respect, subservience, or dedication); *vatsalya-bhāva*, or the "calflike mood" (of tender parental or brotherly feelings); *sākhya-bhāva*, or "friendly mood" (of feelings of friendship); *mādhurya-bhāva*, or "sweet mood" (of delight between lovers). These should ultimately develop into *rasa* or the tasting of the pure *bliss of intimate love-participation in *God.

*Tantrism has a well-known classification of practitioners into three fundamental types. Thus, a distinction is made between the "beastly disposition" (*pashu-bhāva*), the "heroic disposition" (*vīra-bhāva*), and the "divine disposition" (*divya-bhāva*). The word *pashu means "beast" and generally refers to the individual who is fettered to the world of illusion (*māyā*). The predominant quality active in such a person is inertia (*tamas*). However, in some contexts, the word designates a full-fledged initiate of a certain level of spiritual attainment. The disposition of the hero (*vīra*), resulting from a preeminence of the quality of dynamism (*rajas*), is characteristic of the typical spiritual aspirant in the present "dark age" (*kāli-yuga*). The divine disposition is due to a preponderance of the principle of lucidity (*sattva*), and it defines that rare individual who is naturally inclined toward *meditation, *equanimity, and remembering the *Divine.

Bhāva Ganesha Dīkshita is the author of the *Yoga-Anushāsana-Sūtra-Vritti*, also titled *Pradīpikā*. He was a chief disciple of *Vijnāna Bhikshu and probably lived between A.D. 1550 and 1600.

bhāvanā ("cultivation") is sometimes used as a synonym for "meditation" (*dhyāna*).

bhāva-yoga ("Yoga of being"). According to the *Shiva-Purāna* (VII.2.37.9), this is a yogic approach that does not include *mantra* recitation. Cf. *abhāva-yoga*.

bhaya ("fear") is one of the defects (*dosha*) of the ego-personality that need to be overcome. That fear is a universal constant of human experience is recognized by all traditions of *Yoga, as is the possibility of transcending it. Upon full *Self-realization, all fear is extirpated. Cf. *abhaya*.

bhoga ("enjoyment"). In *Classical Yoga, this term stands for "world experience" as the antithesis of emancipation (*apavarga*). The *Yoga-Sūtra* (III.35) defines it as an idea that is based on the nondistinction between the *Self and the most translucent aspect of *Nature, namely the *sattva*. The *Bhagavad-Gītā* (V.22) speaks of the enjoyment that springs from contact with the sense objects as a womb of suffering (*duhkha*).

Bhoja, king of Dhārā, lived between A.D. 1018 and 1060. His personal name was Ranaranga Malla, and he was a worshipper of God *Shiva. He composed a much-acclaimed commentary on the *Yoga-Sūtra* entitled *Rāja-Mārtanda* and is also credited with the authorship of works on *Shaiva philosophy, grammar, ethics, astronomy, and the art of war.

Bhoja-Vritti. See *Rāja-Mārtanda*.

bhoktri ("enjoyer"). According to *Sāmkhya metaphysics, the transcendental *Self is the enjoyer of all things. Thus, the *Maitrāyanīya-Upanishad* (VI.10) asserts that the Self devours "Nature's food" (*prākritam annam*), its food being specifically the "elemental self" (*bhūta-ātman*). In the yogic schools, the *bhoktri* is the *Self as the experiencing subject of mental states. See also *bhoga*; cf. *kartri*.

bhrama ("perplexity"), one of the obstacles (*vighna*) of Yoga, stands for a wandering *mind in need of discipline.

bhrāmarī ("bee") is one of the eight types of breath control (*prāṇāyāma*) of *hatha-yoga*. This technique is described in the *Hatha-Yoga-Pradīpikā* (II.68) as follows: One should inhale while making the sound of a male bee, then exhale slowly (after having retained the air for some time) while making the sound of a female bee. According to the *Gheranda-Samhitā* (V.78ff.), this practice is performed somewhat differently, and is connected with the perception of inner sounds. See also *nāda-yoga*.

bhrānti ("delusion") is one of the ten obstacles (*vighna*) of *Yoga. According to the *Kaula-Jnāna-Nirnaya* (V.2), a medieval work of the *Kaula sect, it is to be overcome through the persistent practice of meditation (*dhyāna*).

bhrānti-darshana ("false vision") is one of the obstructions (*antarāya*) mentioned by *Patanjali. The *Linga-Purāna* (I.9.7) explains it as erroneous knowledge relative to the spiritual goal, one's *teacher, the nature of *knowledge, conduct, and the *Divine.

Bhrigu ("Bhrigu") is one of the sons of the legendary Manu, the ancestor of the human race. He is remembered as a *Vedic seer (*rishi*) who cursed God *Agni turning him into an omniferous deity. He is a member of the *Vedic priestly family of the Bhrigus, who invented the fire *sacrifice. Bhrigu came to be associated with the tradition of *Vaishnavism. He often figures as a *teacher of *Yoga in medieval scriptures.

bhrū-cakra ("brow wheel") is better known as the *ājnā-cakra*.

bhrū-madhya ("brow middle") is the place on the forehead in the middle between the eyebrows. *Yogins are often seen focusing their gaze (*drishti*) on this spot during *concentration. However, the *bhrū-madhya* is also the secret locus in the center of the *head, most frequently referred to as the *ājnā-cakra*, which is a favorite anchor point for the aspirant's attention. The *Tri-Shikhī-Brāhmana-Upanishad* (II.132) regards the *bhrū-madhya* as one of the eighteen vital areas (*marman*) of the *body and as the locus of the "fourth" (*turīya*), that is, the transcendental *Self. Cf. *nāsa-agra*.

bhū-cāra-siddhi or **bhū-cārī-siddhi** ("earth-moving power"), the paranormal ability (*siddhi*) to levitate at will. According to the *Yoga-Tattva-Upanishad* (59), a medieval work, this is one of the benefits of mastery in breath control (*prāṇāyāma*). The *Shiva-Samhitā* (V.88), a late scrip-

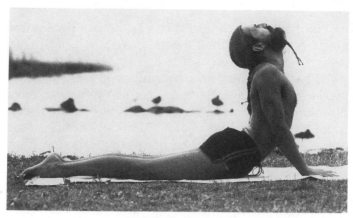

13. *Bhujanga-āsana.*

ture of *hatha-yoga*, also deems it procurable by means of *contemplation upon the *vāna-linga* in the *heart center. See also Levitation.

bhujanga-āsana ("serpent posture"). The Sanskrit word *bhujanga* literally means "crooked limbed" (from *bhuj* + *anga*) and denotes a serpent. This posture (*āsana*) is popularly called "the Cobra." The *Gheranda-Samhitā* (II.42f.), a classic manual on *hatha-yoga*, describes it thus: The body should touch the ground from the *navel down to the toes. Placing the palms on the ground, one should raise the head and shoulders like a serpent. This is said to raise the body temperature and remove *diseases of all kinds, as well as awaken the "serpent power" (*kundalinī-shakti*).

bhujangī ("serpent") is a synonym for *kundalinī.

bhujanginī-mudrā ("serpent seal") is described in the *Gheranda-Samhitā* (III.92f.) as follows: Extending the face a little forward, one should suck in air through the gullet. This is said to quickly cure all abdominal diseases, especially indigestion. See also *mudrā*.

bhukti ("enjoyment") is a synonym for *bhoga*.

bhūmi ("earth") can stand for a variety of things. Thus it denotes (1) the ground on which the yogic practices are performed; (2) the earth element (*prithivī*), (3) the planet earth, and (4) a particular "stage" or "level" of practice.

The last-mentioned connotation deserves comment. *Yoga is a graduated endeavor, and the initiate is thought to progress to ever higher levels of attainment until he or she reaches the final stage (*prānta-bhūmi*), which, according to the *Yoga-Sūtra (II.27), consists in the "sevenfold wisdom" (*saptadha-prajñā*). However, since *progress depends on the individual's capacity and commitment there can be no rigid objective scale, but only models that serve as signposts along the way. One such model is *Patanjali's classification of enstasy (*samādhi*) into four principal types. Although one of *Patanjali's aphorisms (viz. III.6) would seem to imply some kind of natural progression from one enstatic level to the next, the great Yoga master nowhere actually states that a particular sequence must be followed. Sudden leaps to higher levels are in fact admitted by his commentator *Vyāsa. In his *Yoga-Bhāshya (III.6), he remarks that "Yoga itself is the teacher." In the *Tattva-Vaishāradī (I.17), *Vācaspati Mishra compares the *yogin to an archer who first practices with a big target nearby and only later with a smaller target placed at a greater distance. Vācaspati suggests that at first *concentration should involve a "coarse" (*sthūla*) object and later, when the necessary skill has been developed, on objects pertaining to the "subtle" (*sūkshma*) dimension of *Nature.

Vācaspati also mentions four stages of the process of enstatic involution: the *mādhu-mati-bhūmi* ("honeyed level"); the *mādhu-pratīka-bhūmi* ("honey-faced level"); the *vishoka-bhūmi* ("sorrowless level"), and the *samskāra-shesha-bhūmi* ("level consisting of a residuum of subconscious activators"). In the *Yoga-Bhāshya (I.1), moreover, mention is made of five levels of mental activity (see *citta-bhūmi*). See also *atikrānta-bhāvanīya, avasthā, mādhu-bhūmika, prajñā-jyotis, sapta-jnāna-bhūmi*.

bhūta, which is the past participle of the verbal root *bhū* ("to be, to become"), can have several connotations. It can refer to an elemental or disembodied spirit. It can also signify a living being. In many contexts, it denotes the five *elements (*panca-bhūta*) of which the material *cosmos is composed. These are in ascending order: earth (*prithivī*), water (*ap*), fire (*agni*), air (*vāta*), and ether (*ākāsha*). See also *tattva*.

bhūta-ātman ("elemental self") is the individuated self. This concept first appeared in the schools of *Pre-Classical Yoga but is also found in later *Yoga scriptures showing *Vedānta influence. According to the *Mahābhārata epic (XII.245.11), the elemental self resides in the *heart and is a fragment (*amsha*) of the supreme radiance, the transcendental *Self.

bhūta-jaya ("conquest of the elements"). This is one of the paranormal powers (*siddhi*). According to the *Yoga-Sūtra* (III.44), it results from the practice of enstatic constraint (*samyama*) upon the various ontic levels of a given *object.

bhūta-shuddhi ("purification of the elements"). This concept is often used synonymously with *kundalinī-yoga*, which attempts the gradual transformation of the *body into a quasi-divine body (*divya-deha*) endowed with supernal faculties. As the "serpent power" (*kundalinī-shakti*) ascends from the base center to the crown of the *head, it is thought to successively "dissolve" the five elements—earth, water, fire, air, and ether. This is interpreted as a process of gradual *purification. In practice, the ascent of the psychospiritual power leads to a progressive withdrawal of *consciousness from the body, leading to a state of insensitivity and coldness in the trunk and limbs. On the level of the *mind, this spiritual *alchemy has a parallel effect inasmuch as consciousness becomes ever more unified, until the state of formless enstasy (*nirvikalpa-samādhi*) ensues. Now the *yogin's awareness-identity rests in the transcendental *Self, without any bodily awareness.

The process of *bhūta-shuddhi* also has a ritual counterpart whereby the material *elements are symbolically dissolved. The purpose of this *purification is to convert the *body into a temple ready to receive one's chosen deity (*ishta-devatā*). See also *shuddhi*.

bhuvana ("cosmos"). See Cosmos, *jagat*.

bīja ("seed"). In *Classical Yoga, the word denotes the causes of affliction (*klesha*) that are called the "seeds of the defects (*dosha*)," which refers to the subconscious activators (*samskāra*). Furthermore, the term *bīja* can mean the object or prop of *meditation, as in the compounds *sabīja- and *nirbīja-samādhi*. Finally, the word is short for *bīja-mantra*.

bīja-mantra ("seed word"). This is a central concept of *Tantrism. A *mantra* of this category is monosyllabic and so called because it represents the quintessence of more complex *sound combinations. Such "shorthand" *mantras* are characteristically meaningless and have a metalinguistic function. They are thought to represent, and be a part of, specific deities (*devatā*) who are invoked during the *Tantric rituals and with whom the initiate seeks to merge. These mystic phonemes are also associated with the seven psychoenergetic centers (*cakra*) of the *body.

Bile. See *pitta*.

Bileshaya, a great *hatha-yoga* master, is mentioned in the *Hatha-Yoga-Pradīpikā* (I.5), though no further information is given.

bimba ("reflection") is a technical term in the epistemology of *Classical Yoga as interpreted by *Vācaspati Mishra. It denotes the "reflection" of the transcendental *Self-awareness (*caitanya*) in the most lucid aspect of the *mind, namely the *sattva* or *buddhi*. This is also called the "shadow of *Consciousness" (*citi-chāyā*). See also *chāyā, pratibimba*.

bindu ("drop" or "dot"). This word has many different technical connotations in *Yoga. It is occasionally used as a synonym for "source" or "source point" (*bīja*). As such it is the origin of all manifestation, notably all sound (*nāda*). The *bindu* represents the inaudible, transcendental "sound" of the *Absolute, captured in the sacred syllable *om*. It is graphically depicted as the dot in the *ardha-mātra* symbol.
    In *Tantrism and *hatha-yoga*, *bindu* frequently denotes "semen." The loss of semen (*retas*) is considered to be one of the most potent *obstacles to spiritual development, and its preservation is regarded as imperative. The general recommendation is that in order to preserve the semen the *yogin* should abstain from sexual intercourse (*maithunā*). However, even sexually active aspirants are asked to circumvent seminal discharge. According to the *Hatha-Yoga-Pradīpikā* (IV.28), a classic manual of *hatha-yoga*, the stabilization of the semen is effected by means of the stabilization of the mind and the life force (*prāna*). For the movement of the *bindu* is closely connected with the circulation of the life energy, in the form of the *breath. As the *Goraksha-Paddhati* (I.69) declares, so long as the *bindu* remains in the *body there is no need to fear *death.
    A highly recommended practice for the prevention of seminal discharge is the *khecārī-mudrā*, which is said to be effective even during sexual embrace. When the semen has begun to flow down into the genital area, it can be prevented from discharging by means of the *yoni-mudrā*. When the semen has left the penis, it can be sucked back by means of the *vajrolī-mudrā*.
    The scriptures of *Yoga and *Tantrism obviously have a conception of semen that is quite distinct from the modern notion of seminal secretion. It comprises an esoteric dimension that is expressed in the

doctrine of the two types of semen, male and female. The former is called *shukla* or *shukra* (both words meaning "white"), and the latter is called *rajas* (meaning literally "that which is brilliant") of *mahā-*("great")*rajas*. Whereas the white or male *bindu* is situated in the "region of the moon" (*shashi-sthāna*), that is, in the middle of the *head, the red or female *bindu* is to be found in the "genital region" (*yoni-sthāna*).

According to the *Goraksha-Paddhati* (I.72), the union of these two *bindus* is most difficult to achieve. When accomplished, the *yogin* attains to the supreme abode, or *liberation. As the *Yoga-Cūdāmany-Upanishad* (63) states, this union can be brought about through the activation of the "serpent power" (*kundalinī-shakti*), a technique called *shakti-cālana. See also Sexuality.

bindu-jaya ("conquest of the semen"), also called *bindu-siddhi* ("power over the semen"). The *Hatha-Yoga-Pradīpikā* (II.78) considers this to be one of the signs of perfection in *hatha-yoga. See also *vajrolī-mudrā*, *yoni-mudrā*.

Bindunātha is mentioned in the *Hatha-Yoga-Pradipika* (I.7) as an *adept of *hatha-yoga. Judging from his name, he was obviously a master of the *bindu-siddhi*.

Bliss. See *ānanda*, *sukha*.

bodha or **bodhana** ("awakening" or "enlightenment"). This is a common synonym for *moksha* ("liberation"). See also Awakening.

Body. *Yoga, like all esoteric traditions of the world, envisions the human body as a complex hierarchic system of internesting "sheaths" (*kosha*), each vibrating at a different frequency (or degree of subtlety). At the lowest level is the physical body composed of the five material elements (*bhūta*). At the highest level is the universal "body" of the transcendental *Reality, which is pure *Consciousness and unalloyed *Bliss. In between these two extremes are thought to exist a range of intermediary "vehicles" or bodily envelopes that are not normally accessible to our conscious awareness, but their existence is inferable from their various activities. However, these subtle envelopes have been the subject of much introspective exploration by *yogins. Over many centuries, they have developed fascinating models of what has been called esoteric *anatomy. These seek to account for the phenomenology of *altered states of consciousness, notably mystical experiences. Their principal purpose, however, is not to furnish exhaustive descriptions or analyses but to serve as road maps for practitioners traveling on the spiritual *path.

One of the best known yogic models of the subtle dimensions of bodily existence distinguishes seven major psychoenergetic centers (*cakra*). These are thought to be aligned along the spinal axis, and roughly correspond to the nerve plexuses in the physical or "gross" (*sthūla*) body. These centers are connected by means of "conduits" or "channels" (*nādī*) formed of life energy (*prāna*). In fact, to the *yogin's* clairvoyant sight, the person appears as a luminous bubble of energy made up of a dense network of psychoenergetic currents.

Recent studies in *parapsychology and bioelectricity have lent some credence to these models, though these findings remain controversial. Thus, researchers using Kirlian photography have demonstrated the existence of a bioelectric field around living things—a field that disappears only gradually after *death. Researchers studying the meridians of acupuncture have also found positive proof for the existence of bioelectric currents and *cakra*like vortices that cannot be explained by ordinary physiological principles. Mention must also be made of laboratory experiments on out-of-body experiences, which have yielded some evidence in favor of the traditional assumption that *consciousness can operate outside the body. However, there is a need for much more substantive research in all these areas. Perhaps, as medicine outgrows its inherited nineteenth-century materialist paradigm, reputable researchers will be less fearful of entering investigations of this kind. Certainly, the esoteric models of the human body not only offer a far more exciting vision but they are also inherently more plausible than the conventional one-dimensional model of modern medicine. For, however fanciful they may appear in their details, they do justice to the multidimensional nature of existence, as it is becoming obvious through the findings of contemporary physics. See also *deha*, Embodiment, *kāya*, *kosha*, *sharīra*, *tanu*.

Bondage. See *bandha*; cf. Liberation.

Book learning. See *grantha*, *shāstra*.

Bound lotus posture. See *baddha-padma-āsana*.

Bow posture. See *dhanur-āsana*.

Brahma is the creator *God in the classic triad of *Hinduism, the other two Gods being *Vishnu and *Shiva. He is to be carefully distinguished from the *brahman, which is the impersonal *Absolute beyond all distinctions. See also *deva*.

brahma-anda ("brahmic egg") refers to the macrocosm. However, in the *Shiva-Samhitā* (I.91), for instance, the term signifies the microcosm, that is, the human *body. Cf. Microcosm, *pinda-anda*.

brahma-bila ("brahmic cave"). See *brahma-randhra*.

brahma-cakra ("brahmic wheel") is a synonym for *mūlādhāra-cakra*.

brahmacarya ("brahmic conduct") is the mode of life of the *Vedic student called *brahmacārin*. *Brahmacarya* essentially stands for the ideal of chastity. It is called "brahmic conduct" presumably because the *brahman transcends all gender distinctions. The spiritual aspirant is asked to emulate that genderless condition so as to preserve and cultivate the great power inherent in the semen (*bindu*).

Brahmacarya is one of the constituent practices of moral discipline (*yama*). According to the *Yoga-Sūtra* (II.38), the textbook of *Classical Yoga, the *yogin who is firmly grounded in this virtue gains great vitality (*vīrya*). According to the *Bhagavad-Gītā* (XVII.14), it forms part of bodily asceticism (*tapas*). The *Kūrma-Purāna* (II.11.18) defines it as the abstinence from sexual intercourse (*maithunā*) in deed, mind, and speech at all times and in all circumstances. Similar definitions are found in many other works. The *Darshana-Upanishad* (I.13f.) also explains it as the *mind's movement toward the state of the *brahman.

The *Agni-Purāna* (CCCLXXII.9) understands *brahmacarya* as the *renunciation of the eight degrees of sexual activity: fantasizing (*smarana*); glorifying (*kīrtana*) the sex act or the opposite gender; dalliance (*keli*); eyeing (*prekshana*) the opposite gender; talking in secret (*guhya-bhāshana*), that is, love talk; longing (*samkalpa*); the resolution (*adhya-vāsāya*) to break one's vow of chastity, and *kriyā-nivritti*, which is the consummation of the sexual act. According to the *Linga-Purāna* (I.8.17), the above strict definition applies only to anchorites (*vaikhānasa*), forest dwellers (*vānaprastha*), and widowers, whereas householders (*grihastha*) are allowed sexual intercourse with their wives but must practice chastity with regard to other women. See also *vajrolī-mudrā*.

brahma-dvāra ("brahmic gate"), According to the *Shat-Cakra-Nirūpana (3), the "brahmic gate" is situated at the mouth of the *citrinī-nādī and is also called the "place of the knot" (*granthi-sthāna*), meaning the "brahmic knot" (*brahma-granthi*). This opening, which is at the base of the spinal column, is covered by the head of the hidden serpent, the *kundalinī-shakti, and can be broken open by means of the "forceful Yoga" (*hatha-yoga*).

brahma-granthi ("brahmic knot") is the first of the "knots" in the human *body blocking the free flow of life force (*prāna*) along the central channel (*sushumnā-nādī*). It is variously said to be located at the *heart or at the *mūlādhāra-cakra, the lowest psychoenergetic center of the *body. See also *granthi*.

brahma-loka ("brahmic world"), the realm of the *brahman, which is the highest level of existence. See also Cosmos, *loka*.

brahma-muhūrta ("brahmic hour") or the time of sunrise, which is considered ideal for practicing *meditation and especially for rousing the "serpent power" (*kundalinī-shakti*).

brahman is derived from the verbal root *brih* ("to grow" or "to expand") and means as much as "vast expanse." This word is commonly translated as the "*Absolute." In the ancient *Vedas, the term stands for *prayer or *meditation as a means of evoking the universal divine power, also called *brahman*.

It was not until the *Shata-Patha-Brāhmana of the eighth or ninth century B.C. that the word *brahman* acquired its well-known philosophical connotation as the supreme principle behind and above all the various deities (*devatā*) and beings. In this sense, the term *brahman* is sometimes explained in fanciful folk etymology as that which grows (*brihati*) and causes everything to grow (*brihmyati*).

The earliest *Upanishads are unique records of the giant intellectual struggle of the ancient sages to crystallize this concept, which was to become one of the anchor points of *Hindu metaphysics and theology. In the earliest references, *brahman* simply signifies the origin of the *cosmos, the primal entity that procreated the manifold world. A next stage of explanation understood the universe as being identical with that *brahman*. As the *Chāndogya-Upanishad (III.14) puts it: "All this is the *brahman*." This pantheistic conception was subsequently made more explicit in the doctrine of the *brahman* that subsists in everything "as a razor is hidden in a razor case," as the *Brihad-Āranyaka-Upanishad

(I.4.7) declares. Next came the important notion of the identity of the *brahman* with the innermost self (or *Self) in human beings, called *ātman*.

This identity forms the central theme of the *Upanishadic literature and *Vedānta philosophy. The Vedānta schools generally distinguish between a "lower" (*apara*) and a "higher" (*para*) aspect of the *Absolute, and often call the lower aspect the "sound Absolute" (*shabda-brahman*). Cf. Brahma.

brāhmana or **brahmin.** This is the person learned in the *Vedic lore but also, more generally, a member of the first of the four estates (*varna*) of traditional *Hindu society. The brahmins were traditionally the custodians of the sacred knowledge, though, as is evident from the *Upanishads, members of other estates—notably warriors (*kshatriya*)—also played a significant role in the development of *Vedānta and *Yoga. See also Brāhmanism.

Brāhmana is the designation of a work belonging to a particular genre of the sacred literature of *Hinduism, expounding the *Vedic sacrificial ritual and symbolism. The Brāhmanas, the oldest of which date back to about 900 B.C., are exegetical works that seek to explain the archaic theological and ritual speculations of the four *Vedic "collections" (*samhitā*). They elaborated a kind of sacrificial mysticism that subsequently gave rise to some of the speculations in the *Upanishads. See also Brāhmanism, *yajna*.

brahma-nādī ("brahmic conduit"). According to the *Shat-Cakra-Nirūpana* (2) this is a subtle channel situated inside the *citrinī-nādī* that is located inside the *vajrā-nādī* that is, in turn, to be found inside the central conduit (*sushumnā-nādī*) of the *body. In the *Siddha-Siddhānta-Paddhati* (II.27), a medieval work on *hatha-yoga, the "brahmic channel" is said to be the proper object of the practice of the "inner sign" (*antar-lakshya*). See also *nādī*.

brahma-nirvāna ("extinction in the Absolute"). This curious compound is found in the *Bhagavad-Gītā* (II.72), where it stands for the condition of *liberation after *death. Cf. *nirvāna*.

Brāhmanism is a specific phase in the early evolution of *Hinduism. The word designates the priestly culture of late *Vedic times that centered on the esotericism of *sacrifice. See also *brāhmana*.

brahma-randhra ("brahmic aperture") is the opening of the axial channel (*sushumnā-nādī*) at the crown of the *head, corresponding to the *sutura frontalis*. The *Siddha-Siddhānta-Paddhati* (II.8) calls this the "wheel of extinction" (*nirvāna-cakra*). See also *brahma-dvāra*.

brahma-vid ("knower of the Absolute"), a *Self-realized *adept. See also *jīvan-mukta*, *yoga-vid*.

brahma-vidyā ("knowledge of the *Absolute") or *Self-realization. See also *ātma-jnāna*, Enlightenment.

Brahma-Vidyā-Upanishad is a medieval work belonging to the *Yoga-Upanishads. This tract consists of 111 stanzas that deal with the '"*Yoga of sound" (*nāda-yoga*) on the basis of nondualist metaphysics of *Vedānta. Considerable space is given to speculations about the syllable *om* and its three mores. Many *Tantra-type features are referred to, including the "serpent power" (*kundalinī-shakti*), though the text is highly conservative. Mention is made of a *hamsa-yoga*, and *breath control is said to be fivefold. The anonymous author recommends retention (*kumbhaka*) of the *breath with mental *concentration upon the navel (*nābhi-kānda*). He also subscribes to the ideal of radical *renunciation since he enjoins the *adept who has realized the *Self to abandon absolutely everything. It is possible that after stanza fifty-three, a new text begins in which a person named Gautama is instructed once more in the secrets of the *hamsa and related matters.

brahma-vihāra ("brahmic station"). This term refers to a set of four practices well known not only to *Patanjali but also to authorities within *Buddhism. This technique consists of the radiation of friendliness (*maitrī*), compassion (*karunā*), gladness (*muditā*), and equanimity (*upekshā*). According to the *Yoga-Sūtra (I.33), these are to be projected toward all beings and things, regardless of whether they are joyful or sorrowful, meritorious or demeritorious. This practice yields the pacification of *consciousness. As is evident from the *Yoga-Sūtra (III.23), the four *brahma-vihāras* can also be made the theme of *enstatic constraint (*samyama*), in which case the *yogin acquires the respective *powers of friendliness and so on. However, *Vyāsa, an early commentator on the *Yoga-Sūtra, thinks that *upekshā* is unsuitable for this.

Breath, breathing. Early on, humanity appears to have discovered that by manipulating the breath, one can achieve *altered states of consciousness. This knowledge is reflected in the Indo-European languages, where the words for "breath" often also denote "spirit" or "psyche." Our modern civilization has all but forgotten this esoteric connection between *consciousness and the *breath. See also *prāna, svāsha*.

Breath control. See *prānāyāma*.

Bridge. See *cakra-āsana*.

Brihad-Āranyaka-Upanishad ("Great Forest Upanishad") is probably the oldest text of this genre of *Hindu literature and in its earliest portions may date back to the eighth century B.C. This work contains the first clear enunciations of the doctrines of rebirth (*punar-janman*) and liberation (*moksha*).

Brihad-Yogi-Yājnavalkya-Smriti ("Great Codex of the Yogin Yājnavalkya") is a work dealing extensively with ritual worship that was probably composed in the fourteenth or fifteenth century A.D., though some researchers place it in the seventh century A.D. Its unknown author, who is identified with *Yājnavalkya, stresses the practice of *meditation on the sacred syllable *om combined with breath control (*prānāyāma*). The eight "limbs" (*anga*) of *Classical Yoga are mentioned. This scripture must be distinguished from the *Yoga-Yājnavalkya*, which is a shorter and probably earlier text.

Buddha ("Awakened one"). A *hatha-yoga master by this name is mentioned in the *Hatha-Yoga-Pradīpikā* (I.6). He must not be confused with the founder of *Buddhism.

Buddha, Gautama. The founder of *Buddhism is described in the Pali canon as a keen meditator, and the later Sanskrit scriptures of Mahāyāna *Buddhism often refer to him as a *yogin. For a period of time, Gautama studied under two well-known *teachers, and apparently quickly mastered the mystical state that each had put forward as the ultimate form of *enlightenment. Thus, Arāda Kālāma appears to have taught a kind of *Upanishadic Yoga culminating in the experience of the "sphere of no-thing-ness" (*akimcānya-āyatana*). This experience probably corresponds to the formless enstasy (*nirvikalpa-samādhi*) extolled as the highest goal in the *Upanishads. Udraka Rāmaputra, Gautama's other teacher, proclaimed the "sphere of neither consciousness nor unconsciousness" (*naiva-samjnāna-asamjnā-āyatana*) as the most exalted spiritual state.

Unconvinced of the ultimacy of either realization, Gautama took to practicing the fiercest kind of asceticism (*tapas) for a period of six years. However, his efforts proved futile, and he adopted his famous "middle way" between ascetic discipline and the life of a worldling. Remembering a spontaneous experience of *enstasy that had suddenly overwhelmed him in his youth, Gautama began to simply sit in *meditation, resolving not to stir from his seat until he had broken through all conditional forms of *consciousness. After seven days of continuous meditation, he became an "awakened one" (*buddha*), reaching "extinction" (*nirvāna), that is, the cessation of all *desire. Soon afterward, he began to communicate his newly won *enlightenment to others and to share with them his *wisdom about the "four noble truths"— namely that life is suffering (*duhkha); that the *thirst for life is the cause of all suffering; that through the elimination of that innate craving we can go beyond suffering, and that the means of eliminating that thirst for life is the "noble eightfold path" to *liberation discovered by him.

The Buddha's eightfold *path comprises the following practices: (1) "right vision" (*samyag-drishti*), or the realization of the transiency of conditioned existence and the understanding that there is indeed no continuous *ego or self to which we could cling; (2) "right resolve" (*samyak-samkalpa*), or the threefold resolution to renounce what is ephemeral, to practice benevolence, and not to hurt any being; (3) "right speech" (*samyag-vacā*), or the abstention from idle and false talk; (4) "right conduct" (*samyak-karmantā*), consisting mainly in abstention from killing, stealing, and illicit sexual intercourse; (5) "right livelihood" (*samyag-ājīva*), or the abstention from deceit, usury, treachery, and soothsaying in procuring one's sustenance; (6) "right exertion" (*samyag-vyāyāma*), or the prevention of future negative mental activity, the overcoming of present unwholesome feelings or thoughts, the cultivation of future wholesome states of *mind, and the maintenance of present positive psychomental activity; (7) "right mindfulness" (*samyak-smriti*), or the cultivation of awareness of the psychosomatic processes, that is the attentive observation of otherwise unconscious activities; (8) "right concentration" (*samyak-samādhi*), or the practice of certain techniques for the internalization and ultimate transcendence of the individuated *consciousness. This practice comprises the meditative states from sensory inhibition (pratyāhāra) to the various levels of enstatic transcendence (which are called *jhāna* in Pali and *dhyāna* in Sanskrit). But the goal of the eightfold path is *enlightenment, not any higher state of consciousness. The Buddha's teaching can be styled a pragmatic type of *Yoga, which in metaphysical matters favors agnosticism rather than atheism, as often held.

The yogic nature of the Buddha's *path is further obvious from the use of such techniques as postures (*āsana) and breath control (*prānā-yāma). The contribution of *Buddhism to the development of the *Yoga tradition has been considerable, just as the authorities of Yoga have contributed greatly to the unfolding of the Buddhist teachings.

buddhi, the feminine form of *buddha, is one of the key concepts of the traditions of *Yoga and *Sāmkhya, as well as *Vedānta. Its first occurrence is in the *Katha-Upanishad (III.3). In its primary technical meaning, it signifies the first product, or evolute, of *Nature (*prakriti). As such, it is the most refined as well as the simplest form of existence and, by way of further *evolution, gives rise to all other categories (*tattva) of existence—both material and psychic. The buddhi, which is similar to the nous in Neoplatonism, is also called *linga, *linga-mātra, and *sattva.

A second, related connotation of the term buddhi is "wisdom faculty" or "higher mind" in contrast to the lower mind (*manas). In a well-known simile first employed in the *Katha-Upanishad (III.3), the buddhi is said to be the chariot driver, the chariot being the *body and the charioteer being the transcendental *Self. In this sense, the buddhi is the highest or deepest aspect of the human psyche—the birthplace of true *wisdom, or gnosis. Hence in some contexts the word denotes "wisdom." In *Classical Yoga, it simply stands for "cognition."

buddhi-indriya ("cognitive sense"). See indriya.

Buddhism, the spiritual tradition founded by Gautama the *Buddha, can be understood as an elaborate yogic tradition that has developed its own schools of *Yoga. The Buddha's original doctrines—from what we know of them through the Pali canon—suggest an agnostic type of Yoga aimed at achieving the goal of "extinction" (*nirvāna). In later Buddhism, there were several significant developments of a yogic nature, notably the Mahāyāna Buddhist *Yogācāra school of Asanga (fifth century A.D.) and the numerous schools of Buddhist *Tantrism, especially those of Tibet (known as the Vajrayāna), as well as the schools of Chinese Ch'an and Japanese *Zen Buddhism.

buddhi-yoga is a compound that can be met with repeatedly in the *Bhagavad-Gītā*. Thus, according to verse II.49, it consists in one's taking refuge in the "wisdom faculty" (*buddhi*) in order not to hanker after the fruit (*phala*) of one's deeds. In stanza X.10, *buddhi-yoga* is said to be given by the *Lord to those who worship him with fondness. See also Wisdom.

budhyamāna ("awakening one") is an important concept of *Pre-Classical Yoga. The *budhyamāna* is the twenty-fifth principle (*tattva*), which is the principle of conscious existence. When it "awakens," that is, when it realizes its true nature as transcendental *Consciousness, it becomes the *Absolute (called *kevala*). Cf. *abuddha, shad-vimsha*.

Bulb. See *kanda*.

Bull posture. See *vrisha-āsana*.

C

caitanya ("awareness," "intelligence") can stand for the individual *mind as well as the transcendental *Consciousness, the very essence of the *Self. See also *cit*, *citi*; cf. *citta*.

Caitanya (A.D. 1486–1533), or Krishna Caitanya, was the chief revivalist of *Krishna devotion in eastern India. He probably wrote no more than eight devotional verses (called *Shaikshā-Ashtaka* "Eight [Stanzas] of Instruction"). His *bhakti* school of *Vaishnavism is based on the teachings of the *Bhāgavata-Purāna*. He inaugurated the tradition of *go-svāmins*, of which *Bhaktivedanta Swami Prabhupada (d. 1977) of the Krishna Consciousness movement was one of the last great leaders. Caitanya was a man of

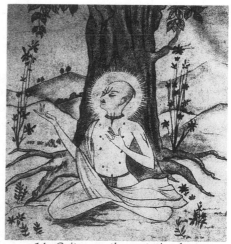

14. Caitanya, the ecstatic adept.

extraordinary charisma and still during his lifetime was revered as an *incarnation of God *Krishna. See also *bhakti-mārga*, *bhakti-yoga*.

71

cakra ("wheel") is derived from the verbal root *car* ("to move"). Apart from its obvious secular meaning, this Sanskrit term has four principal esoteric connotations. First, it denotes the "wheel of becoming" (*bhava-cakra*), or "round of existence" (*samsāra*), that is, the phenomenal *cosmos. Second, it stands for the circle of initiates in the left-hand sexual ritual of *Tantrism where male and female participants sit in a circular arrangement around the *teacher. Third, it refers to a diagram similar to the *yantra* used to determine the right kind of *mantra* for a particular *student or situation. Such diagrams are described, for instance, in the *Mantra-Yoga-Samhitā*. Fourth, the word *cakra* denotes the psychoenergetic vortices forming the major "organs" of the *body composed of life energy (*prāna*). These esoteric structures are also often referred to and graphically depicted as "lotuses" (*padma, kamala*).

Most schools of *Yoga and *Tantrism propose that there are six principal centers (*shat-cakra*), with a seventh center being thought of as transcending bodily existence. These seven centers are in descending order: (1) The *sahasrāra-cakra* ("thousand-spoked wheel") at or above the crown of the *head; (2) The *ājnā-cakra* ("command wheel") in the center of the head, between and behind the eyebrows; (3) the *vishuddha-cakra* ("pure wheel") at the throat; (4) the *anāhata-cakra* ("wheel of the unstruck [sound]") at the *heart; (5) the *manipūra-cakra* ("wheel of the jeweled city") at the *naval; (6) the *svādhishthāna-cakra* ("wheel of the self-base") at the genitals; and (7) the *mūlādhāra-cakra* ("root-foundation wheel") at the anus.

Models involving nine, twelve, and more *cakras* are also known. Thus, the *Kaula-Jnāna-Nirnaya* (X), a medieval work, mentions eight centers, which remain unnamed however, and this scripture (III and V) also speaks of "lotuses" with one hundred, ten million, fifteen million, thirty million, and even one billion petals. These belong to the secret centers that play an important role in higher Yoga practice. The *Kaula-Jnāna-Nirnaya* (X) further claims that *contemplation upon these *cakras* leads to the conquest of *death and to the acquisition of paranormal powers (*siddhi*).

A Kashmiri scroll examined by Fausta Nowotny (1958) lists the following twelve centers or lotuses, in descending order, with their respective location and number of petals: (1) the *bhramara-cakra* ("bee wheel") at or possibly above the crown of the *head—number of petals not given; (2) the *sahasra-dala-cakra* ("thousand-petaled wheel") at the crown on the head—one thousand petals; (3) the *pūrna-giri-pītha-cakra* ("wheel of the full mountain seat") at the forehead—twenty-two petals; (4) the *ājnā-cakra* ("command wheel") at the "brow-middle"—two petals; (5) the *balavat-cakra* ("powerful wheel") at the nose—three petals;

(6) the *vishuddha-cakra* ("pure wheel") at the throat—sixteen petals; (7) the *anāhata-cakra* ("wheel of the unstruck [sound]") at the *heart— twelve petals; (8) the *manas-cakra* ("mind wheel") at the center of the *navel—eight petals; (9) the *manipūra-cakra* ("wheel of the jeweled city") at the navel—ten petals; (10) the *kundalinī-cakra* ("wheel of the *kundalinī") at the womb (*garbha*)—number of petals not given; (11) the *svādhishthāna-cakra* ("wheel of the self-base") at the penis— six petals; (12) the *ādhāra-cakra* ("base wheel") at the anus—four petals.

The most common explanation for these psychoenergetic centers proposed by noninitiates suggests a straightforward *identification* with the nerve plexuses known to medical physiology. However, this hypothesis contradicts the verbal and scriptural testimony of yogic authorities. A more moderate and credible opinion suggests that there is a *correlation* between the *cakras* and the structures of the nervous system. According to some scholars, notably Agehananda Bharati (1965), such speculations make no sense because the *cakras* are merely "systematic fictions" or "heuristic devices" to aid the process of *meditation. While not denying the symbolic component of the *cakra* model, transpersonal psychologist Ken Wilber (in John White, 1979) notes that the *cakras* are real insofar as they are associated with distinct sensations or states of *consciousness, just as they appear to be correlated with certain organs. See also *shat-cakra-bheda*.

cakra-āsana ("wheel posture") is a posture (*āsana*) mentioned in the *Varāha-Upanishad* (V.17), where it is described as follows: One should place the left thigh over the right ankle, and the right thigh over the left ankle while holding the body erect. This could be a description of what modern manuals know as the "mountain posture" (*parvata-āsana*), which is performed by assuming the "lotus posture" (*padma-āsana*) and then raising oneself until the *body is balancing on the knees only, while both arms are stretched upward. In contemporary *Yoga practice, *cakra-āsana* signifies the complete backward bend or bridge.

cakrī-karma ("wheel action") is a *cleansing practice of *hatha-yoga. The *Hatha-Ratna-Āvali* (I.28) describes it thus: One should insert half a finger (sometimes stated to be the middle finger) into the rectum and move it around until the anal sphincter muscle is fully stretched. This practice is recommended for the curing of piles, *diseases of the spleen, and indigestion.

Camel posture. See *ushtra-āsana*.

cakshus ("eye"). See *divya-cakshus, indriya, jnāna-cakshus.*

Candīdās (Sanskrit: Candīdāsa, "Servant of [Goddess] Candī") was a leading Bengali *teacher of the *Sahajiyā movement. He lived in the latter half of the fourteenth century A.D. and achieved fame throughout northern India for his numerous love songs, telling of the play between *Rādhā and her divine lover *Krishna and how to use the *body as a medium of prayerful *meditation. His compositions gave rise to a new school of *Vaishnava poetry. Of the thousands of poems attributed to him, about two hundred are said to be authentic. See also *bhakti-mārga.*

candra ("moon"). In *hatha-yoga* and *Tantrism, the "moon" is an esoteric structure in the human *body from which oozes the "nectar of immortality" (*amrita, *soma). The "moon" showers its ambrosia continuously, but in the ordinary mortal this precious liquid is wasted. The *yogin, however, learns to check its flow and employ it in his quest for the transubstantiation of the body. According to the *Yoga-Shikhā-Upanishad* (V.33), a medieval text, the lunar orb is located at the "root of the *palate" (*tālu-mūla*), a location that the *Kaula-Jnāna-Nirnaya* (V.16) cryptically refers to as the "navel" of the *head. The *Shiva-Samhitā* (II.6) assigns the "moon" to a place at the top of "Mount *Meru," that is, at the upper terminal of the spine. This scripture also states that it has eight "portions" (*kalā*), meaning that it is a half-moon, though elsewhere (V.148) it speaks of it as having sixteen "portions," which amounts to a full moon. Furthermore, the *Shiva-Samhitā* (V.146) announces that the "moon" becomes visible (presumably to the inner eye) through continuous *contemplation over a period of three days.

The "moon's" nectar is thought to ooze down into the trunk where it is consumed by the "sun" (*sūrya*) residing in the abdominal region. Bodily inversion techniques like the *shoulder stand or the *headstand are designed to reverse the downward flow of the lunar nectar. The technique of *jālandhara-bandha,* or throat "lock," and the *khecarī-mudrā,* in which the tongue is turned back against the *palate to block the cranial cavity, have the same purpose. This is analogous to the reversal of the "semen" (*bindu*) attempted through such practices as the *vajrolī-mudrā.*

The metaphor of sun and moon is a good example of the magical notion that the *macrocosm is mirrored in the *microcosm. The compound *hatha-yoga* is esoterically explained as the union of sun and moon, which refers to the two great microcosmic structures. Thus, the *yogin attempts to make a true cosmos ("order") out of his inner environment by means of the integrative power of higher *consciousness.

The lunar excretion or *amrita has, even in some *Yoga texts, been prosaically identified as the saliva. Several modern interpreters have seen in it the cerebrospinal fluid. The preservation of this liquid is thought to promote *health and longevity. But, beyond this, the "moon" is, like the cakras, an important reference point for the yogic meditative journey. The *Shat-Cakra-Nirūpana (41) refers to it as the "lunar circle" (candra-mandala), which is situated in the pericarp of the "thousand-petaled lotus (*sahasrāra-cakra). The *Shiva-Purāna (III.5.53) speaks of this region as being of the nature of supreme *Consciousness. Some scriptures call this location the indu- or soma-cakra, which is generally depicted as a lotus of sixteen moon-white petals. This is described as the seat of the higher mind (*buddhi).

candra-grahana ("lunar eclipse") occurs, according to the *Darshana-Upanishad (IV.46), when the life force (*prāna) reaches the abode of the "serpent power" (*kundalinī-shakti) via the left channel (i.e., the *idā-nādī).

Cangadeva was a renowned *hatha-yogin who became a disciple of the young *Jnānadeva who instructed him in sixty-five verses in the Marathi language. These came to be known as the Cangadeva-Pasashthī.

Carpata, one of the great preceptors of *hatha-yoga, is credited with the authorship of the *Carpata-Shataka ("Carpata's Century [of Verses]"), the Ananta-Vākya ("Endless Speech"), and the Carpata-Manjarī ("Carpata's Flower-Ornament"). One of his disciples was Sahila Varma, king of the Camba state (Punjab), who flourished about A.D. 920.

Carpata-Shataka ("Carpata's Century [of Verses]") is an early work on *hatha-yoga ascribed to *Carpata, of which there appear to be several rare manuscripts.

Carpati is mentioned in the *Hatha-Yoga-Pradīpikā (I.6) as a master of *hatha-yoga. It is not clear whether he is identical with the famous *Carpata.

cathurta ("fourth"). In *Vedānta, this is a technical term referring to the transcendental *Self beyond the three states (*avasthā) of *waking, *dreaming, and *sleeping. It is also called turīya or turyā, both words meaning "fourth." In *Classical Yoga, the word caturtha denotes that mode of breathing (*prānāyāma) that goes beyond inhalation and exhalation, namely the total suspension of the *breath known as *kevala-kumbhaka.

Cauranginātha, also known as Caturanginātha, was a younger contemporary of *Goraksha and apparently was the son of King Devapala of Bengal. He is mentioned in the *Hatha-Yoga-Pradīpikā (I.5) as one of the early masters of *hatha-yoga.

Causation. See kārana, nava-kārana, sat-kārya-vāda.

Causation, moral. See karman.

Causes of suffering. See klesha.

cetas ("mind" or "consciousness") is a synonym for *manas.

Chāndogya-Upanishad is one of the oldest scriptures of the *Upanishadic genre, composed perhaps in the seventh or eighth century B.C. It contains, among other things, elaborate speculations about the sacred syllable *om (called *udgītha). The third chapter is essentially an exposition of the "honey doctrine" (*mādhu-vidyā) and the nature of the life force (*prāna). This scripture affords the historian of religion a valuable glimpse of the earliest formative phase of *Hindu metaphysics, when the *Vedic sacrificial ritual became internalized—thus paving the way for the development of *Yoga within the orthodox circles of *Brāhmanism.

Change. See parināma.

Channels. See hitā, nādī.

Charity. See dāna.

Chastity. See brahmacarya.

chāyā ("shadow" or "reflection") has a technical significance in *Classical Yoga. It stands for the "reflection" cast by the transcendental *Self, or *Consciousness, in the highest aspect of the *mind called *buddhi. This concept, which was first introduced by *Vācaspati Mishra in his *Tattva-Vaishāradī (II.17), seeks to explain how *knowledge is possible given the fact that the mind (*manas, buddhi, citta*) is an evolute of insentient Nature (*prakriti*).

In many works of *Post-Classical Yoga, the word signifies the "aura" surrounding the physical *body and which, according to the *Varāha-Upanishad (V.41), should always be perceived by the *yogin. See also *bimba, pratibimba*.

chāyā-purusha ("shadow man") is the shadow cast by the *body, which is used by some *yogins for divining their own and other people's *destiny.

Cidghanānanda, an eighteenth-century writer, composed two works dealing with *diseases arising from faulty *Yoga practice, the *Mishraka and the *Sat-Karma-Samgraha.

cihna ("sign"). Because *yogins experience the world as a psycho-physical process, they believe that certain external signs are indicative of inner states or possibilities. Thus, according to the *Mārkandeya-Purāna (XXXIX.63), the first signs of *progress along the spiritual *path are as follows: enthusiasm (*ālolya*), *health, *gentleness, pleasant odor, scant urine and excrement, beauty, clarity, and softness of voice. Similarly, the *Shiva-Samhitā (III.28f.) states that a sure sign of progress in the initial stage (*ārambha-avasthā*) is the attainment of an "even body" (*sama-kāya*) that is handsome and emits a pleasant scent. Moreover, the *yogin on this level is said to enjoy a "strong (digestive) *fire," to eat well, and be happy, courageous, energetic, and strong, having well-formed limbs. In the *Yoga-Tattva-Upanishad (44ff.), four external signs are mentioned that result from the *purification of the psycho-energetic currents (*nādī*); these are bodily *lightness, radiance (*dīpti*), increase of the "abdominal fire" (*jāthara-agni*), and bodily slimness. The *Yoga-Yājnavalkya (V.21f.) and the *Shāndilya-Upanishad (I.5.4.), for instance, replace the last sign with the manifestation of the inner sound (*nāda*).

The *Yoga scriptures also know of signs that occur immediately prior to, or that follow upon, *Self-realization. Thus the *Mahābhārata epic (XII.294.20) has this stanza: "Like smokeless, seven-flamed [fire], like the radiant sun, like the lightning flash in space—thus the *Self is seen in the self."

In a similar vein, the *Yoga-Shikhā-Upanishad (II.18f.) lists a number of signs that are styled the "gates" to the paranormal powers (*siddhi*), namely the experience in deep *meditation of *light resembling the flame of a lamp, the moon, a firefly, lightning, the constellations, and lastly the sun. See also *pravritti, rūpa, tāraku-yoga*.

cin-mātra ("pure awareness") is a common synonym for *ātman*. It denotes the transcendental essence, which is supraconscious and mind-transcending. See also *caitanya, cit, citi*; cf. *citta*.

cin-mudrā ("seal of awareness"; for euphonic reasons *cit* is here altered to *cin*) is one of the hand gestures (*mudrā*) used in conjunction with certain postures (*āsana*) or in sacred rituals. It is performed by bringing thumb and index finger together, while the remaining fingers are kept extended. See also *yoga-mudrā*.

cintā ("thought") is often used in the sense of "pondering" or "*meditation*," as for instance in the *Maitrāyanīya-Upanishad* (IV.4), where it is said that the *Absolute can be attained by means of asceticism (*tapas*) and wisdom (*vidyā*) or *cintā*. However, in other works such as the *Bhagavad-Gītā* (XVI.11), the word means "concern" or "care."

cit ("awareness" or "consciousness"). This term is widely employed in *Yoga and *Vedānta scriptures to denote the transcendental *Consciousness, or pure Awareness. See also *caitanya, cin-mātra, citi*; cf. *citta*.

citi-chāyā ("shadow of awareness"). See *chāyā, citi*.

citi ("awareness" or "intelligence") is a synonym for *cit*. See also *citi-shakti*.

citi-shakti ("power of awareness") is a phrase found, for instance, in the *Yoga-Sūtra* (IV.34), where it refers to the transcendental *Self that continuously apperceives the contents of the *mind without itself being involved in the mental processes.

citrinī-nādī ("shining channel") is, according to some *Tantric works, a subtle conduit within the central channel (*sushumnā-nādī*). Within it lies the "brahmic channel" (*brahma-nādī*), which is the actual pathway of the psychospiritual force known as the *kundalinī-shakti*. See also *nādī*.

cit-shakti ("power of awareness") is a synonym for *citi-shakti*.

citta ("mind" or "consciousness") is the past participle of the verbal root *cit* ("to be conscious"). This is one of the key concepts of *Classical Yoga. Even though the term is not explicitly defined by *Patanjali, the founder of this *Yoga school, its meaning can be ascertained from its occurrences in his work. Thus the *citta* is a part of insentient Nature (*prakriti*), although it is not treated as a separate ontic category (*tattva*). Instead, the word is used as an umbrella term for a variety of inner processes, primarily the capacity of *attention. It is in a sense the product of the transcendental *Consciousness (*citi*) and the perceived object inasmuch as it is said to be "colored" by both. There exists a multitude of such consciousnesses, and in aphorism IV.15, Patanjali specifically rejects the idealist view of a single consciousness.

The *citta* is thought to be suffused with countless "subliminal activators" (*samskāra*) combining into what are called the "traits" (*vāsanā*). These are responsible for the production of the various psychomental phenomena, in particular the set of five "fluctuations" (*vritti*). In aphorism IV.24, the *citta* is declared to be ultimately geared toward the *liberation of human beings. Upon the realization of the *Self, consciousness (which is really a material phenomenon) is dissolved because *Self-realization presupposes the "involution" (*pratiprasava*) of the primary constituents or "qualities" (*guna*) of *Nature.

Like all other aspects of insentient Nature (*prakriti*), *consciousness undergoes continual change, and from the yogic viewpoint its most important modifications are the five kinds of "fluctuation" (*vritti*): accurate cognition, erroneous *knowledge, *conceptualization, *sleep, and *memory. These must be stopped in order to actualize higher states of awareness. The Sanskrit commentators discuss at great length whether the *citta* corresponds to the size of the *body (which is the *Sāmkhya view) or whether it is really all-pervasive. They settle for the latter alternative and argue that it is only the mental "whirls" (*vritti*) that can be said to contract and expand. *Vācaspati introduces the distinction between "causal consciousness" (*kārana-citta*) and "effected consciousness" (*kārya-citta*), arguing that the former is infinite, which presumably is intended to approximate *Patanjali's concept of "pure I-am-ness" (*asmitā-mātra*).

To explain the cognitive processes, the commentators resort to various metaphors. Thus, the *Yoga-Bhāshya (I.4) compares *consciousness to a magnet that attracts the *objects, and elsewhere (I.41) compares it to a crystal that reflects the color of the object near it. The *Tattva-Vaishāradī (I.7) also speaks of it as a mirror in which the "*light" of the *Self is reflected (see *chāyā*).

Outside the purview of *Classical Yoga, the term *citta* is generally employed in a less technically precise sense and mostly denotes mind in general. This tendency is present already in the commentarial literature on the *Yoga-Sūtra, where citta is often equated with *buddhi.

One of the most remarkable discoveries of the *yogins concerns the intimate relation that exists between consciousness and the breath (*prāna). This discovery is especially emphasized in the literature of *Post-Classical Yoga. For instance, the *Yoga-Shikhā-Upanishad (I.59) likens the mind to a bird tied up by means of the cord of the life force (*prāna). Elsewhere (VI.69), this work states that wherever the "wind" (i.e., the life force) abides in the body, there too dwells consciousness. In the *Laghu-Yoga-Vāsishtha (V.9.73), the mind is defined as "the quivering of the life force (prāna-parispanda)." The general theorem is that by controlling the breath, the mind can be conquered.

citta-bhūmi ("level of consciousness"). See bhūmi.

citta-mātra ("mere mind"). The notion of "mind only" is central to such idealist schools as *Yogācāra Buddhism and also the philosophy embedded in the *Yoga-Vāsistha. According to this doctrine, the world is nothing other than the pure Mind, also called mano-mātra. *Patanjali, a staunch believer in realism, makes a point to refute this teaching. In his *Yoga-Sūtra (IV.16), he argues: "And the *object is not dependent on a single consciousness (eka-citta). This is unprovable. Besides, what could [such an imaginary object possibly] be?"

citta-sharīra ("mind body"). The *Yoga-Vāsishtha (III.22.15) makes a distinction between the "fleshly body" (māmsa-deha) and the "mind body" that neither dies nor is alive at any time, since it is the aspatial *Reality itself. See also deha, linga-sharīra.

Civavākkiyar (Sanskrit: Shivavākya) is one of the great Tamil *adepts of Southern *Shaivism. He probably lived in the ninth century A.D. His poetry, of which over five hundred poems have survived, and the legends woven around his life show him to have been an outspoken rebel against the religious orthodoxy. He rejected the *Vedas and *Āgamas and condemned idol worship, the caste system, and the doctrine of *rebirth. His poetry, which is forceful and forthright, was left out of the *Shaiva canon. Kamil V. Zvelebil (1973), a renowned scholar of Tamil literature, considers Civavākkiyar "a greater poet than *Tirumūlar" (p. 81). His poetry is a clarion call reminding people to discover the great God, *Shiva, who dwells within.

Clairaudience. See *divya-shrotra*.

Clairvoyance. See *divya-chakshus*.

Classical Yoga refers to the philosophical system that has evolved around Patanjali's *Yoga-Sūtra* and its extensive commentarial literature. This school of thought is generally referred to as the *yoga-darshana*, or *rāja-yoga*, which counts as one of the six classical systems of *Hindu philosophy. The other five are *Sāmkhya, *Vedānta (also known as Uttara-Mīmāmsā), *Pūrva-Mīmāmsā, *Nyāya, and *Vaisheshika.

*Patanjali was not the originator of *Yoga. He merely systematized existing knowledge and techniques. Traditionally, *Hiranyagarbha is credited with originating Yoga, though no actual scriptures have survived that could be identified as having been authored by this legendary *adept. *Patanjali's aphorisms (*sūtra) on Yoga appear to have quickly eclipsed other similar compilations, which undoubtedly existed but are now lost.

The *Yoga-Sūtra provided an interpretation of *Yoga philosophy and practice that stimulated others to elaborate Patanjali's metaphysical ideas. He taught a form of radical dualism that remained quite controversial within the fold of *Hinduism. According to him, there are two eternal categories of existence—the transcendental Self (*purusha) and the transcendental world-ground (*prakriti). The former category comprises countless *Selves that are omnipresent, omniscient, and passive spectators of the spectacle of the *cosmos. The latter category, the world-ground, comprises all the manifest and unmanifest dimensions and forms of *Nature, which are inherently dynamic.

Whereas the *Selves are innately conscious, or rather supraconscious, *Nature is essentially unconscious or insentient. It has no purpose in itself but serves the countless *Selves. They are either aware of their transcendental *freedom or they are entrapped in Nature believing themselves to be finite entities. This is possible because in its highest mode of existence, Nature is transparent enough to "reflect" the "*light" of these Selves and thus create the illusion of sentience and intelligence in its evolutes. Thus the *mind (both as *manas and as *buddhi) is the product of this reflection (*chāyā) of *Consciousness in *Nature. The function of *Yoga is to oblige the Self to awaken to its transcendental status through a progressive withdrawal from the forms of Nature. This is accomplished through Patanjali's eightfold *path (which is generally known as *ashta-anga-yoga), particularly the higher stages of meditation (*dhyāna) and enstasy (*samādhi). The supreme goal is known as "aloneness" (*kaivalya), which is the perfect isolation of the Self.

This radical dualism has provoked much criticism within and also outside *Hinduism, and it has definitely prevented Classical Yoga from becoming a more influential philosophical school. The tenor of Hinduism is nondualist, and this is reflected very well in the fact that the schools of *Post-Classical Yoga are without exception informed by the metaphysics of *Advaita-Vedānta rather than Classical Yoga. Patanjali's system can almost be regarded as an interlude in a tradition that was from the outset nondualistic, because the known schools of *Pre-Classical Yoga (with the exception of *Buddhism, if we wish to include it in this category) are all based on *Vedānta-type teachings.

Classical Sāmkhya. See Sāmkhya.

Cleansing practices. See *dhauti, shauca, shodhana*.

Cobra posture. See *bhujānga-āsana*.

codanā ("urging") is a yogic term found in the *Mahābhārata* epic. In one passage (XII.294.11), the *yogin* is counseled to "impel" (*codayet*) himself by means of the ten or twelve *codanās*. This work further specifies that ten or twelve *codanās* are to be practiced in the first watch of the night and a further twelve in the middle of the night after having slept. Nīlakantha, the best known commentator of the great epic, understands these as restraints of the *breath.

Cognition. See *buddhi, drishti, jnāna, prajnā, pratyaya*.

Compassion. See *dayā, karunā*.

Concentration. Yogic concentration differs from ordinary efforts of focusing *attention by its duration, depth, and notably its purpose, which is to transcend the concentrated *mind itself. See also *dhāranā*.

Conceptualization. See *samkalpa, vikalpa*.

Confusion. See *bhrama, moha*.

Consciousness. The nature of consciousness has been a major philosophical concern in the long *history of *Yoga. Most yogic schools subscribe to the view that conciousness is transcendental, that is, not a product of the finite body-mind, much less a mere brain phenomenon. The transcendental nature of consciousness is thought to be philosophically self-evident and "verifiable" by means of the highest yogic condition—the supraconscious enstasy (called *asamprajnāta-samādhi or *nirvikalpa-samadhi). Consciousness is proposed as the ultimate identity of human beings. Hence it is also called the *Self (*ātman or *purusha), which is the *Spirit beyond *body, *mind, and language.

According to the nondualist schools of *Yoga, that supreme Consciousness is utterly blissful (*ānanda) and overwhelmingly real (*sat). It cannot be known, but it can be realized. *Self-realization is the alpha and omega of all approaches of Yoga. See also cintā, cit, citi, citta, manas, prajnā.

Contemplation. See dhyāna.

Contentment. See samtosha, tushti.

Corpse posture. See mrita-āsana, shava-āsana.

Cosmos. The cosmological and cosmographical ideas of *Yoga are those current in the prescientific literature of *Hinduism, especially the *Purānas. Even though *Vyāsa, in his *Yoga-Bhāshya (III.26), outlines the essentials of the extraordinarily rich and imaginative cosmography of the *Hindus, these conceptions do not play a significant role in Yoga practice. However, they form a part of the general stock of knowledge of the educated sections of society.

According to *Vyāsa's cosmographical sketch, the universe is egg shaped (see brahma-anda) and segmented into seven zones or regions (*lokas), which have their own subdivisions. These are in descending order: (1) The satya-loka ("world of truth"), which is inhabited by four groups of *deities who live as long as there are world creations (*sarga); (2) the tapo-loka ("world of asceticism"), which is inhabited by three groups of deities who live twice as long as the gods of the jana-loka; (3) the jana-loka ("world of people"), which is inhabited by four groups of deities who have mastered the *elements and the *senses; (4) the mahar-prājapatya-loka ("mahar world of Prajapati"), which is inhabited by five groups of deities who have mastered the elements and live for a thousand world cycles (*kalpa); (5) the mahā-indra-loka ("world of the great Indra"), which is inhabited by six groups of deities who have acquired the major paranormal powers (*siddhi) and live for a full world cycle (*kalpa); (6) the antarīksha-loka ("world of the midregion"), which extends from the summit of mount *meru, the mountain at the center of the world, to the polestar and which is populated by the planets and stars; (7) the *bhū-loka* ("earth world"), which comprises (a) the earth (*bhūmi*) with its seven continents, which have mount *meru* in their center and which are encircled by the seven seas and the *loka-aloka* mountains (the diameter of this curved disc being estimated at 500 million *yojanas*, or around 4,500 million miles); (b) the seven nether regions (*pātāla*); and (c) the seven hells (*nāraka*).

Clearly, this and other similar models of the universe belong to the realm of mythology. In *Tantrism and *hatha-yoga, such cosmographical concepts as *meru and the seven worlds are descriptive of the microcosmic reality of the *body, as it is experienced during yogic *meditation. Thus, mount *meru* is the spinal axis or axial current (*sushumnā-nādī*) of the life force (*prāna*), while the seven worlds are the seven major psychoenergetic focal points (*cakra*). See also *bhuvana*, *prakriti*, *sarga*, *vishva*.

Cow-muzzle posture. See *go-mukha-āsana*.

Crazy adept. All major religious traditions of the world include the phenomenon of crazy wisdom—spiritual iconoclasm, whose representatives have been called crazy *adepts. For instance, in *Hinduism there is the figure of the *avadhūta*, in Tibetan (Vajrayāna) *Buddhism we have the *lama myonpa*, and in Christianity the "fool for Christ's sake." They seek to communicate spiritual truths by unconventional, even eccentric, means. Their impromptu methods of instructing others are intended to shock, though their purpose is always benign: to reflect to the ordinary worldling the "madness" of his or her unenlightened existence embroiled as it is in suffering and devoid of self-understanding.

The crazy adepts feel free to reject customary behavior and to be subversive, criticizing and poking fun at the worldly as well as the secular establishment. They may dress in bizarre ways or even go about naked, ignoring the niceties of social contact, cursing and using obscene language, and employing stimulants and intoxicants, as well as sexuality. They embody the esoteric principle of *Tantrism that liberation (*mukti*) is coessential with enjoyment (*bhukti*); that the spiritual *Reality is not separate from the world.

Creation. See *sarga*, World ages.

D

dahara ("miniscule") is derived from the verbal root *dabh* ("to hurt, deceive") and refers to the most subtle space within the *heart, or the "heart lotus" (*hrit-padma*), which is the connecting point between the body-mind and the transcendental *Self. The word also has overtones of radiance, since the connected verbal root *dah* means "to burn" or "be burned."

dahara-ākāsha ("miniscule radiance-space") is one of the inner luminous spaces (*ākāsha*) on which the *yogin may *meditate in *tāraka-yoga.

daiva ("fate") is explained in the *Yoga-Vāsishtha* (II.9.4) as the inevitable consequence of one's auspicious or inauspicious deeds (*karman*). However, elsewhere in this work (II.5.18) its existence is denied, and reliance on it is firmly rejected. Instead the virtue of self-exertion (*paurusha*) is recommended. Fate is sometimes listed as one of the obstacles (*vighna*) of *Yoga.

dama ("restraint") is occasionally regarded in the *Mahābhārata* epic (XII.2ff.) as the highest virtue. In the scriptures of *Post-Classical Yoga, it is sometimes grouped with the moral disciplines (*yama*). The *Bhāgavata-Purāna* (XI.19.36) understands it as *sense control (*indriya-samyama*).

dambha ("ostentation") characterizes, according to the *Bhagavad-Gītā* (XVI.4), the person born to a demonic destiny. See also Pride.

dāna ("donation," "generosity," or "charity"). The *Tri-Shikhi-Brāh-mana-Upanishad* (II.33) counts *dāna* among the ten practices of self-discipline (*niyama*), and the *Shāndilya-Upanishad* (I.2.5) explains it as giving with all sincerity wealth that has been acquired by righteous means. According to the *Bhagavad-Gītā* (XVII.20ff.), *dāna* is threefold, depending on the predominance of the three qualities (*guna*) of *Nature. Thus it can be *sāttvika* (when done in the right place and at the right time as one's duty without expecting any reward and for a worthy recipient), *rājasa* (when a return favor is expected or when one hopes for *karmic merit), and *tāmasa* (done without respect or with contempt at the wrong time in an inappropriate place for an unworthy recipient). The philosophy underlying the virtue of liberality is expressed in the *Mahānārāyana-Upanishad* (523), which exclaims that all beings live from the donations of others. Curiously, the *Shiva-Samhitā* (V.4) considers almsgiving to be one of the obstacles (*vighna*) of *Yoga.

Dance. Since ancient times, dance has served as a means of expressing religious or spiritual sentiments and aspirations, and of transcending *body and *mind. *Vaishnavism, for instance, celebrates the famous dance (*rasa-līlā*) of the God-man *Krishna and the shepherdesses (*gopī*). Through Krishna's magic, each woman thought that she was the only one dancing with her beloved Lord— a striking simile of the spiritual aspirant's journey to the *Divine.

Dance has also been used as a metaphor for the rhythm of the *cosmos. This is beautifully captured in the iconographic image of *Shiva as "Lord of Dance" (*nata-rāja*), where the great God is seen dancing rapturously in a surround

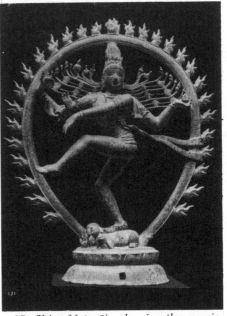

15. *Shiva Natarāja, dancing the cosmic dance.*

of flames, symbolizing the destruction of the universe. The dance itself represents Shiva's five primal activities—creation, preservation, destruction, veiling, and salvific *grace.

Indian dance, like traditional Indian *art in general, can be looked upon as a form of *Yoga. It certainly requires considerable self-discipline and *concentration. Unlike European dancing, Hindu dance involves the entire *body: Every motion is charged with significance, and every pose and gesture is codified in great detail. Thus, the classical texts mention thirteen positions of the *head, thirty-six of the eyes, nine of the neck, and hundreds of hand gestures (*mudrā). See also nriti.

danda-āsana ("staff posture") is mentioned in the *Yoga-Bhāshya (II.46) and is described by *Vācaspati Mishra as follows: One should sit down with the feet stretched out and close together.

danda-dhauti ("cleansing [by means of a] stalk") is one of the forms of "heart cleansing" (*hrid-dhauti). The *Gheranda-Samhitā (I.37f.) describes it thus: One should take a plantain stalk or a stalk of tumeric or cane and introduce it slowly into the gullet, and then draw it out again. This is thought to expel all phlegm (*kapha), bile (*pitta), and other impurities from the mouth and chest. See also dhauti.

Dangerous posture. See sankata-āsana.

danta-dhauti ("dental cleansing") is one of the four forms of cleansing (*dhauti) prescribed in *hatha-yoga. According to the *Gheranda-Samhitā (I.26), it consists of the following practices: cleansing of the teeth (*danta-mūla-dhauti), the tongue (*jihvā-dhauti), the ears (*karna-dhauti), and the frontal sinuses (*kapāla-randhra-dhauti).

danta-mūla-dhauti ("dental root cleansing") is described in the *Gheranda-Samhitā (I.27f.) as follows: Every day in the morning one should rub the teeth with catechu powder or pure earth until all impurities are removed. See also danta-dhauti.

darpa ("arrogance") is universally condemned in the *Yoga scriptures as a character trait that blocks spiritual maturation. See also Pride; cf. amānitva.

darshana ("vision," "sight") can mean "vision" both in the literal and the metaphorical sense. Moreover, it can stand for "viewpoint," as in the expression *yoga-darshana. In the *Mahābhārata epic (XII.232.21), visionary states are regarded as a by-product or "sign" (*cihna) of *progress in *meditation. They are, however, also deemed obstacles (*upasarga) in regard to enstasy (*samādhi). See also ātma-darshana, bhrānti-darshana, siddha-darshana.

Darshana-Upanishad is one of the *Yoga-Upanishads and consists of 224 stanzas distributed over ten sections. Its teachings are expounded by the God-man *Dattātreya to his pupil Samkriti. The fundamental practices of Dattātreya's *Yoga are identical with those introduced in the *Yoga-Sūtra. However, the text is fairly orthodox in style and contents. Much attention is given to the psychoenergetic currents (*nādī) and their *purification, whereas the higher yogic practices are only sketchily described.

Dattātreya is a historical teacher of *Post-Classical Yoga who early on became deified. Dattātreya, whose name means "Datta, son of Atri," was a *crazy-wisdom adept who is mentioned in many *Purānas. He taught an eight-limbed *path (*ashta-anga-yoga), but his name is prominently associated with the *avadhūta tradition. Mythology celebrates him as an incarnation (*avatāra) of God *Vishnu, but *Shiva worshippers also claim him as one of their great spiritual figures. Among other works, he is credited with the authorship of the *Avadhūta-Gītā, the *Jīvan-Mukti-Gītā*, and the *Tri-Pura-Rahasya*, all of which are works espousing *Advaita-Vedānta.

daurmanasya ("depression") is one of the symptoms accompanying the "distractions" (*vikshepa) spoken of in the *Yoga-Sūtra (I.31). *Vyāsa, in his *Yoga-Bhāshya (I.31), explains the word as mental agitation resulting from the frustration of a *desire. According to the *Linga-Purāna (I.9.10), dejection is to be overcome by means of superior dispassion (*vairāgya). Cf. *saumanasya*.

dayā ("sympathy") is sometimes listed as one of the ten practices of moral discipline (*yama). The *Yoga-Yājnavalkya (I.63) defines it as graciousness (*anugraha) at all times toward all beings—in mind, speech, and deed. See also *karunā*.

Dead pose. See *shava-āsana*.

Death. Materialistic philosophies deny that there is any immaterial principle—such as a soul or *spirit—that survives the demise of the physical *body. This one-dimensional view of human nature is vehemently rejected by all schools of *Yoga, including the pragmatic tradition of *Buddhism. In fact, the authorities of Yoga are agreed that it is of acute importance how a person dies. Only complete control of the death process, as effected by full awareness during and after the dropping of the body, guarantees a benign postmortem existence. The grand ideal is to "die," that is, to transcend the ego-illusion, while yet alive, so that death comes as no surprise but is comparable to a simple change of clothes. The esoteric art of conscious dying is hinted at, for instance, in the ancient *Bhagavad-Gītā* (VIII.10; 12f.):

That [practitioner who], at the time of going forth [i.e., death], directs with unmoving mind the life force (*prāna*) to the middle of the eye-brows, while being yoked by love (*bhakti*) and by the power of *Yoga, comes to that supreme divine Spirit (*purusha*).

Controlling all the gates [of the body], confining the *mind in the *heart, fixing the life force in the *head and established in yogic concentration (*dhāranā*), while reciting *om*, the [sacred] monosyllable [signifying] the *Absolute and remembering Me [i.e., *Krishna]—he who [thus] departs, abandoning the *body, goes the supreme course [toward *liberation].

Such a person transcends the law of moral causation (*karma*) and terminates the cycle of repeated births and deaths. This teaching is based on an even older account given in the *Brihad-Āranyaka-Upanishad* (IV.1.f). See also *ātivāhika-deha, jīva, karman, mrityu, para-anta-jnāna*.

Defects. See *dosha, mala*.

deha ("body") is derived from the verbal root *dih* ("to smear, anoint"). Two distinct and contrasting attitudes toward the *body and corporeality in general can be discerned in the spiritual traditions of India (and elsewhere). On the one hand, the body is characterized as an "ill-smelling . . . conglomerate of bone, skin, sinew, muscle, marrow, flesh, *semen, blood, mucus, tears, rheum, feces, urine, *wind, *bile, and *phlegm . . . which is afflicted with *desire, *anger, *greed, *delusion, *fear, *despondency, *envy, separation from what is desirable, union with what is undesirable, *hunger, *thirst, senility, *death, *disease, *sorrow, and the like" (*Maitrāyanīya-Upanishad* I.3).

On the other hand, the *body is elevated to the status of "the temple of God" (*deva-ālaya*), as in the *Maitreya-Upanishad* (II.2). This second, world-affirmative viewpoint is already expressed in the archaic *Chāndogya-Upanishad* (VIII.12.1) where we read: "This body is mortal, o Māghavan. It is subject to *death. Yet it is the resting place of the immortal, incorporeal Self (*ātman*).

In a similar vein, the *Yoga-Vāsishtha* (V.66.32)—almost two millennia later—declares the *body to be a most valuable instrument for discharging one's worldly duties. It is, as the text (IV.23.189f.) affirms, a source of infinite trouble for the spiritually ignorant person, but a fountain of *happiness for the sage who, moreover, does not experience *death as a loss. The body serves him as a chariot and is conducive to his welfare and *liberation. Similarly, the *Mārkandeya-Purāna (39.61) states that the body should be carefully preserved since it is the means of attaining virtue (*dharma), prosperity (*artha), sensual enjoyment (*kāma), and *liberation (*moksha). The *Uddhāva-Gītā (XV.17) compares it to a well-constructed boat that is propelled forward by God *Krishna as a favorable wind and that has one's *teacher as helmsman.

The preservation of the *body and the development of its latent powers (*siddhi) became the primary objective of such *Tantra-based schools as *hatha-yoga. Authorities of this type of *Yoga frequently compare the body to a pot (*ghata) that needs to be well baked in the fire of yogic disciplines. However, this comparison is curiously rejected in the *Varāha-Upanishad (II.25). The *Yoga-Kundaly-Upanishad (I.77) speaks of the transformation of the "material body" (*ādhibhautika-deha) into the "divine body" (ādhidaivika-deha). The purest vehicle, however, is the "superconductive body" (*ātivāhika-deha). As the *Yoga-Shikhā-Upanishad (I.27) explains, the body is ordinarily insentient (*jada) or "uncooked" (apakva) and it must be "energized" (ranjayet) by the *yogin, so that it becomes "cooked" or "ripe" (pakva). In the *Uddhāva-Gītā (X.29), such a ripe body is also called yoga-maya-vapus or a "body fashioned through Yoga," and it is said to be indestructible.

The *Yoga-Vāsishtha (III.57.23) speaks of the "*yogin's body" (yogi-deha) as being invisible even to other yogins. Such a spiritualized body is attributed to many Yoga *adepts, and the idea has provided ample material for folklore and legend. See also dridha-deha, vajra-deha.

dehin ("embodied one") is the individuated self, or human personality. See also jīva, jīva-ātman.

Deity. See deva, devatā, Divine, God.

Delusion. See moha.

desha ("place"). This term denotes both the appropriate environment for yogic practice and special loci for *concentration, such as the psychoenergetic centers (*cakra) and the sensitive places (*marma-sthāna) of the *body.

Proper surroundings are deemed an essential precondition for success in yogic practice. Desha is counted among the constituent disciplines of the fifteen-limbed *Yoga (panca-dasha-anga-yoga). The most general stipulation is that the place should be clean and quiet. Some texts are considerably more specific. Thus, the old *Shvetāshvatara-Upanishad* (II.10) asks that the ground should be level, free from pebbles, gravel, and fire, and that it should be concealed, inoffensive to the ear and pleasing to the eye, as well as protected from the wind. The *yogins* favor secluded spots like mountains, caves, temples, and vacant houses. See also *samketa*.

Desire. See *icchā*, *kāma*.

Desire for liberation. The self-transcending impulse, generally called *mumukshutva*, is the only motivational force that does not lead to *karmic embroilment.

Despair. See *vishāda*.

Despondency. See *daurmanasya*, *vishāda*.

deva ("shining one") can stand for the personal *Divine, such as God *Vishnu, *Shiva, *Indra, *Agni, *Brahma, *Rudra, or the Goddesses *Kālī or *Durgā, or a lower deity comparable to the angels in Christianity. In the latter sense, the *devas* or *devatās* are finite (and unenlightened) entities, though their life span far exceeds that of human beings (see Cosmos). Yet, the *Hindu scriptures uniformly value human existence as higher than the existence of the inhabitants of the heavenly realms (*loka*), because human life affords a unique intensity of experience that can lead directly to spiritual *awakening, or *liberation. See also *Absolute, God, Reality.

deva-datta ("God-given") is one of the ten cardinal psychoenergetic currents (*nādī*) of the *body. According to the *Tri-Shikhi-Brāhmana-Upanishad* (II.82), it resides in the skin and bones and is responsible for *sleep. However, according to the *Siddha-Siddhānta-Paddhati* (I.68), its location is in the mouth, and it is responsible for the knitting of the brows. Most texts assign to it the function of yawning (*vijrimbhana*).

devatā ("deity") is a synonym for *deva*.

deva-yāna ("way of the gods") is the postmortem *destiny that leads one to the Absolute (*brahman*). Cf. *pitri-yāna*.

devī ("Goddess") often refers to the feminine aspect of the *Divine. See also *shakti*.

Devotion. See *bhakti, pranidhāna*.

dhairya ("steadiness") is, according to the *Hatha-Yoga-Pradīpikā (I.16), one of the factors promoting *Yoga. It is counted among the constituent practices of the "sevenfold discipline" (*sapta-sādhana). See also *dhriti*.

dhanam-jaya ("conquest of wealth") is one of the ten cardinal psychoenergetic currents (*nādī) of the *body. Most *Yoga scriptures state that it pervades the entire body and does not leave it even after *death, being responsible for the swelling of the corpse. It is also sometimes thought to cause *phlegm (*shleshma) and hiccupping.

dhanur-āsana ("bow posture") is described in the *Gheranda-Samhitā (II.18) thus: One should stretch the legs on the ground like a stick and catch hold of both feet with one's hands so as to make the *body resemble a bow (*dhanus*). The *Hatha-Yoga-Pradīpikā (I.25) is a little more precise: Grasping the toes with one's hands, one should draw one foot up to the ear as if one were drawing a bow.

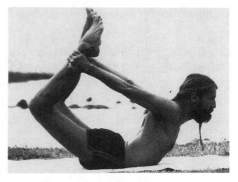

16. *Dhanur-āsana.*

dhāranā ("concentration"), which is also sometimes called *samādhāna* ("collectedness"), is one of the eight "limbs" (*anga) of *Classical Yoga, and is also a component of other versions of the spiritual *path. The *Yoga-Sūtra (III.1) defines it as the binding of consciousness (*citta) to a (single) locus (*desha). It is thus the practice of continuous *attention, which is of the essence of "one-pointedness" (*eka-agratā). The *Amrita-Nāda-Upanishad (15) understands it as the "compression" (*samkshepa*) of the *mind into oneself.

The practice of concentration, which precedes *meditation, is fundamental to the yogic process of introversion. It represents a gathering of one's psychic energy, which is accompanied by a high degree of sensory inhibition (*pratyāhāra*) and a slowing down of thought. Yogic concentration can have a variety of mental objects (*artha*), ranging from the internalized image of a *deity to internalized sound (*nāda*), to a locus (*desha*) within the *body. Deepening concentration leads to meditation (*dhyāna*).

In some contexts, *dhāranā* denotes the retention of the breath. See also *panca-dhāranā*.

dharma, which is derived from the verbal root *dhri* ("to hold, retain"), has many meanings. In *Classical Yoga, the term is primarily employed in the technical sense of "form" or "quality," which is contrasted with the concept of "form bearer" or "substance" (*dharmin*). *Patanjali, the author of the *Yogi-Sūtra (III.13f.), subscribes to the *sat-kārya-vāda, that is, the view that change affects only the form of a thing, not its substance. Thus, he distinguishes between three forms or states of a thing: its "quiescent" (*shānta*) or past aspect; its "uprisen" (*udita*) or present aspect, and its "indeterminable" (*avyapadeshya*) or future aspect. The word *dharma* can also simply stand for "thing" in general.

In the ethical field, *dharma* signifies "righteousness" or "virtue," that is, the moral order, as opposed to *adharma. In *Hinduism, morality is seen as the very foundation of the world. As such, it is considered to be one of the four "human goals" (*purusha-artha). In the *Tattva-Vaishāradī (II.12), *dharma* is explained as that which leads to heaven (*svarga)—rather than to *liberation—and is said to stem from the inclination to perform desirable (*kāmya*) actions. *Vācaspati Mishra, the author of this learned commentary on the *Yoga-Sūtra, even concedes that *dharma* can spring from righteous anger (*krodha*), and he cites the legendary case of Dhruva who took his father's slight as an incentive for performing austerities, which in the end raised him to a position above all others.

Historically, there has been a tension between the ideal of *dharma* and the ideal of *liberation, since the latter is deemed to be above good and evil, virtue and vice. Thus, the *Mahābhārata epic (XII.316.40) has this stanza: "Abandon *dharma* and *adharma*; abandon truth and falsehood. Having abandoned both truth and falsehood, abandon the [principle, i.e., the *mind] by which you abandon [everything]."

That the *yogin should eschew not only vice (*adharma) but also virtue (*dharma*) is, for instance, evident from the *Yoga-Sūtra (IV.7), which makes a distinction between *karma that is black, *kārma* that is white, and the *karma* of the *yogin, which is neither black nor white.

The reason for the *yogin's extraordinary karmic status is his constant transcendence of the ego (*ahamkāra, *asmitā), which experiences itself as the performer of good or evil acts. See also rita.

dharma-megha-samādhi ("enstasy of the *dharma cloud") is the highest level of enstasy (*samādhi) admitted in *Classical Yoga. It follows upon the "vision of discernment" (*viveka-khyāti) and is in turn the precursor to ultimate liberation (*kaivalya). This technical term also occurs in several *Vedānta works, including the Panca-Dashī (I.60), the Paingalā-Upanishad (III.2), and the Adhyātma-Upanishad (38). Its precise meaning is nowhere clearly defined, though many commentators understand the word dharma to denote "virtue" in this context. They may possibly have taken their cue from Mahāyāna *Buddhism, which employs the compound dharma-megha. But why should this elevated *enstatic condition shower virtue upon the *yogin when it precisely signals the concluding phase in his transcendence of dharma and *adharma? In his *Vivarana (IV.29), *Shankara interprets this high-level state somewhat more convincingly as "showering the supreme virtue called 'aloneness' (*kaivalya)." It is, however, more likely that in this context dharma means "constituent" and refers to the *gunas, which, like a faint cloud, still stand between the *yogin and the ultimate condition of *liberation.

The dharma-megha-samādhi is the highest form of supraconscious enstasy (*asamprajnāta-samādhi). It is the final moment in the long and arduous yogic journey, when the primary constituents of *Nature resolve into their transcendental matrix. This "involution" (*pratiprasava) of the gunas coincides with *liberation or *Self-realization.

dharmin ("form bearer") is the unchanging substance as opposed to the changeable form (*dharma). This is a key element of the theory of transformation (*parinama) adopted by *Patanjali in his *Yoga-Sūtra (III.13f.).

dhātu ("constituent") can refer to the three bodily humors—wind (*vāta), gall (*pitta), and phlegm (*shleshma, kapha). It can also refer to the seven constituents that are, for instance, listed in the *Yoga-Bhāshya (III.29): skin, blood, flesh, sinew, bone, marrow, and semen (*shukra). Some schools replace the skin by *rasa (thought to stream from the *heart and sustaining the entire *body) and the marrow by fat. The *Tattva-Vaishāradī (I.30) mentions that the dhātus are so called because they "hold together" (*dhāranā) the physical frame.

Sometimes the dhātu denotes the principal constituent of the body, which is the "nectar of immortality" (*amrita). See also dosha, ojas.

dhātu-strī-laulyaka ("longing for a physical woman") is one of five obstacles (*vighna) mentioned in the *Yoga-Tattva-Upanishad (31). It is presumably the desire to have sexual intercourse (*maithunā) with a flesh-and-blood woman instead of longing to unite with the *Goddess.

dhauti ("washing" or "cleansing") is one of the "six acts" (*shat-karma) of *hatha-yoga. According to the *Gheranda-Samhitā (I.13), it comprises the following four techniques: internal washing (*antar-dhauti); dental cleansing (*danta-dhauti); cleansing of the "heart" (*hrid-dhauti); and rectal cleansing (*mūla-shodhana). The *Hatha-Yoga-Pradīpikā (II.24f.) does not mention these subcategories but describes *dhauti* thus: One should slowly swallow a wet cloth four digits wide and fifteen spans long as instructed by one's *teacher, and then draw it out again. This technique is otherwise known as "cloth cleansing" (*vāso-dhauti). See also *kapāla-randhra-dhauti*.

dhrik-sthiti ("steadiness of vision") is one of the practices of the fifteenfold *path (*panca-dasha-anga-yoga). It is defined in the *Tejo-Bindu-Upanishad (I.29) as that vision, consisting of *wisdom, which sees the world as the *Absolute and which must not be confused with mere gazing at the tip of the *nose. See also *drishti*.

dhriti ("steadiness," "steadfastness") is sometimes counted as one of the ten practices of moral discipline (*yama). The *Shāndilya-Upanishad (I.1.12) understands it as "mental stability" (*cetah sthāpana*) at all times, especially in moments of personal loss. The *Uddhāva-Gītā (XIV.36) explains it as the "mastery over tongue and genitals." The *Bhagavad-Gītā (XVIII.33ff.) distinguishes three types of *dhriti*, depending on the preeminence of the three qualities (*guna) of *Nature. Thus, *sāttvika-dhriti* is that steadiness by which one restrains the *mind, the *breath, and the *senses. *Rājasa-dhriti* is that steadiness by which one holds fast to virtue (*dharma), prosperity (*artha), and pleasure (*kāma) and also clings to their fruits. Finally, *tāmasa-dhriti* is characteristic of the deluded person who is attached to sleep (*svapna), fear (*bhaya), grief (*shoka), dejection (*vishāda), and intoxication (*mada*). See also *dhairya*.

dhvani ("sound") is a synonym for *shabda and *nāda.

dhyāna ("meditation," "contemplation") is a fundamental technique common to all yogic *paths. The *Bhagavad-Gītā (XII.12) places *meditation above intellectual *knowledge, and the *Shiva-Purāna (VII.2.39.28) holds it to be superior to any pilgrimage, austerity, or sacrificial rite. As the *Garuda-Purāna* (222.10) declares: "Meditation is the highest virtue. Meditation is the highest austerity. Meditation is the highest *purity. Therefore be fond of meditation."

In the eightfold path of *Classical Yoga, *meditation precedes *enstasy (*samādhi). *Patanjali, in his *Yoga-Sūtra (III.2), defines it as the "one-directional flow" (*eka-tānatā) of presented ideas (*pratyaya) relative to a single object of *concentration. As such, meditation is a natural continuation or deepening of concentration (*dhāranā). The *Yoga-Sūtra (I.39) maintains that any *object whatsoever can be turned into a prop for the meditative process, though in the *Patanjali-Rahasya (I.39), for instance, the stipulation is made that it should not be a prohibited object, such as a nude female.

*Meditation effects the arrest (*nirodha) of the five kinds of "fluctuation" (*vritti) of *consciousness mentioned by *Patanjali. However, the *Kūrma-Purāna (II.11.40) speaks of a meditation as a "continuum of fluctuations" (*vritti-samtati), with attention resting on a specific locus uninterrupted by other fluctuations. Meditation is marked by an advanced degree of sensory inhibition (*pratyāhāra). Hence the *Mahābhārata epic (XIII.294.16) describes the meditating *yogin thus:

> He does not hear; he does not smell, neither does he taste nor see, nor experience touch; likewise, the *mind ceases to imagine. He desires nothing, and like a log he does not think. Then the sages call him "yoked" (*yukta), "one who has reached *Nature" (*prakritim āpannam*).

Many texts of *Post-Classical Yoga distinguish between a "qualified" (*saguna) and an "unqualified" (*nirguna) meditation. Whereas the former has a concrete *object (such as one's chosen *deity), the latter has no immediate object but is a kind of absorption into oneself. These two categories are also respectively referred to as *mūrti* ("formal") and *amūrti* ("formless") or "partite" (*sakala*) and "impartite" (*nishkala*) meditation. The *Yoga-Yājnavalkya (IX.9f.) gives as an example of the latter type of contemplation the persistent feeling of "I am the *Absolute."

Formal *meditation often contains a strong element of visualization. This is especially true of *Tantrism and *hatha-yoga, where the *yogin is asked to construct elaborate inner environments calling for intense *concentration and imaginative capacity. Usually the object of such detailed visualization is the practitioner's chosen deity (*ishta-devatā). The *God or *Goddess is so vividly imagined that he or she assumes overwhelming psychic reality for the practitioner. The *yogin can next attempt to identify with that deity in the unitive experience of *enstasy until his own *ego identity is obliterated. The underlying idea is that most practitioners find it too difficult to engage the "formless" meditation of imageless absorption.

The *Gheranda-Samhitā (VI.1ff.) makes a distinction between the following three types of meditation: "gross meditation" (*sthūla-dhyāna), "light meditation" (*jyotir-dhyāna), and "subtle meditation" (*sūkshma-dhyāna). The first consists in the contemplation of a concrete form (such as one's chosen deity), and is said to be for beginners; the second consists in the contemplation of different *light phenomena, while the third is equivalent to absorption into the *Self during the performance of *shāmbhavī-mudrā.

Whatever approach one chooses, *meditation continues the potent transformative trend initiated by *concentration. If pursued with adequate rigor, that trend leads to the ultimate obliteration of the subconscious "deposit" (*āshaya), that is, the complete restructuring of one's personal identity—from *ego personality to transcendental Selfhood. Meditation is a stepping-stone to enstasy (*samādhi), and hence must be transcended at a certain point. Therefore, it is not surprising that meditation is, as in the *Shiva-Samhitā (V.4), occasionally reckoned as one of the obstacles (*vighna) of *Yoga.

In some contexts, dhyāna is used in the sense of *samādhi. See also nididhyāsana.

Dhyāna-Bindu-Upanishad, which consists of 106 stanzas, is one of the *Yoga-Upanishads. This tract expounds the "*Yoga of meditation" (*dhyāna-yoga), which is understood to be the *path of meditative introversion by means of the sacred syllable *om, called the *pranava. A sixfold *path (*shad-anga-yoga) is put forward whose constituent practices are posture (*āsana), "breath restraint" (*prāna-samrodha), sense withdrawal (*pratyāhāra), concentration (*dhāranā), meditation (*dhyāna), and enstasy (*samādhi).

The "serpent power" (*kundalinī-shakti) is utilized, though no detailed instructions about its arousal are given, and only the first four psychoenergetic centers (*cakra) of the *body are mentioned and roughly described. The "heart lotus" (*hrit-padma) is given prominence.

dhyāna-mudrā ("seal of meditation") is one of the hand gestures (*mu-drā) used in *Yoga, especially in conjunction with the various *meditation postures. It is performed by resting the open left, palm up, on one's folded legs and placing the right, also palm up, on top, with the tip of the thumbs touching.

The phrase *dhyāna-mudrā* is also used in the *Yoga-Mārtanda* (159) to denote the balance (*samatva*) of the *body during the practice of the "easy posture" (*sukha-āsana*) when one is "inner-minded" even though the eyes are open.

dhyāna-yoga ("Yoga of meditation") is a common compound in the literature of *Yoga. It is frequently used already in the *Mahābhārata* epic. Thus, in one passage (XII.188.1ff.), a fourfold *meditation is taught whose goal is "extinction" (*nirvāna). It con-

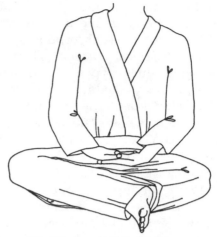

17. *Dhyāna-mudrā, hand gesture of meditation.*

sists in making the *senses into a ball—the phrase is *pindī-kritya*—and sitting like a log, while focusing the *mind on a single point. At the second stage, the mind is said to quiver like a lightning flash in a rain cloud. The mind is further described as tending to roam on the path of the *wind, which presumably means that it is inclined to follow the movement of the *breath, wherefore one should force it back on the path of *meditation. In the course of *meditation, we are told, different types of thoughts arise; these are referred to as *vicāra, *vitarka, and *viveka. While their precise meaning is not clear in this context, these terms have a parallel in the *Yoga-Sūtra.

The *Bhagavad-Gītā* (XVIII.52), a work of *Pre-Classical Yoga, emphasizes that *dhyāna-yoga* must be cultivated in conjunction with dispassion (*vairāgya).

dhyātri ("meditator"), that is, the meditating subject, as opposed to the object of *contemplation, which is called *dhyeya.

dhyeya ("that which is to be contemplated"), or the *object of *meditation. This can be any internalized object whatsoever, including the formless *Absolute itself. See also *ālambana, bīja, desha*.

Diet. See *āhāra, anna, mita-āhāra*.

dīkshā ("initiation") holds a central place in all branches and schools of the *Yoga tradition. According to the *Kula-Arnava-Tantra (X.3), it is impossible to attain *enlightenment without initiation—a sentiment reflected in many other scriptures. This scripture declares: "It is stated in the teaching of *Shiva that there can be no *liberation without initiation and that there can be no such [initiation] without a [qualified] preceptor (*ācārya). Thus is the preceptorial lineage (*paramparā)."

The great importance of *dīkshā* lies in that it consists essentially in the transference of *wisdom (*jnāna) or power (*shakti) from the *teacher to the *disciple. Through initiation, the disciple comes to mysteriously participate in the teacher's state of being and even becomes a part of the teacher's line of transmission (*paramparā). The *guru's lineage is a chain of spiritual empowerment that exceeds the world of space and time.

Both the word *dīkshā* and its underlying concept date back to the *Atharva-Veda, which has the following pertinent stanza (XI.5.3): "Initiation takes place in that the teacher carries the pupil in himself as it were, as the mother [bears] the embryo in her *body. After the three-day ceremony the disciple is born."

Initiation is generally thought to have different degrees. Often a distinction is made between the following three types of initiation: (1) *Mantra-dīkshā in which the *disciple is given an empowered *mantra for *recitation and *meditation; this is also known as *ānavī-dīkshā. (2) *Shakti-dīksha* in which the *teacher activates the disciple's "serpent power" (*kundalinī-shakti) and which, according to the *Shiva-Purāna (VII.2.15.6), requires the teacher to enter the student's body, a feat known as *para-deha-pravesha. (3) *Shiva-dīkshā* is the highest type of initiation, which is given by the teacher's mere touch or glance and upon which the disciple is propelled into the state of enstasy (*samādhi). This is also known as *shāmbhavī-dīkshā.

The process of transmission is frequently referred to as the "descent of power" (*shakti-pāta). See also *abhisheka*.

dīpti ("radiance") or luminosity is associated with many yogic states. Thus, it is listed in the *Yoga-Tattva-Upanishad (45) as one of the signs (*cihna) of the successful cleansing of the psychoenergetic conduits (*nādī).

Disciple. See *shishya*.

Discipline. See *yama, niyama*.

Discrimination or **discernment.** See *vijnāna, viveka, viveka-khyāti*.

Disease. See *roga, vyādhi*.

Dispassion. See *vairāgya, virāga*.

Dissipation. See *avirati*.

Distraction. See *vikshepa*.

Divine. *Hinduism is well known for its astounding variety of meta-physical systems or theologies, which show considerable religious vir-tuosity and philosophical ingenuity. There are first of all the numerous popular deities (*deva, *devatā), such as *Vishnu, *Shiva, *Krishna, *Rāma, *Durgā, and *Kālī. These are worshipped in rural India, and popular imagination views them as superhuman personalities who populate the heavens (*svarga) and who can be petitioned or even coerced through *prayer and magical incantations. The more literate sections of *Hindu society, however, believe that beyond this pantheon of deities abides a single ultimate *Being. In the monotheistic schools like *Vaishnavism, this ultimate *Reality is conceived as suprapersonal. Thus God *Vishnu is celebrated as the "supreme person" (*purusha-uttama), beyond space-time. The pantheistic and panentheistic schools, again, envision the ultimate *Reality to be impersonal, without qualities (*nirguna) and indescribable. They call it the *Absolute (*brahman) or the transcendental *Self (*ātman).

But then there are also philosophical schools like *Classical Sāmkhya, *Mīmāmsā, and *Nyāya that make no reference to a single ultimate *Being but propose a pluralistic metaphysics of countless tran-scendental Selves (*purusha). This is also the position of *Classical Yoga, which postulates a stringent dualism between Nature (*prakriti) and the conscious principle of existence called *purusha*. Like the *Nyāya school, it maintains that the "Lord" (*īshvara) is simply a special kind of transcendental *Self. Probably because of its dualist (or pluralistic) metaphysics and its attenuated concept of *God, Classical Yoga has never become widely influential as a philosophical school, though *Patanjali's systematization of the eightfold yogic *path has served subsequent authorities as a model. The schools of *Pre-Classical Yoga and *Post-Classical Yoga subscribe without exception to the nondualist (*advaita) metaphysics developed in the *Vedānta tradition.

divya-cakshus ("divine eye"), which is also called *divya-drishti*, stands for clairvoyance. It is among the paranormal abilities (*siddhi*) attributed to more advanced *yogins* This is also called "farsightedness" (*dūra-darshana*) in some texts, which is the modern Sanskrit word for "television" as well. See also *kapāla-randhra-dhauti*.

divya-deha or **divya-vapus** ("divine body"). According to the *Hatha-Yoga-Pradīpikā* (IV.71), this lustrous *body is acquired on the first stage of yogic accomplishment, or on the ninth level of the manifestation of the inner sound (*nāda*). Sometimes this term denotes the *ātivāhika-deha*.

divya-samvid ("divine perception") refers, according to the *Yoga-Bhāshya* (I.35), to paranormal sensory activity, such as extremely acute sight or hearing. See also *siddhi*.

divya-shrotra ("divine hearing") or clairaudience is a paranormal ability (*siddhi*) mentioned, for instance, in the *Yoga-Sūtra* (III.41), where it is explained as resulting from the practice of enstatic "constraint" (*samyama*) upon the relation between the ears and space (*ākāsha*).

Dolphin posture. See *makara-āsana*.

dosha ("defect" or "blemish") is a common concept of *Hindu ethics. In the *Yoga tradition, it specifically refers to the five "defects," namely lust (*kāma*), anger (*krodha*), greed (*lobha*), fear (*bhaya*), and sleep (*svapna* or *nidrā*). Sometimes this set is said to consist of passion (*rāga*), delusion (*moha*), attachment (*sneha*), lust, and anger. Occasionally one of them is substituted for faulty breathing (*shvāsa* or *nishvāsa*). In the *Amrita-Nāda-Upanishad* (27), again, seven such blemishes are cited: fear, anger, sloth (*ālasya*), excessive sleep (*atisvapna*), excessive waking (*atijāgara*), overeating (*atyāhāra*), and (excessive?) fasting (*anāhāra*). The *Yoga-Tattva-Upanishad* (12f.) furnishes a list of twenty blemishes that retard one's spiritual *progress, namely lust, anger, fear, delusion, greed, pride (*mada*), passion (*rajas*), birth (*janman*), death (*mrityu*), meanness (*kārpanya*), grief (*shoka*), laziness (*tandrā*), hunger (*kshudhā*), thirst (*trishā*), "thirst for life" (*trishnā*), shame (*lajjā*), anxiety (*bhaya*), sorrow (*duhkha*), dejection (*vishāda*), and excitement (*harsha*). The *Mahābhārata* epic (XII.290.56) suggests that there are even one hundred such defects. It also states (XII.205.18) that all these arise from spiritual nescience (*ajnāna*) and are inborn (*sahaja*). They are *obstacles on the *path.

In the *Yoga-Sūtra (III.50), the term dosha is used only once, where *Patanjali speaks of the "seeds of the defects" (*dosha-bīja), meaning the subliminal "activators" (*samskāra) that generate all psychomental activity. *Patanjali uses the technical term *klesha to refer to the "causes of suffering."

In the medical scriptures of the *Ayur-Veda, the term dosha stands for the three bodily humors, and this usage is occasionally adopted in the *Yoga texts as well. See also dhātu, mala.

Doubt is universally regarded in the spiritual traditions as a great undermining force that saps the practitioner's *enthusiasm and will. It can be overcome by *faith. See also samshaya.

drashtri ("seer") is *Patanjali's term for the *Self in its role as *witness of the flux of psychomental phenomena. It is, as the *Yoga-Bhāshya (II.17) defines it, "the Self conscious of the mind (*buddhi)." See also drishya, sākshin, samyoga.

Dream. Dreaming (*svapna) is an *altered state of consciousness. In the nondualist schools of *Yoga, it is one of the states (*avasthā) that conceal the transcendental *Self. Yet, since dreams are often expressions of the deep structure of one's psychomental life, they can serve as divinatory signs (*arishta). Cf. nidrā, sushupti.

dridha-kāya or **dridha-sharīra** ("firm body"), is a *hatha-yoga term referring to the transformed body of the *adept. See also vajra-deha.

dridhatā ("firmness") is the second constituent of the "sevenfold discipline" (*sapta-sādhana) expounded in the *Gheranda-Samhitā (I.10). It results from the practice of posture (*āsana). According to the *Hatha-Yoga-Pradīpikā (II.13), however, it is effected by rubbing one's perspiration (*sveda) produced in the course of one's exertions in *breath control into the *body.

drishi-mātra ("pure seeing") is a technical expression of *Classical Yoga denoting the very essence of the *Self as the immutable and permanent apperceiving subject of the ongoing mental process. See also drashtri, purusha.

drishti ("view," "opinion," or "gaze"). The *Mandala-Brāhmana-Upanishad (II.2.6) distinguishes three types of gaze during *meditation:

the "new-moon glance" (*amā-drishti*) with the eyes closed; the "first-phase-moon glance" (*pratipad-drishti*) with half-open eyes, and the "full-moon glance" (*pūrnimā-drishti*) with wide-open eyes. Some *postures or techniques of *breath control call for specific eye positions, and the two best known are the gaze at the middle between the eyebrows (*bhrū-madhya*) and the gaze at the tip of the nose (*nāsa-agra*). See also *dhriksthiti*.

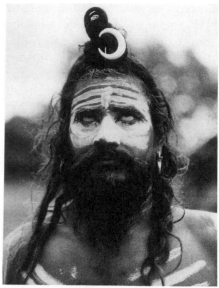

drishya ("that which is to be seen"), that is, the *object. In *Classical Yoga, this is a comprehensive term for Nature (*prakriti*).

18. Yogic gaze (drishti) at the eye-brows.

The *Yoga-Sūtra* (II.18) defines it as having the character of brightness, activity, and inertia, which refers to the three types of primary constituents (*guna*) of Nature. Cf. *drashtri, sākshin*.

duhkha originally meant "having a bad axle hole," but early on the word came to signify "sorrow," "suffering," or "pain." According to the spiritual traditions of India, existence is inherently sorrowful. This doctrine has frequently led Western critics to summarily portray Indian philosophy as profoundly pessimistic. However, this typification is demonstrably misleading, since the avowed goal of Indian spirituality is the perfect transcendence of sorrow or pain. Indeed, most schools of Indian spirituality describe the ultimate *Reality as utterly blissful (*ānanda*). Sorrow, then, pertains only to the ego-ensconced individual, not to the *Self. What more optimistic orientation could there be?

According to *Patanjali's *Yoga-Sūtra* (II.17), the "correlation" (*samyoga*) between the immutable Self and *Nature (or the body-mind), is the cause of the experience of suffering. When that correlation is severed, suffering ceases. Already in the *Bhagavad-Gītā* (VI.23), *Yoga is defined as the "disunion of the union with suffering" (*duhkha-samyoga-viyoga*). Cf. *sukha*.

Durgā ("She Who Is Difficult to Reach") is the cardinal *Goddess of *Hinduism. The *Purānas celebrate her as the divine spouse of God *Shiva, but her historical roots reach back into archaic agricultural religion. Riding on a lion and carrying different weapons, this Goddess is a veritable symbol of destruction. Yet, to her *devotees she is a benign, loving force. See also Kālī.

Duty. See *dharma*.

dvādasha-anta ("ending with the twelfth") is the designation of an esoteric psychoenergetic center (*cakra*) that is held, in some schools of *Shaiva Yoga, to be situated twelve digits *above* the *head. It is commonly equated with the *sahasrāra-cakra*. The expression can also refer to a point in space twelve digits from the tip of the *nose, which is as far as the life force (*prāna*) is thought to extend during exhalation. This space is employed in *tāraka-yoga* to visualize certain *light phenomena. See also *ākāsha*.

dvādasha-ara-cakra ("twelve-spoked wheel") is a psychoenergetic center in the center of the *body known to *Post-Classical Yoga. In some contexts, it denotes the *heart lotus (*hrit-padma*), while in others it refers to the "wheel of channels" (*nādī-cakra*).

dvaita ("duality"). In the schools of *Pre-Classical and *Post-Classical Yoga, which are founded in the metaphysics of *Advaita-Vedānta, the experience of duality is considered to be the result of spiritual nescience (*avidyā*). Cf. *advaita*.

dvandva ("pair") is a common designation for such "pairs of opposites" as heat and cold, light and darkness, or *pleasure and *pain. These bewilder all beings, as the *Bhagavad-Gītā* (VII.27) puts it. According to *Patanjali's *Yoga-Sūtra* (II.48), the *yogin becomes immunized against these dualities through the practice of posture (*āsana*), which includes an element of sensory inhibition (*pratyāhāra*).

dvāra ("gate"). The *Bhagavad-Gītā* (XVI.21) speaks of lust (*kāma*), anger (*krodha*), and greed (*lobha*) as the three gates to hell. More commonly, however, the word *dvāra* stands for the bodily apertures. Already in the ancient *Atharva-Veda* (X.2.31), the *body is likened to a citadel with nine gates. The *Katha-Upanishad* (V.2) speaks of eleven apertures, which, presumably, are the two eyes, two ears, two nostrils, the mouth, the genital opening, the anus, the navel, and the sagittal suture (*vidriti) through which the psyche (*jīva) exits at *death. Occasionally ten such gates are differentiated. The *Amrita-Nāda-Upanishad (26) lists seven gates, but these are esoteric loci in the body, such as the "heart gate" (hrid-dvāra), the "wind gate" (*vāyu-dvāra), which probably refers to the *vishuddha-cakra at the throat, and four unidentified gates located in the *head.

dvesha ("hatred," "aversion"). In *Classical Yoga, this is one of the five "causes of affliction" (*klesha) and is defined in the *Yoga-Sūtra (II.8) as one's dwelling upon what is painful (*duhkha).

However, that hatred can also have a positive spiritual effect is borne out by the story of Shishupāla, the king of Codi, who was released from the grip of the world by virtue of his abiding hatred for God *Vishnu over a period of three lifetimes. As the *Uddhāva-Gītā (IV.22) explains:

On whatever the individual concentrates the *mind fully and intelligently either through attachment (*sneha) or even through hatred—with that he becomes coessential.

Or again: That [*Absolute] sees no distinctions, therefore one should unite [with the Divine] through the bond of enmity or friendship, fear or attachment or desire (*kāma).

These ideas express the position of *samrambha-yoga, one of the most extraordinary developments within *Hinduism. See also rāga.

E

Eagle posture. See *garuda-āsana*.

Earth. See *bhūmi, prithirī*.

Easy posture. See *sukha-āsana*.

Ecstasy, as this Greek-derived word suggests, is a "standing outside" of oneself. It is a nonordinary or *altered state of consciousness that involves a significant shift in one's sense of identity. The experience entails at least a partial transcendence of the *ego, accompanied by extreme blissfulness. Generally speaking, ecstasy conveys emotional rapture and mental exaltation. Since these characteristics do not apply to the typical yogic state of mind-transcending consciousness, Mircea Eliade (1969) and others have proposed to render the term *samādhi as "enstasy" or "enstasis"—a coinage followed here. Enstasy means literally a "standing within" oneself and, ultimately, within one's authentic being, namely the transcendental Self (*ātman, *purusha).

But this distinction is not always clear-cut. There are yogic *samādhis that resemble more ecstasy as commonly understood than *enstasy. However, the general thrust of the yogic states of consciousness is toward the calming of the body-mind so that there is no emotional or intellectual excitation but simple pure Awareness (*cit).

Effort. In some yogic schools, the question is raised about the relationship between personal effort (*prayatna, *yatna) and grace (*anugraha, kripā, *prasāda). The answers range from complete reliance on

106

self-effort to complete reliance on divine intervention. In most cases, however, a middle *path is recommended, whereby a practitioner earns the favor of the *Divine by his or her consistent application to the spiritual process. See also *paurusha*.

Ego. In religious or spiritual contexts, the ego refers to the psychological principle of individuation, whereby a person experiences himself or herself as an individual apart from all other beings. This egoic existence is thought to lie at the root of all human experience of suffering (*duhkha*), and thus the ego is considered to be the principal stumbling block on the spiritual *path.

Two broad approaches to this problem can be distinguished. The first approach seeks to extirpate the ego together with all typically human forms of self-expression. Here the goal is to realize the transcendental *Reality *apart* from the world. This involves the pursuit of extreme inwardness and a radical withdrawal from the world and from participation in human culture. This is the ideal of *abandonment. The second, more integral orientation also seeks *Self-realization through ego-transcendence, but it is basically affirmative of the world. The underlying argument is that if there is only one *Reality it must necessarily include the world, which means that the world and therefore the human personality must be viewed as a valid manifestation of that ultimate Reality. Hence *self-transcendence does not imply ego denial as in the former approach. Rather, the ego-personality is used as an instrument for action in the world, while at the same time it is continually transcended through acts of conscious self-surrender. This ideal is best expressed in the approach of *karma-yoga*. See also *aham*, *ahamkāra, ahamtā, aham-vritti, asmitā, jīva*.

eka ("one") often refers to the singular *Reality, or transcendental *Self, beyond the multiplicity experienced by the *Unenlightened, ego-bound individual.

ekāgratā ("one pointedness") is composed of *eka* ("one, single") and *agratā* ("pointedness"). It stands for the single-mindedness, or focused *attention, which is the very essence of yogic *concentration. Through the practice of one-pointedness, the *mind is prevented from attaching itself to one *object after another. In the *Mahābhārata* epic (XII.242.4), *ekāgrya* (a synonym of ekāgratā), is praised thus: "The 'singleness' (*ekāgrya*) of the *senses and the *mind is the highest [form of] austerity (*tapas*)."

It is *attention's natural tendency to wander. The reason for this constant movement is the vibratory (*spanda*) nature of existence itself. Everything is in continuous flux (*pariṇāma*). The *yogin* attempts to slow down this perpetual motion of *Nature within the *microcosm of his own *consciousness to the point where his true identity, the pure Consciousness (*cit*), becomes obvious to him. See also *ekatānatā*; cf. *sarva-arthatā*.

Ekanātha is a celebrated Marathi *adept who lived c. A.D. 1533–1599. He edited the famous *Jnāneshvarī* and also wrote many original works of his own, notably his commentary on the *Bhagavad-Gītā* and on the eleventh canticle of the *Bhāgavata-Purāna*, as well as his numerous didactic poems (*abhanga*). Ekanātha's approach to *Self-realization combines devotion (*bhakti*), gnosis (*jnāna*), renunciation (*samnyāsa*), and meditation (*dhyāna*). See also Jnānadeva, Nāmadeva.

ekānta-vāsa ("dwelling in solitude") is sometimes counted among the practices of self-discipline (*niyama*).

ekatānatā ("single extension") is the continuity of *ekāgratā* on the level of *meditation (*dhyāna*). It is the continuous flow of "presented ideas" (*pratyaya*).

Element. The five material elements (*bhūta*)—earth, water, fire, air, and ether—are the final products of the process of cosmic *evolution. They form the "coarse" (*sthūla*) dimension of existence.

Elephant seal. See *mātanginī-mudrā*.

Elephant technique. See *gaja-karanī*.

Embodiment. For many spiritual traditions, embodiment is *the* problem to be solved. The reason for this is that embodiment implies the experience of being a specific *body and *mind—an individual, or *ego. Only those traditions, like Mahāyāna *Buddhism, that do not oppose the ultimate *Reality (*nirvāna*) against conditional existence (*samsāra*) have developed a more body-positive and world-positive ethics. For them, embodiment is a unique spiritual opportunity—both in terms of personal *liberation and the exercise of compassion (*karunā*) toward all beings.

Emotion. See Feeling.

Energy. See *bala*, *vīrya*.

Enjoyment. See *bhoga*.

Enlightenment is that condition of the body-mind in which it is perfectly synchronized with the transcendental *Reality. It is identical with *Self-realization. See also *ātma-jñāna*, *bodha*, Liberation, *purusha-jñāna*.

Enstasy. See *samādhi*; cf. Ecstasy.

Enthusiasm, in the form of consistent dedication to the spiritual process, is a basic requirement on the *path to *Self-realization. This must be more than emotional excitement, which tends to be fleeting and unsuited for a long-term commitment to the difficult task of *self-transcendence. Enthusiasm must, rather, be a measure of one's understanding (*jñāna*), or *wisdom, and be borne by a strong faith (*shraddhā*) in the reality of the spiritual process.

Environment. See *desha*.

Envy. See *mātsarya*.

Epic Yoga is the collective designation for the different Yoga schools represented in the *Mahābhārata, one of India's two national epics, the other being the *Rāmāyana. This designation is sometimes used interchangeably with *Pre-Classical Yoga, which, strictly speaking, is a more comprehensive concept. See also History.

Epistemology. See *pramāna*.

Eroticism. See *maithunā*, Sexuality.

Error. See *viparyaya*; cf. *pramāna*.

Ether. See *ākāsha*, *kha*, Space, *vyoman*.

Evil. See *adharma*, *pāpa*; cf. Good, morality.

Evolution signifies the process of unfoldment of forms by stages. Many spiritual traditions postulate a hierarchical series of developmental stages in *Nature. In *Hinduism, it was particularly the schools of *Sāmkhya and Yoga that created comprehensive evolutionary models intended to map out the principal categories (*tattva) of the manifest and unmanifest *cosmos. The purpose of these models is, however, not so much to offer cosmological theories as to serve the involutionary journey of the spiritual aspirant.

Both *Yoga and *Sāmkhya subscribe to a doctrine called *sat-kārya-vāda, which states that the effect (kārya) is preexistent (sat) in the cause. What this means is that all evolving categories of existence are potentially present in earlier categories. Thus, out of the single transcendental matrix (*pranidhāna) of *Nature evolves the category of the *buddhi, or *mahat, which is the unified prephysical and prepsychic field from which in turn emerge the distinct categories of physical and psychic existence. A common illustration of this evolutionary principle is that of an urn (the effect) that was fashioned out of clay (the cause). We can also think of a marble sculpture that preexists in a block of marble and is given shape through the artist's vision and skill.

In the tradition of *Advaita-Vedānta, which has largely adopted the *Sāmkhya account of this cosmogenetic process but which also denies ultimacy to the world of multiple forms, these transformtions from one category into another are considered to be illusory. They are the product of the hypnotizing agency of spiritual nescience (*avidyā). Hence this teaching is known as "phantom development" or vivarta. By contast, Sāmkhya and *Yoga subscribe to a realist philosophy. Their position is known as parināma-vāda or the "doctrine of [real] development." See also parināma, prakriti, sarga.

Equanimity. See sama-darshana, samatva.

Evil. See pāpa, pātaka; cf. punya.

Exaltation. See unmanī.

Excitement. See hatsha.

Existence. See Bhava, Cosmos.

$\mathcal{F}$

Faith, as opposed to mere belief, is a deep-felt trusting attitude toward existence. As such, it is fundamental to all spiritual traditions. Maturation on the yogic *path is unthinkable without faith, especially faith in one's teacher (*guru), who is thought to testify to the reality of the spiritual dimension of life. In the *Bhagavad-Gītā (VII.3), the God-man *Krishna emphasizes the importance of faith (*shraddhā) in this manner: "The faith of every [person] is in accordance with his essence (*sattva), o Bharata [i.e., *Arjuna]. A person (*purusha) is of the form of faith. Whatever his faith, that verily is he." See also *pratīti*.

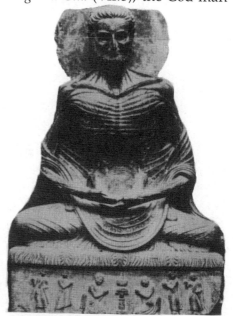

19. Gautama the Buddha during his rigorous fast prior to enlightenment.

Fasting, which is called *upavāsa*, plays a significant role in many religious and spiritual traditions. It is employed as a means of purifying *body and *mind in preparation of higher practices of *self-transcendence, notably *concentration, *meditation, and *enstasy. See also *anāhāra, laghv-āhāra, mita-āhāra*; cf. *atyāhāra*.

111

Fate. See *daiva, karma*.

Fear. See *bhaya*.

Fearlessness. See *abhaya*.

Feeling. It is sometimes thought that the *Yoga tradition, and *Hinduism in general, pays little attention to feelings or emotions. The fact is, however, that the *Hindu authorities have catalogued the entire range of feelings or sentiments that are known to modern psychology. Indeed, the Yoga scriptures refer to affective experiences to be had at the higher levels of enstasy (*samādhi) for which there are no straightforward equivalents in psychology. The enstatic "coincidence with bliss" (*ānanda-samāpatti) is a case in point. Already the *Taittirīya-Upanishad (II.7), which belongs to the genre of early "gnostic" texts, affirms that the "[ultimate *Being] verily is but feeling (*rasa)."

Perhaps what has given rise to the above mistaken impression is the fact that Indian thinkers tend to think more holistically. Thus, in *Yoga the affects are generally treated together with the motivations, which anticipates certain contemporary affecto-motivational theories. This psychological holism is epitomized, for instance, in the *kelsha doctrine of the *Yoga-Sūtra, which identifies the five principal factors governing a person's life—spiritual nescience (*avidyā), which is not merely the absence of right *knowledge but a positive misreading of reality; "I-am-ness" (*asmitā); the "will to survive" (*abhinivesha); attachment (*rāga); and aversion (*dvesha). Attachment and aversion form part of a motivational continuum. The life of the ordinary, unenlightened individual revolves around the pursuit of pleasure and the avoidance of pain. Within this motivational framework, a plenitude of emotions occurs.

The yogic process consists initially in the transmutation of negative emotions into positive feelings—such as compassion (*karunā) or love (*bhakti). This is accomplished through adherence to the principles of moral discipline (*yama) and self-restraint (*niyama). Howver, *Yoga does not stop at the humanistic objective of creating a benign and functional personality. It endeavors to transcend the body-mind and hence also the affective dimension. At the same time, however, it must be emphasized that in most schools the ultimate accomplishment of *Self-realization, or *enlightenment, does not signal the termination of the *yogin's emotional life. Rather, as a fully liberated being, or *adept, he is now able to engage life spontaneously and to freely animate all kinds of emotions without getting bound by them. This is especially evident in the case of the *crazy adepts, who, because their identity rests in the *Self and not in the *ego, are able to activate the entire range of human emotion in order to instruct others. Although the condition of *Self-realization is said to be beyond *good and *evil, the Self-realized adept is essentially a benign, though not necessarily infallible, being. See also Psychology.

Fickleness. See *laulya*; cf. *dhairya*.

Fire. See *agni, jāthara-agni, vaishvānara*.

Fish posture. See *matsya-āsana*.

Food. See *āhāra, anna, anna-yoga*.

Force. See *shakti*.

Fourth. The "fourth" is a *Vedānta designation for the transcendental *Reality. See also *cathurtha, turīya*.

Freedom. All spiritual traditions are in agreement that the ordinary human condition is one of *bondage and that freedom resides in our authentic identity, which is variously called *Self or *Spirit. Conditional existence is governed by the iron law of cause and effect. According to *Hinduism, this is so even in the moral dimension, where our *actions and *volitions determine our future through the mechanism of *karma and *rebirth. So long as we identify with the limited *body and *mind that is called the human "personality," we cannot be free. Freedom reigns beyond the *ego. Thus, the spiritual traditions of India all offer means of transcending the self in favor of the universal Self (*ātman, *purusha). The Self is coessential with radical freedom. This is also often equated with *immortality. Upon *Self-realization, or *enlightenment, the limiting conditions of the body-mind and its environment are no longer experienced as curtailing our essential freedom. The *adept is thus able to act with utter spontaneity (*sahaja) in the world, and to experience its ordinary *pleasures and *pains, without in the least feeling diminished by it in his being. See also Liberation.

Friendliness. See *maitrī*.

Frog posture. See *manduka-āsana*.

G

Gahinīnātha was the *teacher of *Nivrittinātha, the brother and *guru* of the famous Marathi adept *Jnānadeva. He lived in Maharashtra in the twelfth century A.D.

gaja-karanī ("elephant technique") is described in the *Hatha-Yoga-Pradīpikā* (II.38) as follows: One should draw up the *apāna* life force to the throat and then vomit the contents of the stomach. This practice is said to bring the network of psychoenergetic currents (*nādī) gradually under control. This technique is not listed among the "six practices" (*shat-karma), though obviously belongs to this set, and resembles *vamana-dhauti.

gāndhārā- or **gāndhārī-nādī** ("*gāndhārā* channel") is one of the fourteen principal conduits (*nādī) of the life force (*prāna) circulating in the *body. It commences at the "bulb" (*kanda) and extends to the left eye or, as the *Darshana-Upanishad* (IV.22) insists, to the right eye. The *Siddha-Siddhānta-Paddhati* (I.67), again, gives both ears as its termination point. Its position is generally given as being behind the *idā-nādī, but according to the *Varāha-Upanishad* (V.26) it runs between the central channel (*sushumnā-nādī) and the *sarasvatī-nādī.

Ganesha-Gītā ("Ganesha's Song") belongs to what is called the pseudo-Gītā literature. It celebrates the elephant-headed, potbellied God Ganesha ("Lord of the hosts"), who is widely invoked as the remover of *obstacles, as the supreme Godhead. It prescribes a *Tantric

114

type of *Yoga for his worship. The text consists of 414 stanzas distributed over eleven chapters that form a part of the latter portion of the *Ganesha-Purāna*. Most of the verses are identical with those of the *Bhagavad-Gītā*, though the author omits on principal verses focusing on the worship of God *Krishna. This compilation was composed some time between A.D. 900–1300 and it has a commentary by Nīlakantha (c. A.D. 1700) which contains many valuable references to Yoga.

gariman ("heaviness") is one of the classic paranormal powers (*siddhi) ascribed to accomplished *yogins. It is the power to make oneself physically heavy at will.

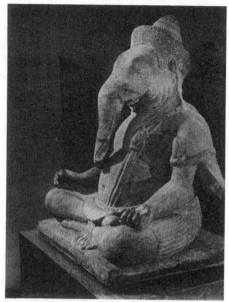

20. *God Ganesha, the remover of obstacles.*

garuda-āsana ("eagle posture") is described in the *Gheranda-Samhitā* (II.37) as follows: Pressing the thighs against the ground, one should keep the *body steady by placing the hands on one's knees. Modern textbooks explain this posture (*āsana) differently: One should stand upright on one leg, wrapping the other leg around the outstretched one. The arms are raised together in front of the body till they are parallel to the ground. Then one should bend them at the elbows and wrap one forearm around the other.

Gauda Abhinanda is the author of the *Laghu-Yoga-Vāsishtha*. He lived in Kashmir in the early tenth century A.D. Some scholars think that he also composed the longer *Yoga-Vāsishtha*, but this seems unlikely.

Gaudapāda is the author of the *Māndūkya-Kārikā*, which is an early exposition of the metaphysics of *Advaita-Vedānta. Often accused of having been a crypto-Buddhist, Gaudapāda's own testimony (IV.99) is that his view is by no means identical with that of the *Buddha. According to tradition, he was the teacher of Govinda who was *Shankara's preceptor. Gaudapāda's *Kārikā* is of interest to *Yoga researchers because it introduces the "intangible Yoga" (*asparsha-yoga).

gāyatrī ("hymnal") is the most famous *mantra of *Hinduism which has been recited daily since ancient *Vedic times. The word also refers to the specific meter in which this *mantra is composed. It runs as follows: *tat savitur varenyam bhargo devasya dhīmahi dhiyo yo nah pracodayāt*, "Let us contemplate that most excellent light of the divine Savitri [the solar God] so that He may inspire our visions." The *recitation of this *mantra was early on assimilated into the *Yoga tradition. See also *ajapa-mantra*.

Gaze. See *drishti*.

Genital control. See *upastha-nigraha*.

Gentleness. See *mādhurya, mārdava*.

Gesture. See *mudrā*.

ghantikā ("bell" or "alligator") is an esoteric structure of the *body, which is mentioned in some texts as being situated at the throat. In most contexts, it would seem to correspond to the uvula. See also *tālu-cakra*.

ghata-avasthā ("state of the 'pot' ") is the second of the four stages (*avasthā*) mentioned in some *hatha-yoga* texts. It is defined in the *Shiva-Samhitā* (III.56) as that stage in which the in-breath (*prāna*), the out-breath (*apāna*), the mystic sound (*nāda*), the "seed" (*bindu*), the individuated self, and the transcendental *Self are all united. According to the *Hatha-Yoga-Pradīpikā* (IV.73), this coincides with the piercing of the "knot of *Vishnu" (*vishnu-granthi*).

ghatastha-yoga ("pot-based Yoga") is the designation given to *hatha-yoga* in the *Gheranda-Samhitā* (I.9). The "pot" (*ghata*) is the *body, which has to be matured in the *fire of *Yoga.

Gheranda-Samhitā ("Gheranda's Collection") is a late seventeenth-century manual on *hatha-yoga* consisting of 351 stanzas distributed over seven chapters. It counts among the three classic scriptures of this school of *Yoga, and the techniques outlined in this tract form the basis of much of contemporary Yoga practice. The teachings are presented in the form of a dialogue between the sage Gheranda, about whom nothing is known, and his disciple Canda Kāpāli. This *Vaishnava work is modeled on the *Hatha-Yoga-Pradīpikā*, and some verses correspond *verbatim* to that manual. Gheranda teaches a "sevenfold discipline" (*sapta-sādhana*) and describes no fewer than thirty-two postures (*āsana*) and twenty-five "seals" (*mudrā*). The most original part of his work is the extensive treatment of the various purification techniques (*shodhana*). He also proposed an interesting classification of the phenomenon of *enstasy (*samādhi*). There are a number of commentaries on this text.

Ghodacolin is mentioned in the *Hatha-Yoga-Pradīpikā* (I.8) as a teacher of *hatha-yoga*. No further biographical information on him is available.

Gītā ("Song"). See *Avadhūta-Gītā, Bhagavad-Gītā, Ganesha-Gītā, Guru-Gītā, Īshvara-Gītā, Uddhāva-Gītā*.

Gītā-Govinda ("Song of Govinda") is an artful composition by the twelfth-century poet Jayadeva. It celebrates the love play between the God-man *Krishna and his favorite shepherdess *Rādhā, and in its strong erotic overtones resembles the most daring medieval Christian writings on bridal mysticism. It is an allegory of the love (*bhakti*) between the *Divine and the human psyche striving for union with the ultimate Lover.

God. See *deva*, Divine, *īsh, īshvara*, Reality.

go-mukha-āsana ("cow-muzzle posture") is described in the *Gheranda-Samhitā* (II.16) as follows: One should place one's feet on the ground with the heels crossed beneath the buttocks. The *body should be kept steady so as to resemble a cow's muzzle. In many other texts, we find this description: One should place the right ankle next to the left buttock and the other ankle similarly next to the right buttock. Modern manuals add that one should reach over one's shoulders with one arm and clasp one's hands.

Good. See *dharma, punya*; cf. *adharma, pāpa*.

gopī ("shepherdess"). Medieval works such as the *Bhāgavata-Purāna* and the *Gītā-Govinda* point to the great love between the God-man *Krishna and the love-sick shepherdesses of Vrindavāna as an example of the intensity of passion necessary in the *Yoga of devotion (*bhakti-yoga*). The *gopīs* had become so distracted by Krishna that they promptly forgot about their husbands and families whenever they heard his magical flute play.

Gopīcandra, or **Gopīcānd,** an eleventh-century king of Bengal whose sensational abdication and conversion of the *Nātha cult is remembered in numerous legends and poems. This event is most articulately presented in the cyclic Hindi poem *Manikcandra Rājar Gan* ("The Song of King Manik Candra").

Gorakh is Hindi for *Goraksha.

Gorakh-Bodh ("Illumination of Gorakh") is an archaic Hindi text, possibly belonging to the twelfth century A.D. It consists of a presumably fictitious dialogue between *Goraksha and his teacher *Matsyendra. It has thirty-three

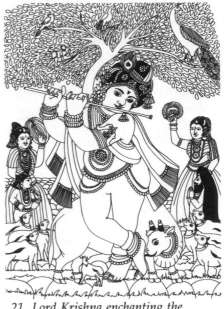

21. Lord Krishna enchanting the shepherdesses (gopī) with his flute play.

verses dealing with such diverse topics as the life of the *avadhūta, the concept of the void (*shūnya), the mystic sound (*nāda), the six esoteric bodily centers (*cakra), the "unrecited recitation" (*ajapa-japa*), which is the *ajapa-mantra, and the doctrine of spontaneity (*sahaja).

Gorakh-Upanishad is an old text of the *Nātha sect. It is composed in mixed Hindusthani and Rajasthani and speaks of the *avadhūta, the doctrine of *kula and *akula, as well as the eight "limbs" (*anga) of *Yoga.

Goraksha or **Gorakshanātha** (Hindi: Gorakhnāth) is the best-known and certainly one of the greatest masters of *hatha-yoga. His probable date is the ninth or tenth century A.D., and he appears to have been a native of the Punjab. He is acclaimed by some as the first writer of Hindi or Punjabi prose and is credited with the authorship of numerous works, including the *Goraksha-Samhitā, the *Amaraugha-Prabodha, the *Jnātā-Amrita-Shāstra, and the *Siddha-Siddhānta-Paddhati.

   Folklore gives varying accounts of Goraksha's origins, but according to traditions in Assam, he belonged to the weaver caste. Most sources are agreed that he renounced the world at an early age and traveled widely as a miracle worker and *teacher. In many parts of northern India, he still commands the respect and veneration as a perfected

adept (*siddha*) and even as a *deity. He was made the patron saint
of Gorkha and was deified early
on, his principal shrine being in
Gorakhpur. The Tibetan sources
speak of him as a *Buddhist ma-
gician. However, the works ascribed to him and his school have
a distinct leaning toward *Shaivism. Goraksha's place of death is
unknown. There are several accounts of his spiritual lineage, but
all unanimously position him
after *Ādinātha (who must be
identified with God *Shiva) and
*Matsyendra.

According to some authorities,
goraksha and *matsyendra* are appel-
lations given to initiates of a certain level of spiritual attainment.

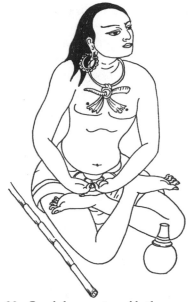

22. *Goraksha, master of hatha-yoga.*

While this may be correct, there is no reason to doubt the historicity
of either personage. Goraksha was one of the luminaries of the tradition of *Nātha sect, though his name is equally associated with the
*Kānphata sect, which he is traditionally said to have founded.

The probable historical relationship between Goraksha and *Matsyendra has been embroidered in numerous legends that depict both
teachers as highly accomplished thaumaturgists. Goraksha appears to
have modified his *guru's* more *Tantric teachings without, however,
abandoning that tradition. There is some truth in Mohan Singh's (1937)
observation that the teachings of Goraksha are to be searched for not
in the *hatha-yoga* scriptures but in the *Samnyāsa-Upanishads that
extol the ideal of *renunciation. Nevertheless, even if Goraksha cannot
be considered as the originator of *hatha-yoga* as we know it from such
works as the *Hatha-Yoga-Pradīpikā* and other earlier texts, there can be
no doubt that he was instrumental in the development of this branch
of *Yoga. Some scholars have suggested that Goraksha reformed the
*Kāpālika sect, which then became the *Nātha sect.

goraksha-āsana ("Goraksha's posture") is described in the *Gheranda-
Samhitā* (II.24f.) thus: One should place the upturned feet between the
knees and the thighs, covering carefully the heels with both outstretched hands, while contracting the throat (*kantha-samkoca*) and

fixing the gaze (*drishti*) upon the tip of the *nose. In the *Hatha-Yoga-Pradīpikā* (I.54), however, this posture is identified with the *bhadra-āsana*.

Goraksha-Bhujanga ("Goraksha's Companion") is a relatively late *hatha-yoga* tract consisting of nine stanzas in praise of *Goraksha, written by Lakshmidhāra.

Goraksha-Paddhati ("Goraksha's Tracks"), which is also known as the *Goraksha-Samhitā* ("Goraksha's Collection"), is one of the many works ascribed to *Goraksha. Many of its 202 stanzas are found in other texts of *hatha-yoga*, and its probable date is the twelfth century A.D. It expounds a sixfold *path (*shad-anga-yoga*) and provides detailed descriptions of the main concepts of esoteric *anatomy. It also contains instructions for the arousal of the "serpent power" (*kundalinī-shakti*). Great emphasis is placed on the recitation of the *pranava* (i.e., *om).

Goraksha-Samhitā ("Goraksha's Collection") is another name for the *Goraksha-Paddhati*. This is also the title of a work on *alchemy ascribed to *Goraksha.

Goraksha-Shataka ("Goraksha's Century [of Verses]") is a tract comprising 101 stanzas and appears to be a fragment of the *Goraksha-Paddhati*.

Goraksha-Siddhānta-Samgraha ("Compendium of Goraksha's Doctrine") is an eighteenth-century work that, as the title suggests, draws on earlier *hatha-yoga* scriptures—some fifty in all.

Goraksha-Vacana-Samgraha ("Compendium of Goraksha's Sayings") is an anonymous work of 164 stanzas with a short appendix of eight verses, which was perhaps authored in the eighteenth century. It opens with the statement that *Reality transcends both dualism (*dvaita*) and nondualism (*advaita*). It teaches a sixfold *path entailing the awakening of the "serpent power" (*kundalinī-shakti*) primarily through the *recitation of the sacred syllable *om combined with *breath control and the ten "seals" (*mudrā*) of *hatha-yoga*. Several verses (150ff.) describe the marks of a radical renouncer (*avadhūta*).

Goraksha-Vijaya ("Goraksha's Victory") is a work on the legendary exploits of master *Goraksha which to this day is sung in ballad form throughout northern India.

Govinda ("Cow Finder"), one of the epithets of *Krishna. In Sanskrit, the word *go* ("cow") also stands for sacred treasure, the philosopher's stone. This usage is already known to the ancient seers of the *Rig-Veda*.

Grace. See *anugraha, kripā, prasāda*.

grahana ("grasping"). In *Classical Yoga, this term denotes the process of cognition, especially sensory perception. Cf. *grahītri, grāhya*.

grahītri ("grasper") is the cognizing or perceiving subject. Cf. *grahana, grāhya*.

grāhya ("to be grasped") is the *object of cognition or perception. Cf. *grahana, grahītri, vishaya*.

grantha ("book"). Spiritual traditions generally deem mere book learning barren in comparison to firsthand experience. Even though the *Yoga tradition has developed an extensive literature expounding sophisticated doctrines, it has never lost sight of the importance of personal commitment and actual practice. The *Mahābhārata* epic (XII.293.25) epitomizes this orientation in the following stanza: "He who does not know the meaning of a book carries only a burden; but he who knows the reality behind a book's meaning, for him the teaching of that book is not in vain."

Some schools of *Yoga, however, are positively antispeculative and decry all forms of learning. This approach is found, for instance, among the followers of the *sahaja* teachings. See also *pandita, shāstra*.

granthi ("knot"). Already the ancient *Chāndogya-Upanishad* (VII.26.2) speaks of the "knots" from which those who know the traditional teachings (*smriti*) are released. The *Katha-Upanishad* (VI.15), again, states that "when all the knots of the *heart here [in the *body] are cut, then a mortal becomes immortal." In this usage, "knot" generally stands for "*desire" or, perhaps, "*doubt," which must be removed before *Self-realization can occur.

Later traditions know of three knots, which are collectively referred to as the *tri-granthi* ("triple knot"). These are "Brahma's knot" (*brahma-granthi*), "Vishnu's knot" (*vishnu-granthi*), and "Rudra's knot" (*rudra-granthi*). They are thought to be located at the *heart, the throat, and the spot between the eyebrows respectively, though according to some authorities their respective locations are the base center (*mūlādhāra-

cakra), the "heart lotus" (**hrit-padma*), and the "command center" (**ājnā-cakra*) in the *head.

These knots are blockages in the axial current (**sahasrāra-cakra*) and prevent the "serpent power" (**kundalinī-shakti*) from ascending to the crown center. The *Yoga-Shikhā-Upanishad (I.113–114) compares their being pierced by the force of the *kundalinī to the piercing of the joints of a bamboo stick by means of a heated iron rod. This process is also known as *vedhaka-traya-yoga* and *shat-cakra-bheda.

Greed. See *lobha*.

Grief. See *shoka*.

grihastha or **grihin** ("householder"). That *Yoga is not exclusively for ascetics who retire to the forest or mountain cave is borne out, for instance, by the *Shiva-Samhitā (V.186), which promises success to the householder who follows the methods outlined in that text. This is the great ideal of the *Yoga of action (**karma-yoga*), which was first announced in the *Bhagavad-Gītā. Cf. *samnyāsin*.

Guilt. See *kilbisha*.

guna ("strand" or "quality"). This word has a great many connotations. Its two most common and connected usages are "quality" and "constituent." In this sense, the term belongs to the technical vocabulary of the *Yoga and *Sāmkhya traditions where it refers to the well-known triad of forces—**sattva*, **rajas*, and **tamas*—that are thought to be the principal building blocks of *Nature. The origin of the *guna* doctrine is obscure, though J. A. B. van Buitenen (1957) has speculated that it may be linked with the archaic *Atharva-Veda (X.8.43), which speaks of the lotus flower with nine *gates, that is, the human *body, covered with three "strands." Van Buitenen has shown that in its earliest conception this doctrine sought to explain the psychocosmological *evolution of the higher *mind, called *buddhi, into the lower mind or **manas*, the senses (**indriya*), and the material elements (**bhūta*).

*Patanjali, in his *Yoga-Sūtra (II.15), pictures these three types of fundamental force—comparable perhaps to the energy quanta of modern physics—as being in continual conflict with each other. As a result of this inherent tension between them, they create the different ontological levels (**parvan*) of reality. The declared goal of *Patanjali's *Classical Yoga is to bring about the "involution" (**pratiprasava*) of the *gunas*, that is, their resorption into the transcendental matrix of Nature (*prakriti*), at least on the personal, microcosmic level.

According to the *Bhagavad-Gītā* (XIII.21), the *gunas* are "born of Nature" (*prakriti-ja*), and they bind the individuated or embodying self (*dehin*) to a particular body (*deha*). In the *Mahābhārata* epic (XII.301.15), *Nature is said to unfold the *gunas* a hundredfold or a thousandfold through its desire and free will and for the sake of cosmic *play. *Patanjali, on the other hand, appears to think of the *gunas* as three types of force or energy whose existence can be deduced from the behavior patterns (*shīla*) of Nature. From the *Yoga-Bhāshya* (II.18), the oldest extant commentary on *Patanjali's aphorisms, we can learn that (1) although the *gunas* are distinct, (2) they are nonetheless inter-dependent and (3) in combination create the phenomenal *cosmos, wherefore (4) everything must be regarded as a "synergization" of these three factors. It was not until *Vijnāna Bhikshu's voluminous *Yoga-Vārttika* (II.18), composed in the sixteenth century A.D., that the *gunas* were conceived as substances existing in infinite numbers and producing the multiple phenomena of the material and the immaterial universe.

The characteristics (*shīla*) of the *gunas* are often described. Thus, *Patanjali, in his *Yoga-Sūtra* (II.18), mentions their respective dispo-sition toward brightness (*prakāsha*), activity (*kriyā*), and inertia (*sthiti*). Other authorities are more explicit but generally emphasize the psy-chological aspects. See also *saguna, tattva;* cf. *nirguna.*

guna-atīta ("transcending the qualities") can refer to both the condition of radical *freedom from *Nature and the person thus free. As the *Bhagavad-Gītā* (XIV.22ff.) puts it, such a person neither rejects nor pines for the manifestations of the three *gunas* but remains the same (*sama*) in *pleasure and *sorrow, honor and disgrace, etc.

gupta-āsana ("concealed posture") is described in the *Gheranda-Samhitā* (II.2) thus: One should conceal the feet between one's knees and thighs and then place the buttocks on one's feet. See also *siddha-āsana.*

guru ("weighty one"). In contrast to most of the hybrid forms of *Yoga taught in the Western world, traditional Yoga is characterized by an intense teacher-disciple relationship that is thought to extend even beyond this lifetime. The *guru*, whose counsel or judgment is "weighty," is the pivot of the entire initiatory structure of Yoga. The following stanzas from the *Shiva-Samhitā* (III.11; 13f.), a late medieval work on *hatha-yoga, illustrate the superlative importance of the guru's role in practically all schools.

> [Only] the *knowledge imparted through the guru's mouth is productive [of *liberation]; otherwise it is fruitless, weak, and the cause of much affliction.

> There is no doubt that the guru is one's father; the guru is one's mother; the guru is God. Therefore he should be served by all in deed, speech, and thought.

> By the guru's favor (*prasāda) everything auspicious for oneself is obtained . . .

Similarly, the *Hatha-Yoga-Pradīpikā (IV.9) declares that without the compassion (*karunā) of a true teacher (*sad-guru), the *sahaja state is difficult to attain. As the *Shiva-Purāna (VII.2.15.38) states, if one's *preceptor is merely "nominal," so is the *liberation that he bestows on the disciple (*shishya). In the *Yoga-Kundaly-Upanishad (III.17), the guru is compared to a helmsman who assists the pupil in crossing the ocean of phenomenal existence in the boat built from his knowledge. The *Advaya-Tāraka-Upanishad (14ff.) has these verses:

> The [true] teacher is well versed in the *Veda, a devotee of *Vishnu, free from envy, pure, a knower of Yoga and intent on Yoga, and always having the nature of Yoga.

> He who is equipped with *devotion to the teacher, who is especially a knower of the *Self, possessing such characteristics [as are mentioned above], is designated as a guru.

> The syllable gu [signifies] darkness; the syllable ru [signifies] the destroyer of that [darkness]. By reason of [his power] to destroy darkness, he is called guru.

> The guru alone is the supreme *Absolute. The guru alone is the supreme way. The guru alone is the supreme knowledge. The guru alone is the supreme resort.

> The guru alone is the supreme limit. The guru alone is supreme wealth. Because he is the teacher of that [nondual *Reality], he is the guru greater than [any other] guru.

The significance of such a *guru* stems from his having realized the *Self. This realization represents a change in his very state of being that spontaneously communicates itself to others, even to the natural environment. The *Self-realized adept is always transmitting his native condition of *liberation, which is the true condition of all beings and things. Thus, he constantly initiates others into the same realization, though they may be slow in experiencing this consciously.

Because of their flawless identification with the transcendental *Reality, such enlightened masters were traditionally approached with the utmost reverence. They were even regarded as embodiments (*vigraha*) of the *Divine. In practice, however, only a small number of teachers alive at any given time are Self-realized. As the *Kula-Arnava-Tantra* (XIII.106ff.) counsels:

O *Devī, there are many *gurus* on earth who give what is other than the *Self, but hard to find in all the worlds is the *guru* who reveals the *Self.

Many are the *gurus* who rob the *disciple of his wealth, but rare is the *guru* who removes the disciple's afflictions.

He is the [true] *guru* by whose very contact there flows the supreme Bliss (*ānanda*). The intelligent man should choose such a one as his *guru* and none other.

The fact so few *gurus* enjoy full *enlightenment has undeniably led to the occasional exploitation of credulous students. Many preceptors expected not only unquestioned *obedience but also constant *service, possibly even a hefty renumeration for this or that initiation (*dīkshā*). For instance, the *Shiva-Samhitā* (V.33) stipulates that one should make over all one's property and livestock to the teacher in exchange for *initiation. Already the *Maitrāyanīya-Upanishad* (VII.8ff.) warns against false teachers who merely deceive the naive.

On the other side, we have warnings against abandoning one's *guru*, which is brought to have dire *karmic consequences. For example, the *Saura-Purāna* (LXVIII.11), a medieval encyclopedic compilation, contains this curselike threat: "May he who deserts his teacher meet with *death. May he who discontinues [the recitation of] the *mantra* [given to him by the teacher] become poverty-stricken. May he who deserts both [teacher and *mantra*] be cast into *hell, even if he be a perfected [*adept]."

One of the most heinous of *sins was to violate the preceptor's bed, for which the only expiation, according to the *Mahābhārata (XII.159.46f.), was *death by embracing a heated female statue of iron, or by self-castration. This capital punishment was presumably felt necessary because of the guru-kula system, where the disciple became part of the teacher's household (kula).

Particularly in medieval times, with the rise of the elaborate and often dangerous psychotechnology of *Tantrism, the guidance of a guru was considered absolutely essential. Perhaps partly in order to counterbalance the excessive authority traditionally granted to the guru and the strong trend toward the deification of spiritual teachers, some *Hindu schools began to emphasize that the real teacher is none other than the transcendental *Self. Thus, the *Uddhāva-Gītā (II.20) states: "The *Self is the teacher of [all] selves, especially of humans, because it guides one to the highest good (shreya) by means of *perception and *inference."

The practice of *guru-yoga and spiritual *transmission is alive even today. The importation of *Yoga and other similar esoteric traditions into the West has raised a number of questions, not least that of the appropriateness of spiritual discipleship and the legitimacy of spiritual authority. See also ācārya, Crazy adept, upādhyāya.

guru-bhakti ("devotion to the teacher") is a requirement on all yogic *paths except (and at least in theory) in the most radical schools of *sahaja-yoga. It is sometimes listed as one of the nine constituent practices of self-restraint (*niyama). The *guru serves the *disciple as a concrete image of the ultimate *Reality, that is, his or her own higher *Self. By constantly thinking about the *guru, the disciple tunes into and indeed participates in the *guru's extraordinary state of being, which is thought to effect a gradual transformation in the disciple. The underlying idea, known in all spiritual traditions, is that one becomes what one makes the focus of one's *attention. The *Yoga-Shikhā-Upanishad (V.53) states: "There is no one greater in the 'three worlds' [i.e., in the total universe] than the guru. It is he who grants 'divine knowledge' (divya-jnāna) and who should be worshipped with supreme devotion (*bhakti)."

That devotion is a form of loving *attachment. Instead of being attached to ordinary things, the disciple channels all his or her emotive energies toward the *guru. This is expressed through constant service (*seva), *meditation upon the guru, and complete obedience (shushrūshā). This process can be understood in terms of the transference phenomenon known to psychiatry, and therefore it is important that the guru should carefully monitor the disciple's spiritual maturation and ensure that he or she does not become neurotically dependent on the teacher but is truly set free. See also *guru-pūjā*.

guru-cakra ("teacher's wheel") is a synonym for **ājnā-cakra*.

Guru-Gītā ("Song about the Guru") is a popular *Hindu work of 352 stanzas that forms part of the Sanatkumāra-Samhitā in the second section of the *Skanda-Purāna*. It is presented as a dialogue between God Maheshvara (i.e., *Shiva) and his divine spouse Pārvatī.

guru-pūjā or **-pūjana** ("guru worship") is the mental or bodily worship of one's *teacher, either in person or in the form of an image (**mūrti*). See also *guru-bhakti*.

guru-sevā ("service for the teacher"), which is listed in the **Shiva-Samhitā* (III.35) as one of the means to success in *Yoga, is fundamental to most schools of Yoga. It is a form of **guru-bhakti* and a concrete way of cultivating *self-transcendence. See also *ācārya-sevana, sevā*.

guru-shushrūshā ("obedience to the teacher") is occasionally counted among the rules of self-restraint (**niyama*), as for instance in the **Linga-Purāna* (I.89.25). The word *shushrūshā* is derived from the verbal root *shru* ("to hear") and means the "desire to listen" to the *teacher. See also Obedience.

guru-yoga is the spiritual discipline of submitting to the *guru's* will in all matters. See also *guru*.

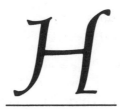

hala-āsana ("plough posture") is described in modern manuals of *hatha-yoga*. It is performed by lowering one's legs from the shoulder stand (*sarva-anga-āsana*) to the ground behind one's *head.

hamsa is usually translated as "swan," but more precisely this designation refers to the wild goose (*Anser indicus*), whose high flight has inspired the ancient Indians to make it the symbol of the sun and, later, of the luminous transcendental *Self (*ātman*), as well as a certain type of renouncer (*samnyāsin*) who has realized that Self.

In the scriptures of *hatha-yoga*, the word *hamsa* frequently stands for the individual self (*jīva*), especially in its aspect as life force (*prāna*) and its external aspect, the *breath. Thus already the *Shvetāshvatara-Upanishad* (I.6) states that the *hamsa* flutters about in the *brahma-cakra*, which here means the lower nature of *God. Elsewhere (III.18), this text declares that although the *hamsa* is embodied in the "nine-gated city," it hovers to and fro outside the *body. This may be the source of the later notion that it leaves the body (in the form of the breath) to a distance of thirty-six digits via the left and the right path (i.e., the nostrils).

In the *Yoga-Upanishads, speculations about the *hamsa* abound. Thus, according to the *Hamsa-Upanishad* (5), the *hamsa* is said to pervade all bodies as fire pervades wood or oil pervades sesame seed. The *Kaula-Jnāna-Nirnaya* (XVII.23), again, states that the *hamsa* is in the shape of a coil extending from the feet to the top of the *head and is also known as *vāma*, which can mean "beautiful," "crooked," and "left." In other words, it is identical with the "serpent power" (*kundalinī-shakti*), the hidden spiritual energy of the body. The *Pāshupata-Brāhmana-Upanishad* (I.25), however, states that the *hamsa* circulates between the left arm and the right hip, whereas the *Yoga-Shikhā-Upanishad* (VI.35) teaches that it moves up and down within the central channel (*sushumnā-nādī*) of the body.

The word *hamsa* is often explained as the sound that is produced by the *breath, the ejection of *prāna causing the sound *ha* and its re-entry into the *body the sound *sa*. This spontaneous sound is widely known as the *ajapa-mantra*, *ajapa-gāyatrī*, or *hamsa-mantra*. The body is thought to automatically recite this mantric sound 21,600 times a day. The *Yoga-Shikhā-Upanishad* (VI.54) counsels that this sound should be recited in reverse, namely as *so'ham*, which means "I am He." This is the "wedge" (*kīlaka*) spoken of in the *Hamsa-Upanishad* (10) by which the door to *liberation can be forced open.

Hamsa-Upanishad ("Swan Upanishad") is one of the *Yoga-Upani-shads and consists of twenty-one short sections expounding in a very condensed fashion the theory and practice of the *hamsa*. The text is in the form of a conversation between Sage *Sanatkumāra and his pupil Gautama. The teaching propounded here is a form of *kundalinī-yoga*. The text mentions eight functions of the *hamsa* but actually describes twelve. These are related to the "lotus of the heart" (*hrit-padma*). It also gives a description of the ten levels of manifestation of the inner sound (*nāda*).

hamsa-yoga ("Yoga of the swan") is an expression found, for instance, in the *Nāda-Bindu-Upanishad* (5) where it stands for the *recitation of the sacred syllable *om*.

hāna ("cessation"). In *Classical Yoga, this term is specificially used to denote the discontinuation of the "causes of affliction" (*klesha*).

Happiness. The pursuit of happiness is endemic to human life. Ordinarily, it takes the form of one's search for pleasurable (*sukha*) experiences and one's simultaneous avoidance of painful (*duhkha*) experiences. But, from a spiritual point of view, neither sensual nor emotional nor intellectual pleasure can ultimately satisfy a person. Only the recovery of one's true identity, as the transcendental *Self, guarantees the end of our incessant thirst (*trishnā*) for ever-new plea-surable experiences. In other words, we tend to look for happiness in the wrong places—either in external things or in internal states—whereas the nature of the Self is inherent *bliss, or *ānanda*. At least this is the teaching of most nondualist schools of *Yoga, though this idea is also implicit in dualist conceptions of the Self, as in *Classical Yoga. For, why would anyone want to realize the Self, or the *Absolute, if that realization were connected with pain or even a mediocre experience? The universal testimony of the *adepts is that recovering one's true identity is the most rewarding of all possible human aspirations (*purusha-artha). See also Joy, sukha.

Hara ("Robber," "Remover") is an epithet of God *Shiva as the destructive aspect of the *Divine. In modern terms, he is the principle of entropy.

Hari ("He Who Is Tawny") is one of God *Vishnu's or *Krishna's many names.

Hariharānanda Āranya (A.D. 1869–1947) was a Bengali *adept who wrote, among other works, the *Yoga-Kārikā and the *Bhāsvatī commentary on the *Yoga-Sūtra. He was the founder of the Kapila Matha in Bihar, one of the last remaining schools in the tradition of *sāmkhya-yoga.

harsha ("excitement") is widely regarded as an undesirable emotional state and is something grouped with the "defects" (*dosha) preventing *progress on the yogic *path.

hasti-jihvā ("elephant tongue") is one of the fourteen principal channels (*nādī) of the life force (*prāna) of the *body. It is generally stated to be located to the rear of the central channel (*sushumnā-nādī) and to extend to the right eye. According to the *Darshana-Upanishad (IV.14), however, it is situated behind the *idā-nādī and to extend to the big toe of the right foot. The *Yoga-Yājnavalkya (IV.44), again, insists that it is connected to the toes of the left foot, while the *Siddha-Siddhānta-Paddhati (I.67) has it proceed to the ears.

hasti-nishadana ("elephant seat"). This is a sitting posture (*āsana) mentioned but not further described in the *Yoga-Bhāshya (II.46). See also nishadana.

Hatha-Ratna-Āvali ("String of Jewels on Hatha[-Yoga]") is a work of Shrīnivāsa Bhatta who lived in the mid-seventeenth century A.D. His *teacher was a certain Ātmārāma. This is a work of 397 verses expanding in masterly fashion on the information contained in the

Hatha-Yoga-Pradīpikā. It appears to have at least one commentary. Shrīnivāsa also wrote works on *Vedānta, *Nyāya, and *Tantra.

Hatha-Sanketa-Candrikā ("Moonlight on the Conventions of Hatha [-Yoga]"). This eighteenth-century work was authored by Sundara Deva, son of Vishvanātha Deva, belonging to the Kashyapa clan (*gotra*) of Benares. The author quotes profusely from other works, and his text runs into some three thousand stanzas. Remarkably, this text contains no references to the *Gheranda-Samhitā*.

Hatha-Tattva-Kaumudī ("Moonlight on the Principles of *Hatha [-Yoga]*") is a work of Sundara Deva, who also authored the *Hatha-Sanketa-Candrikā*. One known manuscript of this text comprises 121 folios.

hatha-yoga ("forceful Yoga"), also called *hatha-vidyā* ("science of *hatha*"), is the type of *Yoga specific to the *Kānphata sect, though this designation is also applied in general to the vast body of doctrines and practices geared toward *Self-realization by means of perfecting the *body. As such, *hatha-yoga* is an important aspect of the pan-Indian movement of *Tantrism. The historical roots of this eclectic Yoga are varied. On the one side, it is anchored in the Tantric *Siddha cult with its *kāya-sādhana ("body cultivation"); on the other side, it was inspired by *alchemy (*rasāyana*). It also receied vital stimuli from *Shaivism, *Shaktism (in the form of the *kundalinī doctrine), *Advaita-Vedānta, and even Vajrāyāna (Tantric) *Buddhism. There also appears to be a strong link with the "practice of the (inner) sound" (*nāda-anusandhāna*), as described in the *Samnyāsa-Upanishads, esoteric Vedānta works dealing with *renunciation.

The most popular teacher of *hatha-yoga*, who is widely celebrated as its inventor, is *Goraksha of the ninth or tenth century A.D. He was a member of the *Nātha tradition in which *body cultivation played a crucial role. Many Western scholars consider *hatha-yoga* to be the product of a period of cultural decline, and even in India it came under attack early in its development. For instance, it is clearly rejected in the *Laghu-Yoga-Vāsishtha (V.6.86; 92), which maintains that it merely leads to *pain. The most formidable critic of *hatha-yoga* was *Vijnāna Bhikshu, a sixteenth-century savant and *Yoga practitioner. Some of his criticisms, especially against the magical undercurrents present in this yogic approach, are undoubtedly justified. Nevertheless, we must guard ourselves against a wholesale condemnation of this tradition, which clearly has spawned some outstanding *adepts. The label "de-

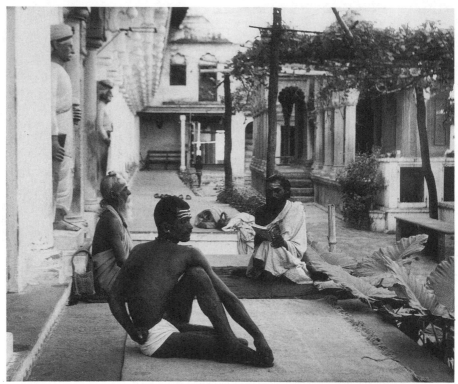

23. A practitioner of hatha-yoga in Benares.

cadent Yoga" (J. H. Woods, 1966) lacks credence. Notwithstanding occasional excesses and aberrations, its body-positive orientation exemplifies the integral spirit of *Tantrism at its best. Like all *Tantric schools, it purports to be a teaching for the difficult conditions of the present "dark age" (*kāli-yuga).

Hatha-yoga can also not be dismissed as an "easy" way. This is hinted at in the word *hatha* itself, which means "force" or "forceful." In the *Jīvan-Mukti-Viveka* (I, p. 156), it is explicitly contrasted with what its author, *Vidyāranya, calls "gentle Yoga" (*mridu-yoga*). He characterized the two approaches thus: One can lead an animal into its stall either by enticing it with some fresh grass or by whipping it. The first way is better; the second merely causes the animal to panic. Similarly, equanimity (*samatva) toward friend and foe is the easy method of subduing the *mind. The other, difficult method is that of breath control (*prānāyāma) and sensory inhibition (*pratyāhāra). This shows a bias against *hatha-yoga* that is common among followers of the *Vedānta tradition, which tends toward world negation and denial of the *body.

The word *hatha* also has a deeper, esoteric significance. Thus, its two component syllables, *ha* and *tha*, are frequently explained as standing for the microcosmic "sun" (*sūrya) and "moon" (*candra) respectively, while *yoga* is the "union" (*aikya) between these two principles.

Hatha-yoga is often contrasted with *rāja-yoga, the "royal" eightfold path of *Patanjali, also known as *Classical Yoga. However, this distinction is relatively recent and perhaps was first introduced by *Vijñāna Bhikshu. From the beginning, *hatha-yoga* included the higher yogic stages of *concentration, *meditation, and *enstasy. Yet, in the *Gheranda-Samhitā (I.1), the *Hatha-Yoga-Pradīpikā, and the *Shiva-Samhitā (V.181)—the three most widely used manuals—*hatha-yoga* is presented as a "stairway" to *rāja-yoga. The *Hatha-Yoga-Pradīpikā (IV.104) proffers the following metaphor: Reality (*tattva) is the seed, *hatha-yoga* the soil, and indifference (*udāsīnya*) the water that together promote the growth of the legendary wish-fulfilling tree (*kalpa-vriksha*), which is the sublime condition of *unmanī, or mind transcendence.

But *hatha-yoga* does not seek mere transcendental experiences. Its objective is to transform the human *body to make it a worthy vehicle for *Self-realization. *Embodiment is understood as a genuine advantage, and *enlightenment is thought to have definite bodily repercussions. As the *Shiva-Samhitā (II.49) affirms: "When the body, obtained through *karma, becomes the means of 'extinction' (*nirvāna), then the 'burden' (*vahana*) of the body is fruitful, not otherwise." Or, in the words of the *Gheranda-Samhitā (I.8): "Like an unbaked urn left in water, the [bodily] vessel is ever [so soon] decayed. Baked well in the fire of Yoga, the vessel becomes purified [and enduring]."

In the *Yoga-Shikhā-Upanishad (I.161ff.), we find these stanzas:

He whose body (*pinda) is unborn and deathless is liberated in life (*jīvan-mukta). —Cattle, cocks, worms, and the like verily meet with their *death.

How can they attain *liberation by shedding the body, o Padmaja?— The life force [of the *yogin] does not extend outward [but is focused in the axial channel, or *sushumnā-nādī]. How then can the shedding of the body [occur]?

The liberation that is attainable by shedding the body—is that liberation not worthless? Just as rock salt [is dissolved] in water, so "Absoluteness" (*brahmatva*) extends to the body [of the enlightened being].

When he reaches the [condition of] "non-otherness" (ananyatā), he is said to be liberated. [But others continue to] distinguish different bodies and organs.

The *Absolute has attained "embodiment" (dehatva), even as water becomes a bubble.

Thus, the *hatha-yogin strives after *liberation via the creation of a "yogic body" (*yoga-deha) immune to *disease and free from the limitations that characterize the ordinary flesh body. The yogic body is said to be endowed with "super senses" (atīndriya) and powers far beyond the capabilities of the normal person. According to the *Yoga-Shikhā-Upanishad (I.134), hatha-yoga removes the "dullness," or impurity, resulting from the "defects" (*dosha). This is mentioned as the second level of yogic attainment, the first being the obliteration of all diseases (*roga). The third level is reached when the "moon" (*candra) showers forth the "nectar of immortality" (*amrita), whereupon the body becomes youthful and the *yogin acquires a variety of psychic powers (*siddhi).

The body of the enlightened *adept is really the universal Body, and hence it is said that he can assume any form or shape at will. This transubstantiated body is also styled *ātivāhika-deha, or "super-conductive body." It is an omnipresent, luminous vehicle. This is explained in the *Yoga-Bīja (53ff.) thus:

The [*yogin's] body is like the *ether, even purer than the ether. His body is more subtle than the subtlest, coarser than any coarse [object], more insensitive [to pain, etc.] than the [most] insensitive.

The [body of] the lord of *yogins conforms to his will. It is self-sufficient, autonomous, and immortal. He entertains himself with play wheresoever in the three realms [i.e., on earth, in the "midregion," and in the celestial worlds].

The *yogin is possessed of unthinkable powers. He who has conquered the senses can, by his own will, assume various shapes and make them vanish again.

The *adepts of hatha-yoga are thus not only *enlightened masters but also magical theurgists, considered on a par with the world creator.

Hatha-yoga's philosophy of the *body is most elaborately discussed in five of the six chapters of the *Siddha-Siddhānta-Paddhati, an early work ascribed to master *Goraksha. This body-oriented approach has led to a plethora of inventions in yogic technology, notably in the areas of cleansing practices (*shodhana, *dhauti), postures (*āsana), and breath control (*prānāyāma). Generally, *hatha-yogins accept the eightfold *path outlined by *Patanjali, though they have greatly developed some of its aspects. The *Gheranda-Samhitā, however, puts forward a "sevenfold discipline" (*sapta-sādhana). In the *Yoga-Tattva-Upanishad (24ff.), again, hatha-yoga is presented as having the following twenty "limbs" (*anga), of which the first eight coincide with those of the eightfold path: moral discipline (*yama); self-restraint (*niyama); posture (*āsana); breath control (*prāna-samyama); sense withdrawal (*pratyāhāra); concentration (*dhāranā); meditation (*dhyāna); enstasy (*samādhi); the "great seal" (*mahā-mudrā); the "great lock" (*mahā-bandha); the "great piercer" (*mahā-vedha); the "space-walking seal" (*khecarī-mudrā); the "water pipe lock" (*jālandhara-bandha); the "upward lock" (*uddīyāna-bandha); the "root lock" (*mūla-bandha); the "practice of the prolated *pranava" (dīrgha-pranava-samdhāna); listening to (i.e., study of) the teachings (*siddhānta-shravana); the "vajrolī seal" (*vajrolī-mudrā); the "amarolī seal" (*amarolī-mudrā); and the "sahajolī seal" (*sahajolī-mudrā).

The "locks" (*bandha) and "seals" (*mudrā) are all designed to control and regulate the flow of life force (*prāna) in the *body. Mastery of the life force is fundamental to all schools of hatha-yoga. Hence *breath control (*prānāyāma) is given such prominence in the scriptures. In the *Amaraugha-Prabodha (4), hatha-yoga is virtually defined as that *Yoga which involves the regulation of the *breath. The underlying idea is that control of the breath implies control of the *mind, for the two are intimately connected.

The *hatha-yogin's primary objective is to intercept the oscillating current of the life force within his own *body. Normally, the life force circulates along the left and the right channel (*nādī) maintaining the bodily activities and producing all the phenomena of ordinary *consciousness, be it awake or asleep. The *hatha-yogin seeks to focus this innate bodily force and prevent it from dissipating. He endeavors to redirect it along the central axis of the body, called *sushumnā-nādī. This is thought to arouse the body's dormant psychospiritual energy, which is known as the "serpent power" (*kundalinī-shakti), and to guide it progressively from the basal center (*mūlādhāra-cakra) to the "thousand-spoked wheel" (*sahasrāra-cakra) at the top of the *head. The crown center is considered to be the seat of the transcendental God *Shiva. The union of the feminine principle in the form of the *kundalinī-shakti with Shiva, the masculine principle, yields the temporary state of nondual *Self-realization, or nirvikalpa-samādhi.

This enstatic realization is held to be more complete than the *sa-

mādhi that results from mere *meditation, as in the *Vedānta tradition, for example, because it includes the body's reality. In *hatha-yoga* and *Tantrism in general, *enlightenment is a matter of the illumination of the whole *body. This approach is epitomized in the Tantric saying that *liberation (*mukti*) and enjoyment (*bhukti*) are perfectly compatible.

The literature of *hatha-yoga* is fairly extensive and barely researched. Very few texts have been edited or translated. Especially, we are still in the dark about the earliest history of this tradition. The two most popular manuals are the *Hatha-Yoga-Pradīpikā* and the *Gheranda-Samhitā*. Other works, in alphabetical order, are the *Amanaska-Yoga, *Amaranātha-Samvāda, *Amaraugha-Prabodha, *Ānanda-Samuccaya, *Brihad-Yogi-Yājnavalkya, *Carpata-Shataka, *Gorakh-Bodha, *Gorakh-Upanishad, *Goraksha-Bhujanga, *Goraksha-Paddhati, *Goraksha-Shataka, *Goraksha-Siddhānta-Samgraha, *Goraksha-Vacana-Samgraha, *Goraksha-Vijaya, *Hatha-Ratna-Āvali, *Hatha-Samketa-Candrikā, *Hatha-Tattva-Kaumudī, *Jnāna-Amrita, *Jyotsnā, *Nava-Shakti-Shatka, *Sat-Karma-Samgraha, *Shiva-Samhitā, *Shiva-Svarodaya, *Yoga-Bīja, *Yoga-Kārnikā, *Yoga-Mār-tanda, *Yoga-Shāstra, *Yoga-Vishaya, and *Yoga-Yājnavalkya. Possibly one of the oldest texts is the *Siddha-Siddhānta-Paddhati. In addition to these works, there are also twenty-one *Yoga-Upanishads.

Hatha-Yoga-Pradīpikā ("Light on the Forceful Yoga") is the most widely used manual on *hatha-yoga*. It was authored by Svātmārāma Yogin, who lived some time in the mid-fourteenth century A.D. This work seeks to integrate the physical disciplines with the higher spiritual goals and practices of *rāja-yoga*. Its great popularity can be gauged from the numerous Sanskrit commentaries written on it, notably those by Umāpati, Mahādeva, Rāmānanda Tīrtha, and Vrajabhūshana. The best-known commentary is the *Jyotsnā* of Brahmānanda. The *Hatha-Yoga-Pradīpikā* comprises four chapters totaling 389 couplets, though the numbering varies from edition to edition. Some manuscripts have an additional chapter of twenty-four stanzas, though this supplement seems to belong to a later period.

Significantly, Svātmārāma does not systematize the yogic *path, but he furnishes many fundamental definitions of core techniques. He describes as many as sixteen postures (*āsana*), most of them variations of the cross-legged sitting posture. For those who suffer from disorders of the bodily humors (*dosha*), the "six acts" (*shat-karma*) are prescribed. These purificatory practices are to be engaged prior to *breath control. Svātmārāma distinguishes eight types of breath control, which he calls "retentions" (*kumbhaka*). These are thought to arouse the "serpent power" (*kundalinī-shakti*). This esoteric process is also aided by the ten "seals" (*mudrā*), which include the three "locks" (*bandha*) of the throat, the stomach, and the anus. However, the text also contains descriptions of the *amarolī-mudrā* and *sahajolī-mudrā*. A prominent feature of Svātmārāma's teaching is "worship through sound" (*nāda-upasāna*) by means of which the condition of mental "absorption" (*laya*) is achieved.

hatha-yogin is a practitioner of the "forceful Yoga" (*hatha-yoga*). In the *Hatha-Yoga-Pradīpikā* (IV.79), he is sharply contrasted with the *rāja-yogin* thus: "[There are those who are] only performers of *hatha* [-yoga], without knowledge of *rāja-yoga*. These practitioners I deem deprived of the fruit of [their] efforts."

This distinction is, however, not meant to apply to all *hatha-yogins*.

Hatred. See *dvesha*, *samrambha*.

Head. The head is a frequent locus of *concentration. Already the *Bhagavad-Gītā* (VIII.12) states that the life force (*prāna*) should be driven into the head. The *Yoga-Sūtra* (III. 32) speaks of a "light in the head" (*mūrdha-jyotis*), upon which the *yogin* should focus his *attention for the practice of enstatic "constraint" (*samyama*) that yields the "vision of the adepts" (*siddha-darshana*). The head is also the location of several important psychoenergetic centers (*cakra): the *dvādasha-anta-*, *sahasrāra-*, *ājnā-*, and *tālu-cakra. Cf. Heart.

Headstand. See *shīrsha-āsana*, *viparīta-kāranī*, *sarva-anga-āsana*.

Health (*ārogya*), which is understood as the harmonious interaction of the three bodily humors (*dosha*), is deemed desirable on all spiritual *paths, presumably because *illness has an adverse influence on one's *attention. However, it is a precondition rather than the goal of *Yoga, even *hatha-yoga. Cf. *roga*, *vyādhi*.

Heart. In the spiritual traditions of India, as elsewhere, the "heart" refers not so much to the physical organ as to a psychospiritual structure corresponding to the heart muscle on the material plane. This spiritual heart is celebrated by *yogins* and mystics as the seat of the transcendental *Self. It is called *hrid, hridaya*, or "heart lotus" (*hrit-padma*). It is often referred to as the secret "cave" (*guha*) in which the *yogin* must restrain his *mind. In some schools, notably Kashmiri

*Shaivism, the word *hridaya* applies also to the ultimate *Reality. See also *anāhata-cakra*, *marman*.

Heaven. See *svarga*.

Hell. See *nāraka*.

Hero. See *vīra*.

Heroic posture. See *vīra-āsana*.

himsā ("harm" or "violence"). According to Vyāsa's *Yoga-Bhāshya* (II.34), there are eighty-one types of violence, depending on whether harm is done, caused to be done, or approved; whether its source is *greed, *anger, or *delusion; whether that impulse is mild, moderate, or vehement (each of which degree has again three forms of intensity). The general principle is that the very intention to harm another being is wrong and is harmful to the intender. Violence breeds violence. The ideal held high in *Yoga is thus nonviolence, or *ahimsā.

Hindu denotes a member or aspect of *Hinduism.

Hinduism is the name given to the dominant culture of India that, in theory at least, is based on the sacred tradition of the brahmins (*brāhmana*). The designation is rather problematic, since "Hindu" describes an amorphous mass of ideas, practices, institutions, and attitudes. What they have in common, however, is a shared history reaching back to the time of the *Rig-Veda and earlier still to the indigenous *Indus civilization. Hinduism came about as a result of a slow but steady process of osmosis between the cultures native to the Indian peninsula and the culture of the immigrant peoples hailing from the steppes of southern Russia and speaking an archaic form of Sanskrit. These seminomads, who called themselves *ārya* ("noble folk"), were the originators of the four *Vedic hymn "collections" (*samhitā*) known collectively as the *Veda. The *wisdom and lore contained in these scriptures greatly influenced subsequent developments.

The following eight periods can usefully be distinguished in the evolution of Hinduism: (1) The Vedic Age (c. 1800–1000 B.C.), epitomized by the teachings of the *Rig-Veda and the other three hymnodies. (2) The Brahmanical Age (c. 1000–800 B.C.), marked by the composition of the *Brāhmana ritual literature. (3) The Upanishadic Age (c. 800–500 B.C.), marked by the teachings embedded in the early *Upanishads,

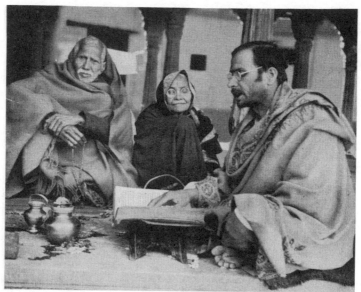

24. *Hindu religious ceremony involving recitation from the sacred texts.*

the first full-fledged mystical communications on Indian soil of which we have knowledge. During this era, *Buddhism and *Jainism emerged as well. (4) The Epic Age (c. 500 B.C.–A.D. 200), so called because of the composition and influence of the *Mahābhārata* epic, which contains the famous *Bhagavad-Gītā*, the earliest and most beautiful work on *Yoga. (5) The Classical Age (A.D. 200–800), characterized by the crystallization of the earlier traditions into philosophical schools and the triumph of *Advaita-Vedānta. This is the period of the composition of the *Yoga-Sūtra*, the textbook of *Classical Yoga. (6) The Tantric Age (A.D. 900–1500), marked by the creation of a new cultural style representing a synthesis of a variety of approaches and embodied in the vast literature of the *Tantras. This period also saw the emergence of *hatha-yoga*. (7) The Sectarian Age (A.D. 1500–1700), captured in the ascendancy of the *bhakti* movement, which was the culmination of the monotheistic aspirations of the two great sectarian cultures of Hinduism—*Vaishnavism and *Shaivism. (8) The Modern Age (A.D. 1700–), marked by the collapse of the Mughal Empire and the establishment of British rule in India and, then, in 1947, India's independence. In the late nineteenth century, Hinduism entered a great renaissance, which brought its teachings to many Western countries.

The conglomeration of religious cultures known as Hinduism claims today over 660 million adherents worldwide. It is important to know that not all Hindu schools of thought acknowledge the Vedic revelation (*shruti*). For instance, the *Tantras purport to be a teaching for the present "dark age" (*kāli-yuga*) in which the religious doctrines and practices of the *Veda are no longer useful. Similarly, in South India millions of adherents of *Shaivism have replaced the four *Vedas with the *Tirukkural*, a poetic compilation mostly dealing with ethical matters and dating approximately from the sixth century A.D.

Hiranyagarbha ("Gold Germ") is hailed in the *Yogi-Yājnavalkya-Smriti* (cited in the *Tattva-Vaishāradī* I.1) as the original propounder of *Yoga. The same claim is made in the *Mahābhārata* epic (XII.337.60). Most scholars assume that Hiranyagarbha is an entirely mythological figure. In the archaic *Rig-Veda* (X.121), he stands for the supreme Lord of all beings who upholds *heaven and earth. In subsequent times, *hiranya-garbha*—"golden germ" or "golden womb"—came to designate the "first-born" entity in the evolutionary series, as taught in *Vedānta but also in some schools of *Pre-Classical Yoga. According to the *Mahābhārata* (XII.291.17f.), the *hiranya-garbha* is none other than the higher mind, that is, the *buddhi* of the *Sāmkhya tradition or the *mahān* of the *Yoga tradition. Other synonyms are *virinca* ("the extended"), *vishva-ātman* ("all-self"), *vicitra-rūpa* ("multiform"), *eka-akshara* ("the one immutable"), and, in *Classical Yoga, *linga-mātra ("pure sign").

Despite this psychocosmological connotations, however, it is likely that there was a sage called Hiranyagarbha, for a person by that name is remembered as having authored a textbook on Yoga (*yoga-shāstra*). Thus, according to the *Ahirbudhnya-Samhitā* (XII.31ff.), a work belonging to the *Pāncarātra-Vaishnava tradition, Hiranyagarbha composed two "collections on Yoga" (*yoga-samhitā*). This *Samhitā* even supplies an apparent and rather sketchy list of their contents, which appear to echo certain notions found in the *Yoga-Sūtra*.

History. The history of *Yoga is barely known, firstly because of the paucity of available materials and secondly, because the Indians, unlike the Chinese, have not kept reliable chronologies until the modern age. The following six phases in the unfolding of Yoga can be distinguished: (1) *Proto-Yoga* of the ancient period, which can be deduced from the archaeological evidence of the *Indus civilization (c. 2500–1800 B.C.) and also from the descriptions in the hymns of the four *Vedic collections. (2) *Pre-Classical Yoga*, which started with the *Upanishads (c. 800 B.C.) expounding a form of sacrificial mysticism based on the internalization of the brahmanical ritual. These efforts led to the development of a rich contemplative technology involving early yogic concepts and practices based on the *Vedānta metaphysics of non-dualism. (3) *Epic Yoga (c. 500 B.C.–A.D. 200), which evolved in the era of the middle *Upanishads and the *Mahābhārata epic. Here we witness a proliferation of schools and doctrines that for the most part continue to espouse nondualism. Yogic teachings developed in close association with *Sāmkhya ideas. Because many of these developments are recorded in the *Mahābhārata, this phase of *Pre-Classical Yoga can also be called *Epic Yoga. (4) *Classical Yoga (starting c. A.D. 200), which has its source in the *Yoga-Sūtra of *Patanjali and was developed over several centuries through an extensive commentarial literature. Its metaphysical foundations are no longer those of *Vedānta, but it avows a strictly dualistic interpretation of reality. (5) *Post-Classical Yoga (c. A.D. 200–1900), which continued the nondualist teachings of *Pre-Classical Yoga, ignoring for the most part the dualistic philosophy of *Patanjali but making occasional use of his delineation of the eightfold path (*ashta-anga-yoga) and his fine definitions. This is the period of the *Yoga-Upanishads and the scriptures of *Tantrism and *hatha-yoga. (6) Modern Yoga (starting c. A.D. 1900), which is epitomized in the *Integral Yoga of Sri *Aurobindo and the many schools of *hatha-yoga.

hitā ("salutary") is an early synonym for *nādī. According to the *Brihad-Āranyaka-Upanishad (II.1.19), there are 72,000 "salutary" rays or channels of the life force (*prāna) that extend from the *heart to the pericardium (puritāt). However, according to the Prashna-Upanishad (III.6), these 72,000 hitās branch off from the 101 *nādīs.

homa ("offering") is a ritual sacrificial offering, which is sometimes counted among the practices of self-restraint (*niyama).

Householder. See grihastha.

hrī ("modesty") is occasionally regarded as one of the practices of self-restraint (*niyama), and sometimes it is counted among the constituents of moral discipline (*yama).

hrid ("heart") can denote both the physical *heart and the spiritual organ so called, as well as the transcendental *Self. In some contexts, it even stands for the chest cavity.

hrid-ākāsha ("heart ether") is the esoteric, radiant space of the *heart, where the transcendental *Self can be experienced. See also hrit-padma.

hridaya ("heart") is a synonym for **hrid*. The three syllables of this word—*hri, da,* and *ya*—are explained in the **Brihad-Āranyaka-Upanishad* (V.3.1) as conveying the ideas of *bringing* a gift, *receiving* a gift, and *going* to heaven. See Heart.

hridaya-granthi ("heart knot") is a synonym for **vishnu-granthi.* See also *granthi.*

hrid-dhauti ("heart cleansing") is a technique of **hatha-yoga,* which is described in the **Gheranda-Samhitā* (I.36ff.). It consists of three practices, namely **danda-dhauti* ("cleansing by means of a stick"), **vamana-dhauti* ("cleansing by vomiting"), and **vāso-dhauti* ("cleansing by means of a piece of cloth").

hrit-padma ("heart lotus"), which is also called the *hridaya-pundarīka* or the **anāhata-cakra.* According to the **Goraksha-Paddhati* (II.68), it is "radiant like lightning." It is described as having eight or twelve petals. See also Heart.

Humility. See *amānitva.*

Hunger. See *kshudhā.*

Hypnosis. Some **Yoga researchers, notably Sigurd Lindquist (1935) have argued that many of the yogic practices, including the postures (**āsana*) but especially the higher meditative and **enstatic states, are based on self-hypnosis. This explanation is, however, reductionistic and not borne out by a careful study of the yogic literature. Besides, the yogic authorities themselves carefully distinguish between hypnosis and higher spiritual phenomena. As a case of hypnosis, the **Mahābhārata* epic (XIII.40f), for instance, relates the story of Devasharman, who asked his disciple Vipula to protect his wife Ruci from the charms of God Indra while he, Devasharman, was on a pilgrimage. Vipula promptly gazed into Ruci's eyes and transferred his mind into her body, rendering her immobile. When Indra, enamored with her beauty, arrived at the hermitage, Ruci was unable to respond, because Vipula had "bound all her senses by the bonds of Yoga."

The condition of enstasy (**samādhi*), though it is preceded by sensory inhibition (**pratyāhāra*), does not amount to a diminished state of consciousness. This is emphasized throughout the spiritual literature of **Hinduism as well as **Buddhism and **Jainism. See also Psychology.

I

icchā ("will"). See *kāma*.

icchā-rūpa ("will-form") is the magical ability to assume any shape whatsoever. Hindu legends are filled with stories of **yogins* who are able to drop their *body at will and take possession of another body. Thus the traditional biography of *Shankara, the famous expounder of *Advaita-Vedānta, recounts how he animated the corpse of a recently deceased king in order to learn the bedroom arts so that he might win a doctrinal contest against an opponent, Mandana Mishra, which he did. See also *kāma-avasāyitva, para-deha-pravesha*.

icchā-shakti ("will power") is not ordinary will power but, according to some schools of *Shaivism, the first of the three aspects of the divine power, the other two being **jnāna-shakti* and **kriyā-shakti*. The *icchā-shakti* is the impulse toward manifestation within the unmanifest principle of power (**shakti*). According to some schools, the "supreme power" (**parā-shakti*) first gives rise to the "power of consciousness" (**cit-shakti*) and the "power of bliss" (*ānanda-shakti*).

idā-nādī ("channel of comfort") is one of the three primary ducts or currents (**nādī*) of the life force (**prāna*) circulating in the human *body according to esoteric *anatomy. It is situated to the left of the axial channel called **sushumnā-nādī*, which runs vertically from the psychoenergetic center (**cakra*) at the base of the spine to the crown of the *head. The *idā-nādī* is generally thought to commence in the "bulb" (**kanda*) and to extend to the left nostril. It coils around the central

143

channel and is associated with the cooling energy of the "moon" (*candra*). The *Shiva-Samhitā* (II.25) curiously states that the *idā* terminates at the right nostril, but this medieval *hatha-yoga* text gives divergent positions for most other esoteric structures, perhaps in order to deliberately mislead the uninitiated.

The word *idā* dates back to the *Rig-Veda* (I.40.4) where it denotes "libation" or "oblation." It is also the name of the female deity of *devotion. The word is connected with the feminine noun *id*, one of whose meanings is "comfort." Thus the technical term *idā-nādī* could be interpreted to be the comforting channel—comforting because it cools the *body during the heat of the day. The *idā* current of the life force corresponds on the physical level to the parasympathetic nervous system. It must, however, not be confused with it. Cf. *pingalā-nādī*.

Ignorance. See *avidyā, ajnāna*.

ijyā ("sacrifice") is sometimes counted as one of the constituent practices of self-restraint (*niyama*). It refers to offering oblations as part of a more ritualistic *Yoga practice. See also *bali*, Sacrifice.

Illness. See *roga, vyādhi*; cf. Health.

Illusion. See *māyā*.

Immortality is often equated with the condition of *liberation, or *enlightenment, in which case it signifies immortality of the spirit, or transcendental *Self. However, traditions like *hatha-yoga* and *alchemy aspire to bodily immortality, though here the *body is understood to be radically transformed. See also *amrita*.

Impurity. See *dosha, mala*; cf. Purity.

Inattention. See *pramāda*.

Incarnation. See *avatāra*.

Individuality. See *ahamkāra*, Ego, *jīva*.

Indra ("Ruler"). During the most ancient period of *Hinduism, God Indra was the principal *deity, the ruler of the *Vedic pantheon. He has often been characterized as a rain god, or god of thunder and lightning. However, it is clear from certain hymns of the *Rig-Veda* that the Vedic people also saw in him a spiritual power, granting flashes of inner illumination. He is also related to *indu* ("juice"), meaning the ambrosial fluid or **soma*, as well as the esoteric "moon" (**candra*) that is thought to ooze that precious liquid in the human *body. See also *deva*.

indriya ("pertaining to *Indra"). This term refers to the sense organs, which are the most powerful influence in the life of the ordinary mortal. As the **Agni-Purāna* (373.20) puts it succinctly: "The senses are all that which [leads to] *heaven or *hell. [A person goes] to heaven or hell, [depending on whether the senses are] restrained or active."

The **Bhagavad-Gītā* (II.62f.) offers the following analysis of the play of *attention:

> When a man thinks of *objects, contact with them occurs. From that contact springs desire (**kāma*), and from desire anger (**krodha*) is bred.

> From anger comes bewilderment (*sammoha*), from bewilderment disorder of the memory, and from disorder of the memory the destruction of wisdom (**buddhi*). On the destruction of *wisdom [a person] is lost.

The **Bhagavad-Gītā* (II.65f.) then recommends the following attitude:

> Although moving with the senses among objects, [the person with] a well-governed self, disjoined from passion (**rāga*) and aversion (**dvesha*), under the control of the *Self, approaches serenity (**prasāda*).

> [On reaching] serenity, there arises for him the obliteration of all *suffering. For the clear minded, the wisdom faculty (**buddhi*) is at once firmly grounded.

According to the *Sāmkhya tradition, which is widely accepted on this point by other schools, there are eleven sensory instruments. These can be arranged into three groups: (1) the cognitive senses (*jnāna-* or *buddhi-indriya*) composed of eyes (*cakshus*), ears (*shrotra*), nose (*ghrāna*), tongue (**rasa*), skin (**tvac*); (2) the conative senses (*karma-indriya*) composed of voice (*vāc*), hands (*pani*), feet (*pāda*), anus (*pāyu*), and genitals (*upastha*); and (3) the lower mind (**manas*). Although these designations suggest physical organs, the *indriyas* are rather their intrinsic capacities.

In the *Mahābhārata* epic (XII.195.9), the five (cognitive) senses are compared to lamps set on high trees that illumine things and produce *knowledge. They entice *attention to focus on external reality rather than the *Self. Hence the *yogin is constantly counseled to practice sensory restraint (*indriya-jaya). In the *Katha-Upanishad (III.3f.), the *body is likened to a chariot and the senses to unruly horses that need to be checked. Another popular metaphor for the process of sensory inhibition (*pratyāhāra) is that of a tortoise withdrawing its limbs. See also bhūta, buddhi, Cosmos, Evolution, tanmātra.

indriya-jaya ("conquest of the senses") is the capacity to control the outflowing of *attention through the sensory pathways. According to the *Yoga-Sūtra (II.41), such mastery is one of the benefits of cultivating perfect purity (*shauca). *Patanjali also speaks of the "obedience" (vash-yatā) of the senses as a result of the constant practice of sense withdrawal (*pratyāhāra).

indriya-nigraha ("sense restraint") is sometimes counted among the practices of moral discipline (*yama). It is equivalent to *pratyāhāra.

indu-cakra ("wheel of the nectar"), also called *shodasha-cakra, is an esoteric psychoenergetic center (*cakra) located in the *head above the *manas-cakra. It is generally thought to have sixteen petals of moon-white color, and to be the seat of the higher mind (*buddhi). See also Indra.

Indus civilization. This ancient civilization, which was discovered in the early 1920s, existed along the Indus river in the Punjab and extended for over one thousand miles from north to south. Its origins are obscure. The large, well-organized cities of Harappā and Mohenjo Daro, which have been excavated, appear to date from the middle of the third millennium B.C. This civilization appears to have come to an abrupt end about 1500 B.C., and this event is generally associated with the invasion of the *Vedic tribes that had crossed the Hindukush mountains. Some scholars conjecture that, after the destruction of the big cities, the Indus people migrated to the southern tip of the Indian peninsula.

Since the pictographic Indus script has not yet been deciphered, it is difficult to get a clear idea of the religious world of this great civilization. However, the archaeological evidence suggests that the Indus people were, like the later *Hindus, very pollution conscious and engaged in a variety of rituals of *purification. Particularly remarkable is the absence of weapons in the more than sixty excavated sites. This could point to a strict morality of nonharming (*ahimsā), which would be extraordinary for that historical period. Apart from architectural clues, there are above all the over two thousand terra-cotta seals featuring inscriptions and artistic motifs that convey some idea of the mythological and religious notions current in that civilization. One seal in particular has attracted the attention of *Yoga researchers. It shows a horned deity seated cross-legged in the fashion of the later *yogins, surrounded by animals. The figure has been tentatively identified as God *Shiva in his role as *Pashupati, or Lord of Beasts.

Other evidence, suggesting an early Goddess cult and fertility beliefs, indicates a remarkable continuity between the Indus civilization and later *Hinduism. It is plausible that some of the constituent elements of *Yoga, especially in its more *Tantric aspect, should have derived from that civilization. However, Yoga has many roots, and certainly its emergence as a full-fledged tradition did not occur until about 500 B.C., long after the demise of that ancient civilization. See also *Pre-Classical Yoga.

Inference. See *anumāna*.

Initiation. See *abhisheka*, *dīkshā*.

īrshyā ("jealousy") is a synonym for *mātsarya*.

īsh, īsha, īshāna ("ruler"). The theistic schools of *Hinduism often describe the *Divine as the ruler of the world and the individual body-mind. One of the most beautiful expressions of this idea is found in the *Īsha-Upanishad*, a work belonging to the pre-Christian era. See also *īshvara*.

īshitritva or **īshitva** ("lordship") is one of the classic paranormal powers (*siddhi) granting the accomplished *adept sovereignty over *Nature. According to the *Yoga-Bhāshya* (III.45), this power allows the adept to create, rearrange, or even destroy the material elements (*bhūta).

ishta-devatā ("chosen deity"). Since it is difficult to relate to the transcendental *Reality in abstract terms, many *Hindu practitioners choose to worship the *Divine in the form of one of the many deities (*deva) known in *Hinduism, such as *Vishnu, *Krishna, *Shiva, or the Goddess *Kālī. These are thought to be actual spiritual forces, not merely products of the religious imagination. They can be invoked and approached for grace (*prasāda). According to the *Yoga-Sūtra* (II.44), the *yogin can come into contract with his chosen deity especially by immersing himself into the study (*svādhyāya*) of the sacred lore.

īshvara ("foremost ruler," "lord") is a word found already in the ancient *Brihad-Āranyaka-Upanishad* (I.4.8, etc.). In the *Vedānta-inspired schools of *Yoga, it refers to the transcendental *Self as it governs the *cosmos and the individuated being. This is epitomized in the following stanza from the *Bhagavad-Gītā* (XVIII.61): "The Lord abides in the *heart region of all beings, o *Arjuna, whirling all beings by [His] power (*māyā*), [as if they were] mounted on a machine (*yantra*)."

In the *Epic Yoga schools of the *Mahābhārata*, the *īshvara* is also referred to as the "twenty-fifth principle," since he transcends the twenty-four principles or evolutionary categories (*tattva*) of *Nature. In *Classical Yoga, the *īshvara* is defined as a special Self (*purusha*). This specialness consists in that the Lord was at no time embroiled in the play of Nature, whereas all other Selves will, at one time, have been or become caught up in the illusion of being embodied and thus bound to the mechanisms of Nature. Specifically, the *īshvara* is said to be untouched by the "causes of affliction" (*klesha*), action (*karman*), action's "fruition" (*vipāka*), and the subconscious "deposits" (*āshaya*). The Lord's freedom is eternal.

This view has led to theological difficulties, since *Patanjali also regarded the *īshvara* as the first "teacher." How can an utterly transcendental *Self possibly intervene in the spatiotemporal world? In his *Yoga-Bhāshya* (I.24), *Vyāsa tries to deal with this issue. He explains the *īshvara's* teaching role in terms of the Lord's assumption of a perfect medium, which Vyāsa calls *sattva* ("beingness"). *Vācaspati Mishra compares this to the role played by an actor who nevertheless is aware that he is not identical with the character of his role. He also emphasizes that this is possible because the Lord's *sattva* is devoid of any trace of *rajas and *tamas. Vyāsa further explains that the Lord appropriated such a perfect *sattva* vehicle for the "gratification of beings" (*bhūta-anugraha*). Both exegetes further insist that the proof for this belief is to be found in the sacred scriptures, which are manifestations of that perfect *sattva. See also *anugraha, bhāgavat, prasāda*.

Īshvara-Gītā ("Song of the [divine] Ruler") is one of the imitations of the *Bhagavad-Gītā*. It consists of eleven chapters with a total of 497 stanzas and is a part of the *Kūrma-Purāna* (II.1–11). It is presented as a conversation between God *Shiva and a group of sages. This scripture (II.40) defines *Yoga as "one-mindedness" (*eka-cittatā*) and emphasizes the interrelation between Yoga and wisdom (*jnāna). Thus we find the following stanza (II.3), for instance: "Wisdom springs from Yoga [practice]; Yoga derives from wisdom. For him who is dedicated to Yoga and wisdom, nothing is unattainable."

It is through the favor (*prasāda) of *Shiva that extinction (*nirvāna) is reached. The spiritual *path is the eightfold Yoga (ashta-anga-yoga) taught by *Patanjali.

Īshvara Krishna is the author of the *Sāmkhya-Kārikā, which is to *Classical Sāmkhya what the *Yoga-Sūtra is to *Classical Yoga. He lived probably after *Patanjali, some time in the fourth century A.D.

īshvara-pranidhāna ("devotion to the Lord") is one of the constituents of self-restraint (*niyama). The *Yoga-Bhāshya (I.23) explains this practice as a special kind of love (*bhakti) or intention (abhidhyāna) by which the Lord (*īshvara) becomes inclined to favour the *yogin. Elsewhere (II.1;32) in this commentary, it is explained as the offering up of all actions to the supreme teacher, that is, the *īshvara, and as the renunciation (*samnyāsa) of the fruit (*phala) of one's *actions.

īshvara-pūjana ("worship of the Lord") is sometimes counted among the practices of self-restraint (*niyama). The *Darshana-Upanishad (II.8) explains it as a *heart devoid of passion (*rāga), speech not tainted by untruth, and *action free from harm (*himsā).

J

jādya ("dullness"). According to the *Yoga-Shikhā-Upanishad (I.134), the ordinary *body suffers from "dullness," which can be removed through the practice of *hatha-yoga. The *hatha-yogin seeks to draw the life force (*prāna) up into the central channel (*sushumnā-nādī), which is said to render his body lustrous. This practice also gives him the ability to "walk in space" (khecara). See also *khecarī-mudrā.

jagat ("world"). See Cosmos, vishva.

Jaigīshavya is a prominent *teacher of *Epic Yoga whose views on *Sāmkhya and *Yoga are quoted several times in the *Yoga-Bhāshya (e.g., III.18), the oldest available commentary on the *Yoga-Sūtra of *Patanjali. In the Matsya-Purāna (180.59), he is said to have attained "aloneness" (*kaivalya) after kindling the "fire of Yoga" by means of *meditation. His didactic conversation with Asita Devala is recorded in the *Mahābhārata epic (XII.222.4ff.). He is also attributed with the authorship of the Dhāranā-Shāstra ("Textbook on Concentration"), a late work that is more akin to *Tantrism than *Yoga.

jāgrat ("waking") is one of the five states (*avasthā) of *consciousness. It is the ordinary *waking state marked by a sharp awareness that has, however, a narrow focus. By contrast, the condition of *enstasy is characterized by suprawakefulness that has no focus because the limiting *ego is absent in it. Whereas the former type of consciousness is inherently dis-eased, the latter is experienced as whole and indescribably blissful (*ānanda).

Jainism is the spiritual tradition founded by Vardhamāna Mahāvīra, an older contemporary of Gautama the *Buddha. The historical roots of Jainism, however, go back to a hoary past. Thus, the Jaina scriptures speak of a lineage of twenty-four "ford makers" (*tīrthankāra*), or *adept teachers, of whom Mahāvīra was the last. The spirituality of Jainism has preserved many archaic features, and it tends toward ascetic rigor. It has greatly influenced the development of the ethical aspects of *Yoga, especially the virtue of "nonharming" (*ahimsā*) and the teachings on moral causation (*karma*). Later Jaina writers have articulated ideas and practices that are rather similar to *Hindu Yoga. Thus the renowned scholar Haribhadra (c. A.D. 750) has made use of some of the codifications of *Patanjali. Among his over fourteen hundred works are several trea-

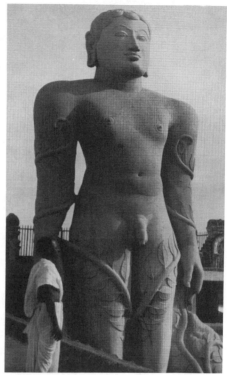

25. Gomateshvara, the nude "ford-maker" of Jainism.

tises on Yoga, notably his *Yoga-Bindu* ("Seed of Yoga") and *Yoga-Drishti-Samuccaya* ("Collection of Yoga Views"). Hemacandra, in his seventh-century work *Yoga-Shāstra* ("Yoga Compendium"), also availed himself of some of the formulations found in Patanjali's *Yoga-Sūtra*.

jala ("water") is one of the five material elements (*bhūta*). The *Yoga-Shikhā-Upanishad* (V.50) mentions that *concentration upon the water element bestows the paranormal power (*siddhi*) of never being overcome by that element. See also *ap*.

jālandhara. See *Jālandhari*.

jālandhara-bandha ("water pipe lock") is an important practice of *hatha-yoga* consisting in the "contraction of the throat" (*kanthasamkocana*), which is achieved by placing the chin on the chest, usually

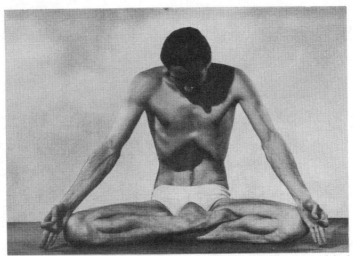

26. *Jālandhara-bandha (throat lock) combined with the upward lock (uddīyāna-bandha).*

after inhalation. In the *Gheranda-Samhitā* (III.13), a medieval work on *hatha-yoga*, this technique is praised as a "great seal" (*mahā-mudrā*). It is practiced in conjunction with a variety of postures (*āsana*) and "seals" (*mudrā*). According to the *Goraksha-Paddhati* (I.79), this *bandha* "binds" the network of channels (*sirā*) and prevents the ambrosial liquid (*amrita*) from flowing into the trunk. It is also thought to cure *diseases of the throat.

jālandhara-pīṭha ("water pipe seat") is a synonym for *vishuddha-cakra*.

Jālandhari ("Net Bearer") was a famous master of *hatha-yoga* and prior to his *renunciation of the world was allegedly ruler of Hastinapur in northern India. He is said to have initiated King *Bhartrihari. According to some traditions, he was also called Hadipā (Hadipāda), who is known to have initiated King *Gopicandra of Bengal. In other legends, Jālandhari is remembered as the teacher of Kānha, Mīna, Caurangi, Carpati, and several other well-known adepts (*siddha*). According to Tibetan sources, he was born a shūdra in Sindh, learned and taught *Yoga and *Tantra at Oddiyāna and Jālandhara in the north-west of India. Before settling in Bengal, he is further said to have visited Nepal.

jala-vasti ("water syringe") is one of two forms of *vasti. The *Gheranda-Samhitā* (I.46f.) describes it as follows: One should immerse oneself in water up to the *navel and while performing the "raised posture" (*utkata-āsana) should contract and dilate the anal sphincter muscle. This is thought to cure urinary disorders, digestive troubles, and "cruel wind" (krūra-vāyu). Cf. shushka-vasti.

jana-sanga ("contact with people"). Socializing is, according to the *Hatha-Yoga-Pradīpikā (I.15), one of the factors by which *Yoga is foiled. See also sanga.

japa ("recitation") is defined in the *Yoga-Yājnavalkya (II.12) as the "repetition (*abhyāsa) of *mantras in accordance with the rules." This is an extremely old practice belonging to the earliest developments of *Yoga. It probably grew out of the meditative recitation of the sacred *Vedic texts, which required the utmost *concentration of the priest, since each holy word had to be accurately pronounced lest it should adversely affect the sacrificial ritual (*yajna).

The *Yoga-Sūtra (I.28), the textbook of *Classical Yoga, recommends the recitation of the sacred syllable *om for the removal of all obstacles (*antarāya). This recitation should naturally lead over into the contemplation (*bhāvanā) of the inner significance of this *mantra. Mindless repetition of words has no desirable effect. Japa, like all other practices of *Yoga, is to be performed with great attentiveness and dedication. According to the *Mahābhārata epic (XII.190), a person who fails to be intent on the meaning of the words he recites is destined to go to *hell.

Japa can be practiced verbally or mentally. In the former case, a mantra can be "whispered" (upāmshu) or "voiced" (ucca, elsewhere called vācika). According to the *Yoga-Yājnavalkya (II.15f.), whispered recitation is a thousand times better than voiced japa, whereas mental (mānasa) recitation is a thousand times better than whispered japa. However, *meditation is stated to be a thousand times better than even mental japa. The *Linga-Purāna (I.85.106) makes the point that recitation in one's home is good. But recitation in a cow pen is a hundred times better and on a riverbank a thousand times better than japa at home. But, the text notes, in the presence of God *Shiva, recitation is infinitely efficacious. See also hamsa.

japaka ("reciter") is a practitioner of *japa, a japa-yogin.

jāthara-agni ("belly fire") is both the digestive heat in the stomach area and, on the esoteric level, the "sun" (*sūrya) that devours the divine nectar (*amrita) dripping from the "moon" (*candra) in the *head. Some techniques of *hatha-yoga, such as *vahni-sāra-dhauti, *shushka-

vasti, and **viparīta-kāranī*, are specifically designed to stimulate that abdominal "fire." Indeed, the anonymous author of the **Yoga-Tattva-Upanishad* (45) values increased digestive heat as a sign (**cihna*) of the successful cleansing of the channels (**nāḍī*) through which the **life force circulates. See also *vaishvānara*.

Jealousy. See *mātsarya*.

jihvā-bandha ("tongue lock"). See *mahā-bandha*.

jihvā(-mūla)-dhauti ("cleansing of the tongue's [body]") is also called *jihvā-shodhana* ("purification of the tongue"). This practice forms part of what is known as "dental cleansing" (**danta-dhauti*). The **Gheranda-Samhitā* (I.29f.) describes it as follows: One should rub and clean the tongue by means of the index, middle, and ring fingers. Then one should massage it with butter and milk and thereafter slowly pull it out with the help of an iron tool. This should be done daily with diligence at sunrise and again at sunset. Gradually, the tongue's tendon (here called **lambikā*) becomes elongated, which is said to remove aging, **disease, and even **death. See also *khecarī-mudrā*, *lambikā-yoga*.

jīta-indriya ("he whose senses are conquered") is often used to refer to a master of **Yoga. See also *indriya*.

jīva ("life," "alive") roughly corresponds to what is called the psyche or, as the **Mahābhārata* epic (XII.180.30) puts it, "the mental fire." This is the individuated self (**jīva-ātman*) as opposed to the transcendental Self (**parama-ātman*). The **Laghu-Yoga-Vāsishtha* (V.10.18) calls it the mind (**citta*) that does not know **Reality and hence is afflicted with **suffering. According to the schools of **Vedānta, the numerous individuated selves are the product of an illusion. Their multiplicity, which stems from spiritual nescience (**avidyā*, **ajñāna*), is not ultimately true. Upon **enlightenment, the seeming diversity of existence melts away, and there is only the singular transcendental **Self (**ātman*).

In the **Goraksha-Paddhati* (II.35), an old **hatha-yoga text, the *jīva* is compared to a bull who is "triply bound" and "roars a mighty roar." The phrase "triply bound" suggests the individual's experience of confinement by the three primary constituents (**guna*) of **Nature. The **Shiva-Purāna* (I.16.99f.) defines the *jiva* as "that which decays from the moment of birth" and as "that which is born enmeshed and entwined." For the same reason, the **Gheranda-Samhitā* (III.50) styles it an "animal" (*pashu*) so long as the spiritual force, or **kundalinī-shakti*, is still dormant and not yet awakened. The *Kaula-Jnāna-Nirnaya (VI.7) states that the individual is called jīva while it abides in the *body, whereas it is the supreme *Shiva upon release from the bodily fetters. In the moment of *death, the jīva is generally thought to escape through the crown of the *head (in the case of *yogins) or through other bodily orifices (in the case of those who are spiritually unprepared).

There is a close relationship between the jīva and the life force (*prāna) as *breath—a relationship that has been carefully studied in *hatha-yoga. Thus, in the *Goraksha-Paddhati (I.38f.), we find this important verse:

Even as a ball struck by a club flies up, so the psyche (jīva), struck by *prāna and *apāna does not stand still. Under the influence of prāna and apāna, the psyche rushes up and down through the left and right paths [i.e., through the *idā- and *pingalā-nādī], and because of this moving to and fro cannot be seen.

Even as a hawk tied to a rope can be brought back again when it has flown off, so the psyche bound by *Nature's "strands" (*guna) is pulled about by prāna and apāna.

It leaves [the body] with the sound ha and it enters with the sound sa—both sounds being continually recited [and forming the *hamsa-mantra].

The *Yoga-Vāsishtha (appendix to VI.50.2ff.) has this fascinating division of jīvas into seven types depending on their spiritual maturity and power: (1) the svapna-jāgara ("dream-waking"): he whose *dreams are the waking world of others; (2) the samkalpa-jāgara ("imagination-waking"): he whose imagination is so powerful that it creates a waking world for others; (3) the kevala-jāgara ("sole waking"): he who experiences the waking state for the first time; a "new soul"; (4) the cīra-jāgara ("long waking"): he who has experienced the *waking state for many lifetimes; an "old soul"; (5) the ghana-jāgara ("solidified waking"): he whose repeated evil *actions have reduced him to a state of relative unconsciousness; (6) the jāgrat-svapna ("waking dream"): he for whom the world perceived in the waking state is but a *dream; (7) the kshīna-jāgara ("dwindled waking"): he for whom the waking world has ceased to exist as an apparently independent *creation because he has realized the transcendental *Self.

Elsewhere (III.94.2ff.), this scripture proposes a twelvefold classification of jīvas on the basis of the interplay of the primary constituents (*guna) of *Nature. All such schemas serve the principal purpose of driving home the point that the *waking state, which is so highly valued in our modern civilization, does by no means express the ultimate human potential. Rather it reflects a particular degree of awareness that is characterized by a certain level of moral and spiritual maturity. See also Actor, *dehin, hamsa*.

jīva-ātman ("living self"), the individuated *consciousness or psyche (*jīva*). According to *Vedānta and the *Vedānta-based schools of *Pre-Classical and *Post-Classical Yoga, *liberation consists in the merging of the individuated self with the transcendental or supreme *Self (*parama-ātman*).

jīvan-mukta ("living liberated") refers to the *adept who is *liberated, or *enlightened, while he or she is still embodied. This is the grand ideal of those spiritual schools of *Hinduism that subscribe to *non-dualism, or the teaching that upon *Self-realization the distinction between transcendence and immanence collapses: The world is seen to arise in and as the *Divine. Hence, *liberation is not an otherworldly alternative that implies disembodiment. The *Bhagavad-Gītā (II.56f.) proffers this description of a *jīvan-mukta*:

> [He whose] *mind is unagitated in suffering (*duhkha*), devoid of longing during pleasure (*sukha*), and free from passion (*rāga*), fear (*bhaya*), and anger (*krodha*)—he is called a sage (*muni*) steadied in the vision [of the *Self].

> He who is unattached toward everything, who does not rejoice at whatever auspicious [events] happen to him, nor hate whatever inauspicious [events occur]—his wisdom (*prajñā*) is well established.

Thus, the *jīvan-mukta*'s continual immersion in the *Self expresses itself in his stoic attitude toward existence, which allows him to recognize the same (*sama*) in all things. However, his *equanimity also has more positive, outgoing characteristics. He is, above all, a compassionate being. This is made clear in the following stanzas from the *Bhagavad-Gītā (XII.13ff.), where the God-man *Krishna instructs Prince *Arjuna:

> [He who feels] no *hatred toward any being, [who is] friendly and compassionate . . . [that] *yogin who is ever content, self-controlled, of firm resolve, with *mind and wisdom (*buddhi*) offered up in Me, who is My *devotee—he is dear to Me.

He from whom the world does not shrink and who does not shrink from the world and who is free from exultation, *anger, *fear, and agitation, is dear to Me.

In the *Yoga-Vāsishtha (V.77.7ff.), composed over a millennium after the above Gītā verses, we find these memorable stanzas:

He does not concern himself with the future, nor does he abide [exclusively] in the present, nor does he recall [i.e., live in] the past, but he acts out of the Whole.

Sleeping, he is awake. Awake, he is like one asleep. Performing all [necessary] actions, he "does" nothing whatsoever inwardly.

Inwardly always renouncing everything, without inner *desires and performing externally what has to be done, he remains [completely] balanced (*sama).

Remaining perfectly happy and experiencing enjoyment in all that is expected [of him], he performs all *actions while abandoning the misconception of doership.

[He behaves] as a boy among boys; an elder among elders; a sage among sages; a youth among youths, and as a sympathizer among the well-behaved afflicted.

[He is] wise, gracious, charming, suffused with his *enlightenment, free from pressure (kheda) and distress, an affectionate friend.

Neither by embarking on the performance of action nor by abstention, nor by [such concepts as] bondage or emancipation, underworld or *heaven [can he be perturbed].

[For,] when the objective world is perceived as the unitary [*Reality], then the mind fears neither *bondage nor emancipation.

Some schools claim that the jīvan-mukta is capable of shape shifting and that he therefore enjoys *immortality. However, for most authorities his physical *body is by no means incorruptible, but *death does not affect his existential status as a free being in the least.

jīvan-mukti ("living liberation") is the condition of a *jīvan-mukta. Cf. videha-mukti.

Jīvan-Mukti-Viveka ("discernment about living liberation") is a remarkable *Vedānta text by Vidyāranya Tīrtha, a fourteenth-century scholar and spiritual practitioner. This comprehensive work offers a detailed discussion of the yogic path from a Vedāntic point of view. Vidyāranya cites a great many scriptures, and his work contains illuminating commentaries particularly on the *Yoga-Vāsishtha and the *Yoga-Sūtra.

jnāna ("wisdom," "knowledge") is a word that is applied in both sacred and secular contexts. It can stand for learning, or conceptual *knowledge, and also for higher, intuitive insight and *wisdom, or gnosis. Occasionally, *jnāna* is even equated with the ultimate *Reality itself.

The *Bhagavad-Gītā (XVIII.20ff.), the most important work of *Pre-Classical Yoga, distinguishes three types of *jnāna* depending on the predominance of one or the other of the three primary constituents (*guna) of *Nature: (1) *sāttvika-jnāna*, whereby one sees the one immutable *Reality in all things; (2) *rājasa-jnāna*, whereby one sees but the composite nature of things, not their underlying unity; (3) *tāmasa-jnāna*, whereby one irrationally clings to a single thing as if it were the whole, without concern for *Reality.

The *Yoga-Vāsishta (III.118.5ff.), composed about A.D. 1100, mentions seven stages or levels (*bhūmi) of *wisdom. The first stage is called *shubha-icchā*, or the impulse toward what is spiritually auspicious. The second is *vicāranā*, or the profound consideration of spiritual teachings. This is followed by *tanu-mānasī*, or the refinement of one's thinking. The fourth is *sattā-āpatti*, or the acquisition of a pure being. The fifth is *asamsakti*, or nonattachment. This is followed by *pada-artha-bhāva*, or the recognition of what truly matters, which is *enlightenment. The final stage is *turya-ga*, or the intuition of the "Fourth" (*turya). These stages of *jnāna* lead to final and irrevocable *liberation. Thus, as is stated in the *Bhagavad-Gītā (IV.36), wisdom is a "raft" (*plava*) by means of which one can cross the "crooked stream of life." As another stanza (IV.38) in this *Yoga classic has it, wisdom is the "greatest purifier on earth."

Sometimes *jnāna* is contrasted with *yoga* (in the sense of specific practices). Thus, the *Tri-Shikhi-Brāhmana-Upanishad (II.19) declares: "Wisdom is brought about by Yoga. Yoga is developed by wisdom." See also *prajñā*, *sapta-jnāna-bhūmi*, *vijnāna*; cf. *ajnāna*, *avidyā*.

Jnāna-Amrita ("Immortal Nectar of Wisdom") is a medieval work on *hatha-yoga ascribed to *Goraksha.

jnāna-bandhu ("friend of knowledge") is an intellectual who studies spiritual matters but fails to convert his interest into living practice.

jnāna-bhūmi ("level of wisdom"). See *jnāna*, *bhūmi*, *sapta-jnāna-bhūmi*.

jnāna-cakshus or **jnāna-netra** ("eye of wisdom"). The transcendental *Self is invisible to the human eye. However, the metaphor of vision has almost universally been employed to describe *Self-realization. In the *Bhagavad-Gītā (XV.10), for instance, it is stated that the Self can be seen through the eye of *wisdom. According to another stanza (XIII.34), this inner eye helps one distinguish between the "field" (*kshetra*) and the "field knower" (*kshetra-jna*), that is, between *Nature and the Self. See also *manas-cakra*.

Jnānadeva, Maharashtra's greatest mystical and poetic genius, lived in the latter half of the thirteenth centuries. He was probably born in A.D. 1275 and died at the young age of twenty-one, apparently by voluntarily dropping his mortal coil while in the state of *enstasy. His *Jnāneshvari*, a comprehensive verse commentary on the *Bhagavad-Gītā, is the first philosophical work in the Marathi language. He also authored the *Amrita-Anubhava* ("Experience of Immortality") and a number of shorter tracts. His spiritual roots lie in the *Nātha tradition on the one side, and the *bhakti movement on the other. In the *Jnāneshvari* (XVIII.1751ff.) he gives his

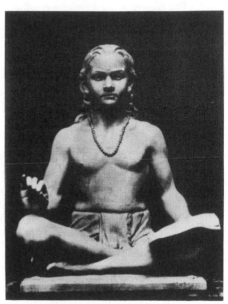

27. *Jnānadeva.*

spiritual lineage as follows: *Shiva, *Shakti, *Matsyendra, *Goraksha, *Gahinī, and *Nivritti (his elder brother).

Jnānadeva's philosophy revolves around the notion that the manifest world is a "sport" (*vilāsa*) of the *Absolute, an expression of the supreme *love of the singular *Reality. He refutes the dualism of *Classical Sāmkhya, the idealism of later *Buddhism, and especially *Shankara's theory of nescience (*avidyā*) as the ultimate cause of the world's existence. Jnānadeva regards *bhakti, instilled with *wisdom, as the alpha and omega of spiritual life. His philosophical position is known as *sphūrti-vāda*, or the doctrine of spontaneous manifestation. Although he was initiated into *hatha-yoga* by his brother, it is clear from some passages in his *Jnāneshvarī* (e.g. XVIII.1138) that he was critical of the techniques and rituals of this branch of *Yoga. His works extol the virtue and liberating power of *devotion.

jnāna-indriya ("cognitive sense"). See *indriya*.

Jnāna-Kārikā ("wisdom activity") is a text of the *Kaula school consisting of 137 verses (*kārikā*) distributed over three chapters. The last chapter describes the proper *environment for the *kaula-yogin*, which includes such places as cave, cremation ground, the confluence of rivers, and crossroads; however, these are interpreted symbolically as locations within the *body.

jnāna-mārga ("path of wisdom") generally refers to the nondualistic approach of the *Upanishads. It is also used synonymously with *jnāna-yoga*. See also Path.

jnāna-mudrā ("wisdom seal") is one of the hand gestures (*mudrā*) used during *meditation. It is performed by having the thumb and index finger touch so that they form a circle, while the remaining three fingers are extended. In the *Brahma-Vidyā-Upanishad* (64), the *jnāna-mudrā* is interpreted symbolically as consisting in the recollection of the *hamsa-mantra* in the state of *enstasy. See also *cin-mudrā, dhyāna-mudrā, vishnu-mudrā*.

Jnānaprakāsha is a South Indian *adept who lived in the sixteenth century A.D. He wrote a commentary on the *Shiva-Jnāna-Siddhi* ("Perfection of Shiva Wisdom"), a thirteenth-century Tamil classic of the *Shaiva-Siddhānta tradition. He is also credited with the authorship of several other works including the *Shiva-Yoga-Sāra* ("Essence of Shiva-Yoga") and the *Shiva-Yoga-Ratna* ("Jewel of Shiva-Yoga"). He understands *yoga* not in the sense of "union" but as a means of realizing one's identity (*sayujya*) with *Shiva, or "Shivahood" (*shivatva*). His *path is that of gnosis (*jnāna*) through *meditation and *enstasy, though he also values *breath control.

jnāna-shakti ("power of wisdom") is one of three aspects of the *Divine. It is intended to account for the fact that the ultimate *Reality is not insentient but supraconscious and the matrix for all levels of manifest awareness or intelligence. Cf. *icchā-shakti, kriyā-shakti*.

jnāna-yoga ("Yoga of wisdom") is one of the principal branches of *Yoga, the others being *bhakti-yoga and *karma-yoga. It is virtually identical with the spiritual *path of *Vedānta, which places a premium on gnosis. Specifically, *jnāna-yoga* consists in the constant exercise of discriminating *Reality from unreality, the *Self from the "non-Self" (*anātman). The compound *jnāna-yoga* is first employed in the *Bhagavad-Gītā (III.3), where the God-man *Krishna tells his pupil *Arjuna: "Of yore I proclaimed a twofold approach in this world, o guileless one—the Yoga of *wisdom for the *sāmkhyas* and the Yoga of action (*karma-yoga) for the *yogins." Here the *sāmkhyas* are not so much the followers of any particular school of *Sāmkhya as what could be called contemplatives. Accordingly, the principal technique of *jnāna-yoga* is *meditation. It is in the simplified inner environment of meditation that *discrimination between the Real and the unreal can be pursued most effectively. *Krishna equates *jnāna-yoga* with *buddhi-yoga, for it is the *buddhi or "wisdom faculty" that makes such discernment possible.

In the fifteenth-century *Vedānta-Sāra* ("Essence of *Vedānta") of Sadānanda, the *path of *jnāna-yoga* is stated to consist of four principal means: (1) discrimination (*viveka) between the permanent and the transient, the Real and the unreal; (2) renunciation (*tyāga) of the enjoyment of the fruit (*phala) of one's *actions; (3) the "six accomplishments" (*shat-sampatti*) consisting of tranquility (*shama*), sense restraint (*dama), abstention (*uparati*) from actions that are not relevant to the maintenance of the body-mind or to the pursuit of *enlightenment, endurance (*titikshā*), mental "collectedness" (*samādhāna*), and faith (*shraddhā); and (4) the "urge toward *liberation" (*mumukshutva*).

Some works, such as *Shankara's brilliant commentary on the *Brahma-Sūtra (I.1.4), speak of a sevenfold *path of *jnāna-yoga*. It consists of the above-mentioned practices with the exception of mental collectedness, and additionally has "listening (*shravana) to the sacred lore, "pondering" (*manana) of the truth of the scriptures, and *meditation or *nididhyāsana. See also *jnāna-mārga*.

jnāna-yogin is a practitioner of *jnāna-yoga*. See also *jnānin*.

Jnāneshvarī ("Goddess of Wisdom"), also called *Bhāva-Artha-Dīpikā* ("Light on the Meaning of Being"), is the major work of *Jnānadeva. He is said to have delivered its nine thousand verses *ex tempore* at the age of fifteen in A.D. 1290.

Jnātā-Amrita-Shāstra ("Compendium on the Immortal Knower") is a rare work attributed to *Goraksha. It consists of 227 verses.

jnānin ("knower") is a synonym for *jnāna-yogin*. The *Tri-Pura-Rahasya* (XIX.16ff.), a late but important *Vedānta work expounding *jnāna-yoga*, distinguishes between three types of practitioners of this *Yoga. The first type suffers from the fault of pride. The second suffers from the illusion of doership, that is, from the assumption of being an ego-personality engaged in acts rather than the *Self beyond *ego and *action. The third and most common type suffers from the "monster" of *desire, that is, from motivations that run counter to the primal impulse toward *self-transcendence. Depending on the practitioner's efforts and personality type, *jnāna-yoga* can manifest differently in different individuals. However, the unknown author of the *Tri-Pura-Rahasya* (XIX.71) is quick to point out that these differences do not mean that *wisdom itself is manifold. Rather, *jnāna* admits of no distinction; it is coessential with *Reality.

In some contexts, the word *jnānin* stands for the individual who ponders the great teachings of the scriptures but cannot really be considered a spiritual practitioner (see *jnāna-bandhu*). The *Yoga-Shikhā-Upanishad* (I.48f.), again, contrasts, the *jnānin* with the *yogin*, arguing that whereas the former does not rid himself of future births, the latter learns to master his *body and hence is assured of *liberation.

Joy. See *ānanda*, Bliss, Happiness, *sukha*.

jyotir-dhyāna ("light meditation") is also called *tejo-dhyāna*. This is one of three kinds of *meditation described in the *Gheranda-Samhitā* (VI.1). It involves *concentration on the esoteric center at the base of the spine where the individual psyche (*jīva-ātman*) is said to be located in the form of *light. An alternative process is concentration on the '"fire" of the *pranava (i.e., *om), visualized at the spot between the eyebrows. Cf. *sthūla-dhyāna*, *sūkshma-dhyāna*.

jyotis ("light"). Since ancient times, the transcendental *Reality has been described as unimaginably luminous. The *Bhagavad-Gītā* (XIII.17) calls that Reality "light of lights beyond darkness." Most *Hindu scriptures make reference to the *light aspect of the *Self. The *Shiva-Samhitā* (V.23) epitomizes this trend in the following words: "He who sees that brilliance unobstructed even for an instant is released from all *sin and reaches the highest estate." See also *tāraka-yoga*.

Jyotsnā ("Moonlight") is the principal commentary on the *Hatha-Yoga-Pradīpikā*. Its author, Brahmānanda, offers many valuable explanations of the ideas and practices of *hatha-yoga*.

$\mathcal{K}$

Kabīr, one of the great medieval *Hindu saints, lived from A.D. 1440 to 1518. He was brought up by a Muslim weaver in Benares but converted to *Hinduism through the influence of Rāmānanda (A.D. 1440–1470). He was also greatly influenced by the female *adept *Lallā, by *Nāmadeva, and not least the teachings of Sufism. Kabīr was at heart a *bhakta, who was very critical of *hatha-yoga. He did not deny that by manipulating the life force (*prāna) one could experience exquisite *bliss. Yet, he saw little value in this because, as he noted, such artificially produced states are exceedingly temporary. He also opposed the caste system and excessive image worship.

kaivalya ("aloneness") is the state of unconditional existence of the *Self. In *Classical Yoga, it refers more precisely to what the *Yoga-Sūtra (II.25) styles the "aloneness of seeing (*drishi)," which refers to the Self's innate capacity for unbroken apperception of the contents of consciousness (*citta). In an alternative definition, the *Yoga-Sūtra (IV.34) explains this as the "involution" (*pratiprasava) of the primary constituents (*guna) of *Nature, which have lost all purpose for the Self that has recovered its transcendental autonomy. According to yet another of *Patanjali's aphorisms (III.55), kaivalya is said to be established when the *sattva (the highest ontological aspect of *Nature) and the *Self are of comparable purity. The *Hatha-Yoga-Pradīpikā (IV.62), a classic manual on *hatha-yoga, defines kaivalya as that which remains after the lower *mind has been "dissolved" through yogic practice. The *Mandala-Brāhmana-Upanishad (II.3.1) speaks of the '"*light of alone-

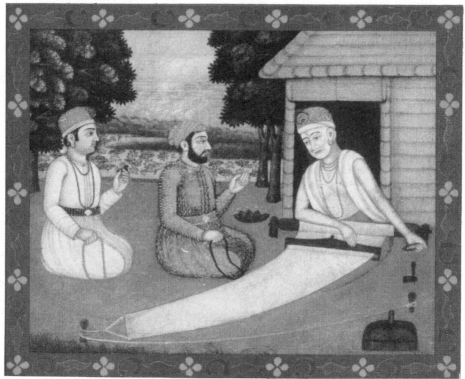

28. Kabīr, the weaver-mystic.

ness" (*kaivalya-jyotis*), which is motionless and full, "resembling a flame in a wind-still place." The **Jīvan-Mukti-Viveka* (II) explains it as "the condition of the isolated (*kevala*) Self, that is, freedom from the *body, etc." which is "obtainable through gnosis (**jñāna*) alone."

In the *Yatīndra-Mata-Dīpikā* (VIII.16f.), a seventeenth century *Vedānta work, *kaivalya* is contrasted with **moksha*, or *liberation, as follows:

> The seekers after liberation are of two kinds: the followers of *kaivalya* and the followers of *moksha*. [That which is] named *kaivalya*, [as reached] through **jñāna-yoga*, is of the nature of realization as distinct from *Nature. They say this realization is a realization without the Lord (**bhāgavat*) . . .

> The followers of *moksha* are of two kinds: the *bhaktas and the *prapannas [for whom the Lord is the ultimate *Reality].

Thus, according to this interpretation, *kaivalya* is founded in a dualistic metaphysics, whereas the metaphysical underpinning of the ideal of *moksha* is distinctly theistic. Historically speaking, however, *kaivalya* originated in the schools of *Epic Yoga, which were panentheistic, and the term continued to be used as a synonym for *moksha* in many of the schools of *Post-Classical Yoga.

Kākacandi Īshvara is mentioned in the *Hatha-Yoga-Pradīpikā* (I.7) as an *adept of *hatha-yoga*. He is credited with the authorship of a *Tantra work on *alchemy bearing his name.

kāka-mata ("crow doctrine") is referred to in the *Yoga-Shikhā-Upanishad* (I.144) and is explained in *Upanishad Brahmayogin's commentary on this text as the doctrine that Maheshvara (i.e., *Shiva) is the "master of illusion" (*māyin*), that is, the source of the illusion (*māyā*) that is called the world.

kākī-mudrā ("crow seal") is mentioned in the *Gheranda-Samhitā* (I.22) in connection with the "expelled washing" (*bahish-krita-dhauti*). According to stanzas III.86f., it is performed by shaping the mouth like a crow's beak and then sucking in the air. This work also states that by practicing this technique one becomes free of *disease "like a crow."

kāla ("time," "death"). The principal reason why conditional existence (*bhava*) is experienced as filled with suffering (*duhkha*) is that it is temporal. Time is seen as the great enemy of all creatures. As the *Yoga-Vāsishtha* (I.23.4) puts it: "There is nothing here in this universe that all-voracious time does not devour, like the submarine fire [swallows] the overflowing ocean."

The author of the *Yoga-Vāsistha* (VI.7.34) compares time to a potter who, continually turning his wheel, produces innumerable pots only to smash them whenever he fancies to do so. The *Mahābhārata* epic (XI.2.8; 24) has these two stanzas:

Time pulls along all creatures, even the gods. There is none dear to time, none hateful.

Time "cooks" [all] beings. Time destroys [all] creatures. [When all else is] asleep, time is awake. Time is hard to overcome.

Yet to transcend time is precisely the objective of all spiritual traditions. Hence the *yogin seek to "cheat" time and *death by realizing the transcendental *Reality, which is immortal. The perfected *adept is also called kāla-atīta or "he who has transcended time." This attitude is epitomized in the following verse from the *Hatha-Yoga-Pradīpikā (IV.108): "The yogin yoked through *enstasy . . . is not devoured by time."

Probably under the influence of later *Buddhism, *Patanjali and his commentators have speculated about the nature of time. According to *Classical Yoga, time consists of a series of "moments" (*kshana). This idea of the discontinuous nature of time corresponds with modern quantum-physical notions. The time intervals cannot be perceived in themselves. However, according to the *Yoga-Sūtra (III.52), the *yogin can focus on the reality of time while in the *enstatic condition, which yields *discernment-born wisdom" (viveka-ja-jnāna). The commentaries compare these minute intervals of time to the atoms (*parama-anu) of matter. These kshanas are considered to be real, whereas temporal duration is merely a "mental construct" (buddhi-samāhāra).

The term kāla is also used in the scriptures of Yoga to denote the appropriate time for practice. Thus, the *Gheranda-Samhitā (V.8ff.) stipulates that one should not commence practice when the weather is either too hot or too cold, or during the rainy season. The two ideal seasons, therefore, are spring (vasanta) and autumn (sharad). The *Mārkandeya-Purāna (39.47) adds to this that one should also abstain from practicing *Yoga when it is windy or where other extremes (*dvandva) prevail. The *Mahābhārata (XII. 294.9) additionally mentions three occasions when Yoga practice should be interrupted—during urination, defecation, and eating. However, this puritanical prescription is not upheld by other, more body-positive schools. A favorable time for Yoga practice, particularly *meditation, is sunrise, known as "Brahma's hour" (brahma-muhūrta). Some scriptures also recommend the time of sunset and just before and after midnight. See also Cosmos, kalpa, yuga.

kalā ("part") is one of the categories (*tattva) of existence distinguished in Kashmiri *Shaivism, where it stands for secondary or partial creatorship. In *Tantrism and *hatha-yoga, it also refers to the potentiality of *sound. It is often mentioned together with *nāda and *bindu. Kalā signifies the sixteenth part of anything, specificially the moon. Thus a number of medieval works on *Yoga mention the lunar "part" in the "thousand-spoked wheel" (*sahasrāra-cakra). In the *Shat-Cakra-Nirūpana (46), it is called amā-kalā, amā being one of the many synonyms for *candra*, the esoteric "moon" from which drips the "nectar of immortality" (*amrita*). This work (47) also mentions a *nirvāna-kalā* ("part of extinction") within this *amā-kalā*. Such concepts are best understood as attempts to explain specific experiences in *meditation and *enstasy. The experience of the *amā-kalā* is associated with supraconscious enstasy (*asamprajnāta-samādhi*).

Kālāmukha ("black-faced") **sect**. This is a *Tantra-based cult of about A.D. 1000 that is generally regarded as a branch of the *Lakulīsha tradition. Since none of the scriptures of this cult, whose members were fond of learning, have survived, it is difficult to get a clear picture of its metaphysics and spiritual practice. This well-organized sect has frequently and apparently unjustly been accused of indulging in eccentric and obscene rituals similar to those of the *Kāpālikas. The sect got its name from the fact that its adherents wore a striking black mark on their foreheads, indicating their *renunciation of the world.

Kālī, the "black" Goddess, who is portrayed with bulging eyes and protruding tongue, represents the destructive aspect of the *Divine. See also *deva*, Durgā.

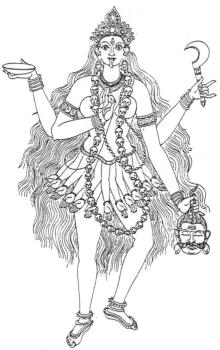

29. *Goddess Kālī.*

kāli-yuga ("dark age") refers to the present eon of spiritual decline. It is traditionally said to have started with the death of the God-man *Krishna in 3006 B.C. This idea is fundamental to *Tantrism, which purports to be a new gospel for the dark age. See also *kalpa*, *yuga*.

kalpa ("usage" or "rule"). *Hindu cosmology knows of world cycles of immense duration. A *kalpa* represents one full day in the life of the Creator, *Brahma. It translates into 4.32 billion human years of twelve million divine years or one thousand "great ages" (*mahā-yuga*). Brahma is thought to live for 36,000 *kalpas*. Each *kalpa* has a "day" and a "night." During the "night" phase, the *cosmos is temporarily dissolved. This dissolution is known as a *pralaya. Since the creation of the present universe, a total of almost two billion years are said to have elapsed, which surprisingly approximates modern computations for our star system.

kāma ("desire") stands for desire or *pleasure in general and the sexual urge, or sensuality, in particular. In the sense of pleasurable experience or objects, kāma is considered to be one of the legitimate goals of human aspiration (*purusha-artha). Yet, from the point of view of the highest human potential, which is liberation (*moksha), it is typically viewed as unworthy of one's pursuit. In fact, together with anger (*krodha) and greed (*lobha), kāma is widely deemed to be one of the three "gates to *hell."

kāma-avasāyitva ("desire dwelling") is the paranormal power (*siddhi) of perfect wish fulfillment. A *yogin endowed with this ability realizes all his desires. The *Yoga-Bhāshya (III.45) wisely observes that this does not mean that the *adept can overthrow the natural order of the universe, as instituted by the Lord (*īshvara). However, this cautionary objection is seldom heeded in the popular *Yoga literature, which abounds in stories of *yogins and ascetics who do not hesitate to set the world topsy-turvy in order to force the gods to do their bidding.

kamala-āsana ("lotus posture") is a synonym for *padma-āsana.

kāma-rūpa ("desire form") is both the geographic region of Assam, a stronghold of *Tantrism, and an esoteric structure of the human *body. In the latter sense, kāma-rūpa refers to the secret locus at the perineum (*yoni). It forms a part of the basal center (*mūlādhāra-cakra) and is represented as a deep red triangle (trikona), also called "triple city" (tripura, traipura). According to the *Shat-Cakra-Nirūpana (8), it has the brightness of ten million suns. It is here that the lower opening of the central channel (*sushumnā-nādī) is found. It is the seat of the "serpent power" (*kundalinī-shakti).

Additionally, kāma-rūpa (sometimes spelled kāma-rūpatva) is the paranormal power (*siddhi) to assume any shape at will. See also icchārūpa.

kampa or **kampana** ("tremor") is a curious yogic phenomenon associated with the arousal of the "serpent power" (*kundalinī-shakti). According to the Yoga-Yājnavalkya (VI.26) and a number of other *hatha-yoga scriptures, trembling occurs during the second stage of breath control (*prānāyāma*). The *Kaula-Jnāna-Nirnaya* (XIV.16) speaks of two degrees—general trembling and violent shaking of the limbs, which is accompanied by the hearing of different inner sounds. The *Mārkandeya-Purāna* (39.56) recommends as a remedy that one should fix the *mind on the image of a mountain (a symbol of steadiness).

kanda ("bulb"), which is sometimes spelled *kānda*, is the point of origin of the network of channels (*nādī*) along or through which the life force (*prāna*) circulates in the *body. Some schools specify its location as being at the base of the spine, corresponding to the position of the perineum (*yoni*), others as being in the "middle of the body" (*dehamadhya*). It is unanimously said to be egg shaped, though the *Hatha-Yoga-Pradīpikā* (III.113) describes it as having the appearance of a "rolled cloth." Its size is often given as nine digits long and four digits wide, and it is generally stated to be soft and white. It is also known as *kanda-yoni* and *kanda-sthāna*. The *Yoga-Kundaly-Upanishad* (I.49) mentions a *kanda* near the ankles, by which this text probably means a sensitive area (*marman*).

Kānerin is mentioned in the *Hatha-Yoga-Pradīpikā* (I.7) as a master of *hatha-yoga*. Nothing is known about him.

Kānipā, a pupil of *Jālandhari, is the reputed founder of the *Aghorī sect.

Kānphata sect. The Hindi word *kānphata* means "ear splitting," which refers to the custom of slitting the cartilages of both ears to accommodate large earrings (called *darshan* or *kundal* in Hindi). This originally ascetic order is said to have been founded by *Goraksha, who is also credited with the authorship of *hatha-yoga. Today the sect comprises men and women, some of whom are married. Their social status is generally low, and they engage in occultism, dream interpretation, and psychic healing.

During the late sixteenth century A.D., the order experienced the destruction of many of its temples at the hands of the Sikhs. There are still numerous Kānphata monasteries (*matha*) found scattered throughout India. Each belongs to one of the original twelve subdivisions of the order. Two levels of initiation (*dīkshā*) are generally recognized: First there is a probationership of up to six months, during which the student lives in confinement to test his or her resolution. This is followed by the candidate's formal acceptance as a disciple, at which time he or she receives a *mantra* and the *yogin's* garb. In the second stage of initiation, the disciple's ears are pierced, which is thought to stimulate a particular current (*nādī) of the *life force associated with the acquisition of magical power.

There is no question that the Kānphatas were instrumental in the development of *hatha-yoga. They produced a fairly extensive literature on this type of *Yoga, though today very few of its members are literate. Undoubtedly many texts are lost forever. See also Nātha sect, Siddha cult, Tantrism.

kantha-bandha ("throat lock") is a synonym for *jālandhara-bandha, which is also occasionally called kantha-mudrā ("throat seal") and kantha-samkoca ("throat contraction").

kantha-cakra ("throat wheel") is a synonym for *vishuddhi-cakra.

Kanthadi is mentioned in the *Hatha-Yoga-Pradīpikā (I.6) as an *adept of *hatha-yoga. Nothing is known about him.

kānti ("beauty"). Physical beauty is sometimes considered one of the signs (*cihna) of successful *Yoga practice. It is the result of enhanced *prāna activity in the *body.

kapāla-bhāti ("skull brightening") is one of the "six acts" (*shat-karma). The *Gheranda-Samhitā (I.55), a favorite manual on *hatha-yoga, describes it as consisting of three practices, which are said to remove phlegm (*kapha). They are the "left process" (*vāma-krama), the "inversion" (*vyutkrama), and the "process [of the sound] shīt" (*shīt-krama). According to the *Hatha-Yoga-Pradīpikā (II.35), kapāla-bhāti simply consists in rapid breathing similar to the "bellows" (*bhastrikā), which is recommended as a means of curing disorders (like corpulence) resulting from a surplus of phlegm. See also sīt-karī.

kapāla-kuhara ("cranial cavern") is the cavity in the skull into which the backturned tongue is inserted in the practice of the *khecarī-mudrā.

kapāla-randhra-dhauti ("cleansing of the skull opening") is a part of dental cleansing (*danta-dhauti) in *hatha-yoga. The *Gheranda-Samhitā (I.34f.) describes it thus: One should rub with the thumb of the right hand the depression in the forehead near the bridge of the *nose. It further states that this practice, which should be done daily in the morning, after meals, and in the evening, induces "divine sight" (divya-drishti), or clairvoyance. See also divya-cakshus.

kāpālika is mentioned in the *Hatha-Yoga-Pradīpikā (I.8) as a master of *hatha-yoga. His historicity is uncertain.

Kāpālika sect. This *Shaiva cult, which may have originated in the south of India in the first centuries A.D., belongs to the more eccentric manifestations of *Hindu spirituality. The name "Kāpālika" means "skull bearer" and is explained by the curious practice of carrying a human skull, which serves as a food bowl. The Kāpālikas' other distinguishing mark is a club (khatvanga). This sect can be considered as belonging to *Tantrism, as its practitioners consume meat and wine, and engage in sexual rites (*maithunā). No scriptures of this religious school are extant. See also Goraksha; Cf. Kālāmukha, Kānphata.

Kapālin is mentioned in the *Hatha-Yoga-Pradīpikā (I.7) as a master of *hatha-yoga. Nothing is known about him.

kapha ("phlegm"), also called *shleshma, is one of the three humors (*dhātu) recognized by native Hindu medicine (*Āyur-Veda), many of whose principles came to be adopted in Yoga. Phlegm is described as heavy, cold, oily, sweet. Cf. pitta, vāta.

Kapila is traditionally believed to be the founder of the *Sāmkhya tradition, though in later texts, such as some of the *Purānas, he is hailed as a great *yogin. It is likely that there were several historical personages of that name. The word kapila appears already in the *Rig-Veda (X.27.16), where it stands for the color "reddish-brown." It is in the *Shvetāshvatara-Upanishad (V.2) that the seer (*rishi) Kapila is mentioned. Kapila, the Sāmkhya authority, is widely celebrated as the author of the Sāmkhya-Sūtra, but this work appears to date from c. A.D. 1400. Kapila's actual teaching can no longer be reconstructed, though it was in all likelihood a panentheistic doctrine revolving around the concepts of Self (*purusha) and Nature (*prakriti). The southern recension of the *Mahābhārata epic includes a probably fictitious dialogue between Kapila and his chief disciple Asuri.

kārana ("cause"), as opposed to "effect" (kārya). See also karma, kartri, nava-kārana, sat-kārya-vāda.

karma or **karman** ("action"). This word denotes *action in general. The *Bhagavad-Gītā (XVIII.23ff.) distinguishes three fundamental types of acts, depending on the *actor's inner disposition: (1) Sāttvika-karman, which stands for actions that are prescribed by tradition, performed without attachment by a person who does not hanker after the "fruit" (*phala*); (2) *rājasa-karman*, which is performed out of ego-sense (*ahamkāra*) and in order to experience *pleasure; (3) *tāmasa-karman*, which is performed by a deluded, or confused, individual who has no concern for the moral and spiritual consequences of his or her deeds.

A further meaning of *karman* is "ritual act." But more specifically, *karman* (or *karma*) refers to the moral force of one's intentions, thoughts, and behavior. In this sense, *karma* often corresponds to *fate, as determined by the quality of one's being in past lives and the present life. The underlying idea is that even the moral dimension of existence is causally determined. As the *Shiva-Samhitā* (II.39), a late *hatha-yoga* scripture, puts it: "Whatever is experienced in the world—all that is springs from of *karma*. All creatures have experiences in accordance with [their] *karma*."

The *Gheranda-Samhitā* (I.6f.), a popular manual on *hatha-yoga*, has these two stanzas:

> Through good and bad deeds the "pot" (*ghata*) [i.e., the body] of living beings is produced; from the *body, *karma* arises. Thus [the circle] revolves like a waterwheel (*ghatī-yantra*).

> As the waterwheel moves up and down powered by the bullocks, so the psyche (*jīva*) passes [repeatedly] through life and death, powered by *karma*.

The doctrine of *karma* is intimately connected with the idea of rebirth (*punar-janman*). Both teachings first surfaced in India, as far as we can tell, during the age of the earliest *Upanishads.

Generally, *karma* is thought to be of three kinds: (1) *Sancita-karma*, or the total accumulated stock of karmic deposits (*āshaya*) awaiting fruition; (2) *prārabdha-karma*, which has come to fruition in this life (e.g., our bodily constitution); (3) *vartamāna-* or *āgāmi-karma*, which is *karma* acquired during the present lifetime and which will bear fruit in the future. The *Yoga-Sūtra* (III.22) distinguishes between moral retribution that is "acute" (*sa-upakrama*) and "deferred" (*nirupakrama*). *Vyāsa, in his *Yoga-Bhāshya* (III.22), imaginatively likens the former type to a wet cloth that is spread out to dry quickly, and the latter type to wet cloth rolled into a ball, which only dries very slowly.

All *karma*, whether "good" or "bad," is considered to be binding. *Karma* is the mechanism by which conditional existence maintains itself. Notwithstanding the sweeping influence of *karma*, the philosophers and sages, with few exceptions, have not succumbed to fatalism.

On the contrary, their thinking has revolved around the question of how this nexus of moral causation can be escaped. All spiritual *paths start from the assumption that the law of moral retribution, which is comparable to what modern physics calls a natural law, can be transcended. Thus, in his *Yoga-Sūtra (IV.7), *Patanjali states that karma is fourfold, which is explained in the *Yoga-Bhāshya as follows: Karma can be "black," "black and white," "white," and "neither white nor black."

In order to outwit the iron law of karma, one has to transcend the very *consciousness that generates mental and physical *actions and their consequences. In other words, one must go beyond the *ego-personality, the illusion that one is an agent (*kartri). This philosophy is beautifully epitomized in the teaching of *karma-yoga in the *Bhagavad-Gītā. Realizing that life is synonymous with activity, the God-man *Krishna taught that mere abstention from action does not lead to *liberation, or *enlightenment. Hence he recommended the path of "action transcendence" (*naishkarmya-karman). Only acts done without postulating a subjective center—the *ego—are nonbinding. By constantly cultivating a self-transcending disposition, the vicious circle of karmic existence can be intercepted. Thus, future karma is prevented, whereas past karma is simply allowed to play itself out as it will. Spiritual practice is thought to be capable of diffusing otherwise severe physical karma. For instance, karma that would ordinarily cause a car accident may be neutralized in a dream experience of that predestined accident, and so on.

karma-indriya ("action organ"). See indriya.

karma-yoga ("Yoga of [self-transcending] action") was first communicated under this name over two thousand years ago in the *Bhagavad-Gītā, though it undoubtedly existed prior to this scripture. The Gītā introduces this *path as one of the two "ways of life" (*nishthā) taught by *Krishna, the other being *sāmkhya-yoga. Karma-yoga encourages an active life, though from an ingenious perspective: All work must not only be appropriate, which for the most part means allotted to one by one's position in life, but it must also be performed in the spirit of an inner sacrifice (*yajna). Only then are one's actions not karmically binding.

According to the Matsya-Purāna (52.5f.), karma-yoga is a thousand times better than *jnāna-yoga, which here means the path of *meditation and *renunciation. However, in the *Uddhāva-Gītā (XV.7), karma-yoga is introduced as the first step toward *jnāna-yoga. It is intended for those who are not "disgusted" with actions and who still entertain all kinds of desires. *Karma-yoga* is sometimes also called **kriyā-yoga*. See also Action, *karma*.

karmin ("worker") is a synonym for *karma-yogin*, the spiritual practitioner who follows the *path of *karma-yoga*.

karna-dhauti ("ear cleansing") is one of the practices of **danta-dhauti*. According to the **Gheranda-Samhitā* (I.33), it should be done with the index and ring fingers. Regular daily practice leads to the perception of inner sounds (**nāda*).

kārpanya ("meanness") is sometimes listed as one of the "defects" (**dosha*) on the spiritual *path.

kartri ("actor, agent"). This is one link in the "action nexus" (*karma-samgraha*), the other two being the object (**kārya*), and the causal process (**kārana*) itself. The **Bhagavad-Gītā* (SVIII.26ff.) distinguishes three types of agents: (1) The *sāttvika-kartri*, who is free from attachment, steadfast, dedicated, unchanged by success or failure, and who does not utter "I"; (2) the *rājasa-kartri*, who hankers after the fruit (**phala*) of his actions, is passionate, greedy, impure, subject to elation and depression, or of a violent nature; (3) the *tāmasa-kartri*, who is undisciplined, vulgar, obstinate, deceitful, base, slothful, despondent, and procrastinating. See also Action, Actor, *karma*.

karunā ("compassion") is mentioned, for instance, in the **Yoga-Sūtra* (I.33) as a positive emotion to be projected. *Patanjali probably borrowed this term and the practice for which it stands from *Buddhism. In certain schools of *Shaivism and also in *Rāmānuja's school of *Vaishnavism, *karunā* stands for divine *grace. See also *dayā*.

Katha-Upanishad is probably the oldest verse *Upanishad, which, in its earliest portions, dates back to the fifth century B.C. It is also the first Upanishad to contain explicit *Yoga and *Sāmkhya ideas. These are crafted onto an ancient narrative in which the student Naciketas is initiated into the higher mysteries by the God of Death (*Yama). The second chapter, which appears to be a self-contained unit, expounds a type of *Epic Yoga, consisting in the "firm binding of the *senses." In one verse (II.12), the compound *adhyātma-yoga* occurs, the goal of which is the realization of the transcendental Self (**purusha*). The general tenor of this work is panentheistic.

katthana ("boastfulness"). According to the *Yoga-Tattva-Upanishad* (3), this is one of the five "obstacles" (*vighna*) of *Yoga. See also *abhimāna*; cf. *mauna*.

kaula is short for *kaula-mārga* ("path relating to the *kula*"). This spiritual approach is extolled in the *Kula-Arnava-Tantra* (II.13–14; 20–21) as follows:

> Just as the footprints of all creatures are lost in an elephant's footprints, so the [philosophical] viewpoints of all people are [absorbed] in the *kula* [teaching].

> Just as iron is never comparable with gold, so the *kula* teaching should never be likened to any other [teaching].

> Riding on the vehicle of the *kula* teaching the most excellent person goes across the island [of this world] to *heaven and [then] obtains the jewel of *liberation.

> In all other [philosophical] viewpoints, people attain to liberation through prolonged *practice. However, in the Kaula [school], [they are liberated] instantly.

Fundamental to the practice of the Kaula school is the divinization of the *body through stimulating the flow of the "nectar of immortality" (*amrita*). In the *Kaula-Jnāna-Nirnaya* (XIV.94), this ambrosial liquid is stated to be the "true condition of the Kaula." The term *kaula* also applies to a practitioner of the spiritual *path of the *Kaula sect. According to the *Akula-Vīra-Tantra* (version B; 43), there are two classes of *kaulas*: the *kritaka-* ("artificial") *kaulas*, who know the "serpent power" (*kundalinī-shakti*) and seek to manipulate it to gain *enlightenment, and the *sahaja-* ("spontaneous") *kaulas*, who have achieved identity with *Shiva and abide perpetually in the state of *samarasa*. See also Adept, *kula*, Spontaneity.

Kaula-Jnāna-Nirnaya ("Ascertainment of Kaula Knowledge") is an ancient *Tantric work ascribed to *Matsyendra. It is the oldest known source about the *kaula-mārga* taught by him. According to the colophon, this work comprises one thousand verses but all the available manuscripts, dating back to the mid-eleventh century A.D., appear to be incomplete. The first chapter, most of which is missing, deals with the process of cosmic *creation. The second chapter discusses macrocosmic and microcosmic dissolution (*laya, *pralaya). The third chapter outlines the different bodily locations (*sthāna) for *meditation and also speaks of the true nature of the phallus (*linga) and how it is to be worshipped. This is followed by a lengthy treatment of the paranormal powers (*siddhi) accruing from spiritual practice. The next three chapters deal with the hidden bodily centers (*cakra) and various esoteric processes, including the *khecarī-mudrā. The eighth chapter introduces rituals of *worship of the different kinds of female power (*shakti). The next chapter is a list of teachers of this particular school. The tenth chapter discloses the "seed-" or *bīja-mantras for the various *cakras. This is followed by dietary and behavioral considerations. The thirteenth chapter is dedicated to a discussion of the means of *liberation, especially the esoteric teaching of the *hamsa. The remaining eleven chapters deal with all kinds of esoteric processes for initiates.

Kaula sect. The beginnings of this school within the broad movement of *Tantrism may reach back to the fifth century A.D. Traditionally, *Matsyendra is venerated as its founder, though it appears that he merely founded the *yoginī-kaula* branch in Assam. Be that as it may, by the time *Abhinava Gupta wrote his learned works on Kashmiri *Shaivism in the tenth century A.D., the Kaula tradition was well established, looking back on a long history.

In consonance with the *Siddha tradition, the *kaulas believe that *enlightenment is a bodily event and that the body's structures, if rightly manipulated, would yield *Self-realization. The central mechanism of this process is the "serpent power" (*kundalinī-shakti), also known as the *kula. The body-positive orientation of the *kaulas* included the employment of *sexual rites (*maithunā), a feature of many *Tantric schools.

The literature of the Kaula sect, which was probably very comprehensive, is poorly preserved and very little researched. The most popular work is undoubtedly the *Kula-Arnava-Tantra. Another less well-known, but for the historian more significant, treatise is the *Kaula-Jnāna-Nirnaya.

kaushala ("skill"). In the *Bhagavad-Gītā (II.50), *Yoga is defined as "skill in action." See also *buddhi-yoga, karma-yoga*.

kāya ("body") is a synonym for *deha and *sharīra.

kāya-sampat ("perfection of the body") is mentioned in the *Yoga-Sūtra (I.45) as resulting from the total "conquest of the elements" (*bhūta-jaya), and consists in beauty, gracefulness, strength, and "adamantine robustness" (vajra-samhananatva). See also Body, kāya-siddhi.

kāya-shuddhi ("body purification"). See Purification, Purity.

kāya-siddhi ("perfection of the body") is, according to the *Yoga-Sūtra (II.43), one of the results of asceticism (*tapas). As the *Yoga-Bhāshya (II.43) explains, such perfection is demonstrated in the acquisition of the eight major paranormal powers (*siddhi), as well as by such paranormal abilities as clairvoyance (dūra-darshana) and clairaudience (dūra-shravana). See also Body, kāya-sampat.

Keshidvāja is a teacher of *Epic Yoga. In the *Agni-Purāna (379.25), he defines *Yoga as the "union" (*samyoga) of the mind with the *Absolute (*brahman).

keshin ("long-haired one") is a *Vedic type of ecstatic to whom a whole hymn is dedicated in the *Rig-Veda (X.136). Some scholars have seen in the keshin a forerunner of the later *yogin. He appears to represent a mystical culture distinct from the sacrificial ritualism of the Vedic "seers" (*rishi).

kevala ("alone"). This adjective is sometimes used as a noun to denote the *Self. According to the *Yoga-Tattva-Upanishad (12f.), this term refers to the psyche (*jīva) "devoid of the twenty defects (*dosha)."

kevalata or kevalatva ("aloneness") is a synonym for *kaivalya.

kevalī-bhāva ("condition of aloneness") is a synonym for kaivalya used in the *Yoga-Vāsishtha (III.4.53). This concept is found already in the *Mahābhārata (XII.306.77), where it is stated that he who has "become alone" (kevalī-bhūta), sees the twenty-sixth principle (i.e., the *Self).

kevala- or kevali-kumbhaka ("absolute retention") is one of the forms of breath control (*prānāyāma) in *hatha-yoga. The *Hatha-Yoga-Pradīpikā (II.73) defines this technique as the retention of the *breath without inhalation and exhalation. This work (II.72) also stipulates that one should practice *sahita-kumbhaka so long as one is not accomplished in kevala-kumbhaka. The *Gheranda-Samhitā (V.89) explains it thus: "When the breath is confined to the 'pot' (ghata) [i.e., the *body], this is kevala-

kumbhaka." This text (V.92f.) further specifies that one should start by retaining the breath between one and sixty-four times. This should be done every three hours or, if this is not possible, five times a day (in the early morning, at noon, twilight, midnight, and in the fourth quarter of the night), or three times (morning, noon, and evening). One should also try to increase the duration of each retention daily.

kevalin ("he who is alone") denotes the transcendental *Self. The term is used, for instance, in the *Yoga-Bhāshya* (I.24), which states that there are numerous *kevalins* who have severed the three "fetters" (*bandhana*), which perhaps refers to the bonds of the three types of primary constituent (*guna*) of *Nature. The *kevalins* are the liberated *adepts who have perfectly recovered their transcendental Selfhood.

kha ("hole" or "space/ether") is a synonym for *ākāsha.

Khanda is mentioned in the *Hatha-Yoga-Pradīpikā* (I.8) as an *adept of *hatha-yoga. No further biographical information is available about him.

khecari-mudrā ("space-walking seal"). This word is derived from *kha and the verbal root *car* ("to move"). It stands for one of the principal "seals" (*mudrā*) of *Tantrism. Already hinted at in the pre-Christian *Maitrāyanīya-Upanishad* (VI.20), this technique has immense importance in *hatha-yoga where it is used in conjunction with *breath control. In the *Gheranda-Samhitā* (III.25ff.), we find the following description: One should cut the tongue's frenum and move the tongue constantly, milking it with butter and pulling it out by means of an iron implement. When the tongue has been elongated to the point where it can reach the spot between the eyes, one is fit for the *khecari-mudrā*. In this technique, the tongue is turned back and slowly inserted into the "skull cavity" (*kapāla-kuhara*). This produces all kinds of sensations, including a whole range of tastes—from saltish to bitter to sweet—as the ambrosial liquid (*amrita*) begins to flow abundantly. One's gaze (*drishti*) should be fixed on the middle of the forehead. This *mudrā* is said to prevent fainting (*mūrchā*), *hunger, *thirst, lassitude (*ālasya*), *disease, ageing, and even *death. It is also stated to create a "divine body" (*deva-deha*). Such a transubstantiated, beautiful *body is immune to the *elements and to snake bites.

The *Hatha-Yoga-Pradīpikā* (III.34) advises that one should cut the frenum only a hair's breadth at a time and rub the tongue with powdered rock salt (and yellow myrobalan). This procedure should be done every seven days, until the frenum is completely severed after about six months. This scripture (III.41) also explains that both the tongue and the *mind must move into the "space" (*kha) for this *mudrā to be effective. Stanza III.42 makes the further point that by this technique the *semen is prevented from falling even when one is embracing a passionate women. The *yogin who is skilled in this practice is claimed (III.44) to conquer *death within fifteen days. Another verse (IV.49) has it that the khecarī-mudrā should be practiced until the "Yoga sleep" (*yoga-nidrā) sets in. The *Shāndilya-Upanishad (I.7.15) defines the khecarī-mudrā as the state in which the *breath and *mind have come to rest upon the "inner sign" (*antar-lakshya).

The anonymous author of the *Yoga-Kundaly-Upanishad (II.44), which devotes a long section to the "science of the khecarī" (khecarī-vidyā), observes that while performing this technique one should also block the nostrils with a small plug made out of gold, silver, or iron wrapped with a thread soaked in milk. This work also makes the anatomically doubtful claim that some *yogins can extend their tongues to the crown of the *head, though some practitioners have succeeded in elongating their tongue by two inches and more. See also lambikā-yoga.

khecaratva ("space-walking") is variously understood as either *levitation or an out-of-body experience, which books on *occultism call "astral travel." This paranormal ability (*siddhi) is also called khe-gati. See also ākāsha-gamana, lāghava.

khyāti ("vision"). See anyatā-khyāti, viveka-khyāti.

kilbisha ("guilt") is a synonym for *dosha. See also klesha, pāpa.

kīrtana ("chanting"). Singing songs of praise in the ritual *worship of one's "chosen deity" (*ishta-devatā) is one of the "limbs" (*anga) of *bhakti-yoga. This practice tends to lead more often to *ecstasy rather than *enstasy.

klesha ("trouble," "affliction"). This word is found already in the *Mahābhārata epic, where it is generally used in the sense of "toil" or "struggle." However, there is at least one passage (XII.204.16) that suggests a more technical use of the term: "As seeds roasted in fire do not sprout again, so the *Self (*ātman) is not bound again by the kleshas [once they have been] burnt by means of wisdom (*jnāna)."

Here the term stands for what has been called the "causes of affliction." Presumably reiterating an earlier tradition, *Patanjali distinguishes five such causes: nescience (*avidyā*), "I-am-ness" (*asmitā*), attachment (*rāga*), aversion (*dvesha*), and the "will to live" (*abhini-vesha*). These factors, which can be compared to the "drives" of an earlier generation of psychologists, provide the cognitive and motivational framework for the ordinary individual enmeshed in conditional existence (*samsāra*) and ignorant of the transcendental *Self. As the *Yoga-Sūtra* (II.12) states, these *kleshas* are the root of the *karmic "deposit" (*āshaya*) in the subconscious. Their effects are felt not only in one's present life but they also determine the quality of one's future *rebirths. According to the *Yoga-Sūtra* (II.4), the *kleshas* exist in various states. They can be (1) "dormant" (*prasupta*), that is, exist in the form of "subliminal activators" (*samskāra*) ready to manifest as psychomental activity; (2) "attentuated" (*tanu*), that is, temporarily prevented from taking effect by way of *concentration or other yogic techniques; (3) "intercepted" (*vicchinna*), which is the case when one kind of *klesha* blocks the operation of another; and (4) "aroused" (*udāra*), that is, fully active. According to *Patanjali, it is the purpose of *kriyā-yoga* to achieve the "attenuation" (*tanū-karana*) of these *kleshas*. Ultimately, the *kleshas* are completely obliterated through the realization of the "cloud-of-dharma" enstasy (*dharma-megha-samādhi*).

In the *Yoga-Bhāshya* (I.8), the following alternative designations are furnished: "darkness" (*tamas*); "delusion" (*moha*); "great delusion" (*mahā-moha*); "the dark" (*tāmisra*); and "the pitch dark" (*andhatāmisra*). Another name for *klesha* is "error" (*viparyaya*). See also *aklishta, dosha, klishta*.

klishta ("afflicted"). This is the past participle of the root *klish*, from which the noun *klesha* is derived. *Patanjali looks upon the five types of mental activity (*vritti*) as being either "afflicted" or "nonafflicted" (*aklishta*). The *Yoga-Bhāshya* (I.5) explains the former as "caused by the *kleshas*," but the *Mani-Prabhā* (I.5) offers the more convincing interpretation of "resulting in *bondage."

Knots. See *granthi*.

Knowledge. See *jnāna, prajnā, vidyā, pramāna*; cf. *ajnāna, avidyā, viparyaya*.

Korantaka is mentioned in the *Hatha-Yoga-Pradīpikā* (I.6) as a master of *hatha-yoga*. Nothing is known about him.

kosha ("sheath"). All major spiritual traditions of the world sanction the belief that the physical *body is not the only vehicle in which *consciousness can express itself or in which the spirit, or Self (*ātman), manifests itself. Thus most schools of *Post-Classical Yoga and *Vedānta accept the doctrine of the "five sheaths" (*panca-kosha*), which was first introduced in the ancient *Taittirīya-Upanishad (II.7). This scripture speaks of the five envelopes that occlude the pure *light of the transcendental *Self: (1) the "sheath composed of food" (*anna-maya-kosha*); (2) the "sheath composed of life force" (*prāna-maya-kosha*); (3) the "sheath composed of mind" (*mano-maya-kosha*); (4) the "sheath composed of awareness" (*vijnāna-maya-kosha*), and (5) the "sheath composed of bliss" (*ānanda-maya-kosha*). The last-mentioned envelope is equated in the *Taittirīya-Upanishad with the transcendental *Reality itself, though later schools consider it to still be a fine veil around the Self.

This model is not accepted in *Classical Yoga; yet here, too, the existence of a supraphysical *body is postulated, which is composed of more "subtle" (*sūkshma*) matter-energy than the material body. While the *Yoga-Sūtra does not mention such a body directly, it is implied for instance in the notion that there are highly evolved masters of *Yoga who have merged with the very ground of *Nature. This merging is of exceedingly long duration and is called *prakriti-laya*, and it is a condition of quasi-liberation. Also, the deities (*deva*) exist in some form or another, and the "Lord" (*īshvara*) himself is held to have assumed a highly refined supramaterial condition, called *sattva*, in order to instruct the ancient sages.

However, in one passage in the *Yoga-Bhāshya (IV.10), *Vyāsa distinctly argues that consciousness (*citta*) is all pervasive and that therefore there can be no question of a subtle or "superconductive" (*ātivāhika*) body. This all-pervasive *citta* contracts and expands only in its manifestation as mental activity (*vritti*). Possibly the differences in opinion are the result of taking the concept of *body too literally. We can conceive of a universal field of *consciousness that, seen hierarchically, is yet delimited from another universal field of different quality, such as the highly attenuated *sattva field that certainly *Vyāsa assumes for the *īshvara in his teaching mode. It is possible to speak of such a field as a body.

kraunca-nishadana ("curlew seat") is mentioned in the *Yoga-Bhāshya (II.46), and the *Tattva-Vaishāradī (II.46) unhelpfully observes that for its performance one should study the typical posture of a curlew.

kri-kara (*"kri*-maker"), which is sometimes spelled *kri-kala*, is one of the five secondary forms of the life force (**prāna*) circulating in the *body. It is responsible for causing hunger (**kshudhā*) or sneezing.

kripā ("grace") is a synonym for *anugraha, prasāda*; cf. Effort.

Krishna ("Puller"), the incarnate *God worshipped in the *Vaishnava tradition, is so called because he pulls or attracts devotees' hearts to himself. It is sometimes doubted that there was an actual historical person by the name of Krishna whose teachings are recorded in the *Bhagavad-Gītā and other parts of the *Mahābhārata epic, but this scholarly skepticism is probably unwarranted. The name Krishna first appears in the ancient *Rig-Veda (VIII.74), where it refers to a sage. In another passage (VIII.85), it refers to a monster. A reference that is thought more likely to pertain to the *adept Krishna is contained in the *Chāndogya-Upanishad (XXX.6), where Krishna is called the son of Devakī and the pupil of Ghora Angirasa, a sun priest belonging to the tradition of the *Atharva-Veda. S. Radhakrishnan (1948) pointed out the "great similarity between the teaching of Ghora Angirasa . . . and that of Krishna in the *Gītā*" (p. 28). It appears that this Krishna was the leader of a branch of the Yādava tribe and a much-revered spiritual teacher. In the course of time, he became deified like so many other masters.

In medieval times, Krishna became associated with the exuberant *bhakti movement, a further development of the *bhakti-yoga* first taught in the *Bhagavad-Gītā. His fictitious life story is told in the *Hari-Vamsha* ("*Hari's Genealogy"), an appendix to the *Mahābhārata epic, and then also in the *Bhāgavata-Purāna. There he is celebrated as a full *incarnation (*pūrna-avatāra*) of God *Vishnu.

Krishna, Gopi (A.D. 1903–1984) was born in Kashmir. In 1937, after seventeen years of practicing *meditation while simultaneously pursuing a career as a government employee, Gopi Krishna experienced a sudden awakening of the "serpent power" (**kundalinī-shakti*). For several years, this unleashed psychospiritual power played havoc with his body and mind, until the condition stabilized. His tribulations are recorded in great detail in his autobiography *Kundalini: Evolutionary Energy in Man*. This testimony is the most comprehensive descriptive account of the *kundalinī* phenomenon available. In subsequent years, he wrote many other books, in which he expressed the belief that the *kundalinī* is the mechanism that is responsible for the higher spiritual evolution of humanity. Gopi Krishna did not found a school or move-

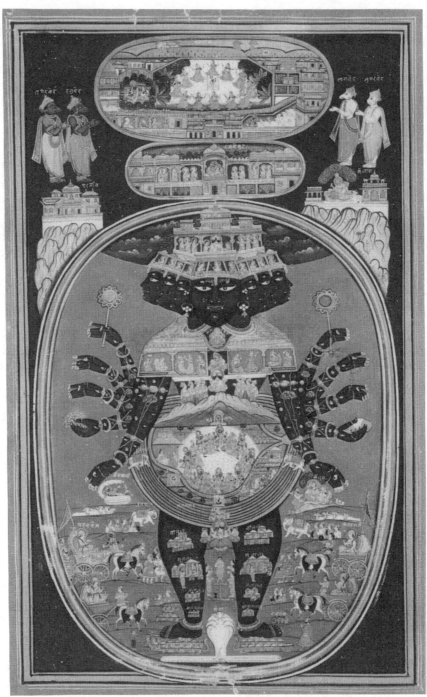

30. Lord Krishna in his universal aspect (vishva-rūpa).

ment, but his work did much to make *kundalinī-yoga* more widely known in the West.

kriyā ("act" or "rite") is often used synonymously with *karman*. In contemporary *Yoga circles, *kriyā* also stands for involuntary movements of the limbs resulting from the arousal of the "serpent power" (*kundalinī-shakti*).

kriyā-shakti ("action power") is that aspect of the *Divine that is the source of all dynamism in *Nature. Cf. *icchā-shakti, jnāna-shakti*.

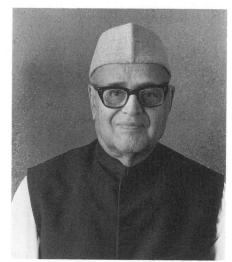

31. Gopi Krishna.

kriyā-yoga ("Yoga of [ritual] action"). In the *Tri-Shikhi-Brāhmana-Upanishad* (II.23), this *path is contrasted with *jnāna-yoga* and equated with *karma-yoga*. It is also said in verse twenty-four to consist in the fixation of the *mind upon a particular object and the adherence of the mind to the moral disciplines enjoined in the scriptures. The last is deemed *karma-yoga* proper.

According to the *Bhāgavata-Purāna* (XI.27.49), *kriyā-yoga* can be either *Vedic or *Tantric ritual practice. Both approaches are said to lead to the *Divine.

In the *Yoga-Sūtra* (II.1), *kriyā-yoga* stands for the *Yoga of transmutative action that obliterates the "subliminal activators" (*samskāra*) through asceticism (*tapas*), study (*svādhyāya*), and devotion to the Lord (*īshvara-pranidhāna*). This Yoga can be contrasted with the *ashta-anga-yoga*, whose "limbs" (*anga*) are expounded in aphorisms II.28–III.8. Even though *Patanjali's Yoga has achieved fame for its eightfold path, it is likely that this particular systematization was merely cited by Patanjali and that his own contribution to Yoga was *kriyā-yoga*.

In modern times, *kriyā-yoga* was taught by Paramahamsa *Yogananda. This approach is presented by his followers as a form of *rāja-yoga*, but it includes concepts and exercises deriving from, or at least similar to, *kundalinī-yoga*.

krodha ("anger") is considered one of the "gates to hell." It is frequently mentioned together with desire (*kāma*) and greed (*lobha*). In a memorable passage in the *Bhagavad-Gītā* (II.63), anger is said to arise from desire and to cause bewilderment (*moha*), which in turn leads to confusion of one's memory, and loss of wisdom (*buddhi*), whereupon a person is completely lost.

kshamā ("patience") is often listed among the moral disciplines (*yama*). In the *Yoga-Yājnavalkya* (I.64), it is defined as equanimity (*samatva*) toward all pleasant and unpleasant things. The *Darshana-Upanishad* (I.16–17) explains it as refraining from agitation when provoked by one's enemies. See also *kshānti, titikshā*.

kshana ("moment" or "instant") is defined in the *Yoga-Bhāshya* (III.52) as the time taken by an atom (*parama-anu*) to shift from one position to another. See also *kāla*.

kshānti ("forbearance") is a synonym for *kshamā*. The *Bhagavad-Gītā* (XIII.7) considers it to be a manifestation of wisdom (*jnāna*).

kshara ("mobile") is a common term in *Epic Yoga for *Nature, which is constantly in flux, while the ultimate *Reality is perfectly stable. Cf. *akshara*.

kshetra ("field") is a term of *Epic Yoga to denote *Nature and/or the body-mind, as opposed to the "field knower" (*kshetra-jna*).

kshetra-jna ("field knower"), also called *kshetrin*, is the transcendental *Self supporting the individual *consciousness. As the *Mahābhārata (XII.212.40) puts it: "That being (*bhāva*) who abides in the *mind is called 'field knower.' "
      The *Yoga-Bhāshya* (II.17) emphasizes that the "field knower" is immutable and inactive. According to the *Bhagavad-Gītā* (XIII.2), the "field knower" of all the "fields" is none other than God *Krishna.

kshudhā ("hunger") is sometimes counted as one of the "defects" (*dosha*) and can, according to some works of *Post-Classical Yoga, be combatted by *shītalī-prānāyāma*.

Kshurikā-Upanishad ("Dagger Upanishad") is one of the *Yoga-Upanishads, a *Vedānta-based tract of twenty-four stanzas dealing principally with concentration (*dhāranā*). Concentration is called the knife or "dagger" (*kshurikā*) by which the *yogin severs the knot of *ignorance. Here *dhāranā is a combination of focusing *mind, breath (*prāna*), and *gaze upon specific locations in the *body, namely the ankles, shanks, knees, thighs, anus, penis, *navel, central channel (*sushumnā-nādī), "heart abode" (hridaya-āyatana), and throat. According to the commentary by *Upanishad Brahmayogin, two further stations are the middle of the eyebrows (*bhrū-madhya) and the *sahasrāra-cakra at the crown of the *head. The text refers to these loci (*desha) as "joints" (*marman) that are to be severed. A similar process is described for the 72,000 currents (*nādī) of the *life force circulating in the body. They have to be "cut off" with the exception of the axial channel (*sushumnā-nādī). The goal of this *Yoga is absorption (*laya) into the *Absolute.

kuhū-nādī ("new moon channel") is one of the fourteen principal channels (*nādī) through which the *life force flows in the *body. According to the *Shāndilya-Upanishad (I.4.9), it is situated to the back and side of the central channel (*sushumnā-nādī) and to extend to the genitals. The *Darshana-Upanishad (IV.8) also places it to the side of the central channel, and the *Yoga-Shikhā-Upanishad (V.26) associates it with the anus and defecation.

kukkuta-āsana ("cock posture") is described in the *Gheranda-Samhitā (II.31) thus: Sitting in the "lotus posture" (*padma-āsana), one should insert the hands between one's thighs and knees and raise oneself, supporting the *body with the elbows.

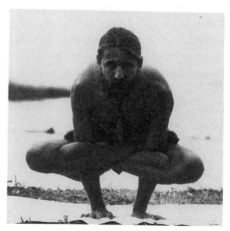

32. Kukkuta-āsana.

kula is a term with many meanings. In ordinary contexts, it stands for "family," "flock," or "home," thus conveying the idea of the familiar. Something of this connotation is preserved in the usage of the term kula in the esoteric schools of *Tantrism, where it refers to the divine power (*shakti), the feminine aspect of the *Absolute. The masculine aspect of the *Divine is known as *akula. To confuse matters, kula is also used to describe the experience of the union between *Shiva and *Shakti, *God and *Goddess, Power and *Consciousness. See also kaula.

Kula-Arnava-Tantra ("Flood of Kula Treatise") is a major text of the *Kaula school consisting of seventeen chapters with a total of 2059 stanzas dealing with *concentration upon various psychoenergetic centers (*cakra*) and the paranormal powers (*siddhi*) resulting from this practice.

kula-kundalinī is a synonym for *kula* and *kundalinī*.

kumbhaka ("potlike"). Breath retention is one of the most direct means of effecting changes in *consciousness—a fact that has been exploited in many spiritual traditions around the world. The term *kumbhaka* can denote both breath control (*prānāyāma*) in general and the key practice of breath retention in particular. In the latter sense, the term *kumbhaka* refers to the fact that during the suspension of the breath the trunk of the *body is filled up with life energy (*prāna*), which is retained as a pot (*kumbha*) retains liquid. But since this technique also stabilizes the *mind, the *Yoga-Tattva-Upanishad* (142) likens *kumbhaka* to a lamp inside a pot that does not flicker because no breeze can reach it.

According to the *Shāndilya-Upanishad* (I.7.13.5), *kumbhaka* is of two kinds—"associated" (*sahita*) with inhalation and exhalation and "isolated" (*kevala*), that is, without either inhalation or exhalation. The latter type of retention is an advanced form of breath control, which should occur without strain. Whereas the *sahita* forms of *kumbhaka* attract the "serpent power" (*kundalinī-shakti*) into the central channel (*sushumnā-nādī*), the "isolated" retention is the principal means of forcing that power up along the spinal axis to the center at the crown. The *Hatha-Yoga-Pradīpikā* (II.72ff.) makes this observation:

> So long as [the *yogin* still aspires to] the attainment (*siddhi*) of the *kevala* [type of breath suspension], he should practice the *sahita* [variety]. —When the breath (*vāyu*) is easily retained, without exhalation and inhalation . . .

> . . . this [type of] breath control is said to be *kevala-kumbhaka*. —When this *kevala-kumbhaka* without exhalation and inhalation is attained . . .

> . . . nothing in the three worlds is difficult for him to obtain. —He who is empowered by means of *kevala-kumbhaka*, through the retention (*dhāranā*) of the breath at will . . .

> . . . attains even to the condition of *rāja-yoga*. There is no doubt about this.

According to the *Shiva-Samhitā (III.53), one must be able to retain the *breath for three ghatikās (i.e., seventy-two minutes) before one can hope to obtain paranormal powers (*siddhis). Elsewhere (III.59), this work states that when one is able to perform kumbhaka for a whole yāma (i.e., three hours) the body becomes so light that one is able to balance on one's thumb (see also *lāghava).

kundalini-shakti ("serpent power") is also called kundalī, kutilangī, bhujanginī, ātma-shakti, avadhūtī, and a host of other names. This mysterious psychospiritual force is a conceptual and practical mainstay of *Tantrism and *hatha-yoga. In the *Hatha-Yoga-Pradīpikā) (III.1), it is hailed as the support of all *Yoga treatises (*tantra). The enigmatic kundalini may have been hinted at already in the *Rig-Veda (X.189) under the name of Vāc Virāj ("Voice Resplendent"), who is described as a "serpent queen" (sarpa-rājnī). In view of the fact that the kundalini experience is claimed to depend on universal structures of the *body, we must assume that it was encountered by mystics throughout the ages. However, it was only with the body-positive esotericism of the *Tantras that this experience was elaborated into a full-fledged conceptual model that then served practitioners as a road map in their efforts to systematically awaken the kundalini power.

On the occult principle that the *body is a microcosm that faithfully reflects the large configurations found in the *macrocosm, the kundalini is envisioned as being the individualized form of the cosmic feminine principle, or *shakti. That divine Force is thought to manifest in the form of the kundalini on the one hand, and the life force (*prāna) on the other. The kundalini is, however, understood as a more fundamental potency in the spiritual process. Perhaps the relationship between the kundalini and prāna can be compared to that of an A-bomb to an H-bomb. It takes the concentrated impact of the prāna force, regulated through *breath control, to trigger the kundalini force and make it ascend along the central conduit of the *body.

The kundalini is pictured as residing in a state of potency, brilliant as a million suns, at the lowest esoteric center (*cakra) of the *body. The kundalini's state of potency is expressed in the notion of its lying coiled—three and a half, five, and eight coils are often mentioned—at the basal center. This hidden serpent closes off the gate to *liberation, which is the lower entrance to the central channel (*sushumnā-nādī). The *Goraksha-Samhitā (I.47ff.) observes:

The serpent power, forming an eightfold coil above the "bulb" (*kanda), remains there all the while covering with its face the opening of the door to the *Absolute.

Through that door the safe door to the *Absolute can be reached. Covering with the face that door, the great Goddess is asleep [in the ordinary person].

Awakened through *buddhi-yoga together with [the combined action of] *mind and *breath, she rises upward through the *sushumnā like a thread [being pushed through] a needle.

Sleeping in the form of a serpent, resembling a resplendent cord, she, when awakened by the Yoga of *fire [i.e., mental concentration and breath control], rises upward through the *sushumnā.

Just as one may open a door with a key by force, so the *yogin should break open the door to *liberation with the kundalinī.

The *Tantric yogin's task consists in obliging the kundalinī to "uncoil" and rise to the "thousand-petaled lotus" at the top of the *head, which is the locus of the static pole of the psychospiritual energy. It is the seat of *Shiva. The resulting reunion of Shiva and Shakti, *God and *Goddess, is celebrated as the supreme goal of Yoga. It manifests in a radical switch in *consciousness, obliterating the sense of individuation and flooding the *body with divine nectar, the kula-amrita (or *soma), which is experienced as unsurpassably blissful (*ānanda).

The ascent of the kundalinī from the base *cakra to the *head is associated with a variety of psychic phenomena, notably heat and light (*jyotis) but also different kinds of sounds (*nāda). According to the *Yoga-Shikhā-Upanishad (I.114f.), the constant stimulation of the kundalinī produces a sensation in the central channel similar to that of ants crawling up the spine. Some of these physiological side effects can be greatly disturbing, especially when the kundalinī awakening has occurred spontaneously and without adequate preparation, or *purification. They have been vividly described by Gopi *Krishna (1971), a modern kundalinī "victim" who gradually learned to master this power. He described his experience as follows:

> Suddenly, with a roar like that of a waterfall, I felt a stream of liquid light entering my brain through the spinal cord.
>   Entirely unprepared for such a development, I was completely taken by surprise; but regaining self-control instantaneously, I remained sitting in the same posture, keeping my mind on the point of

concentration. The illumination grew brighter and brighter, the roaring louder, I experienced a rocking sensation and then felt myself slipping out of my body, entirely enveloped in a halo of light (pp. 12–13).

The final realization of the *Tantric *yogin* is thought to be more complete than that of the *rāja-yogin* because it includes the *body. In other words, it is not merely a mind-transcending state but illumines the body itself: The body is experienced as the body of the *Divine. In this way, the *Tantric *yogin* combines the ideal of liberation (*mukti) with the ideal of "enjoyment" (*bhukti). See also *granthi*.

kundalinī-yoga is the *Tantric discipline involving the deliberate arousal of the *kundalinī-shakti. See also *bhūta-shuddhi*.

kūrma ("tortoise") is one of the five secondary forms of life force (*prāna). According to the *Tri-Shikhi-Brāhmana-Upanishad (II.82), it circulates in the skin and bones and is responsible for the closing (and opening) of the eyes, which is its widely accepted function.

kūrma-āsana ("tortoise posture") is described in the *Gheranda-Samhitā (II.32) thus: One should place the crossed heals under the scrotum and keep the *body, *head, and neck aligned. The *Hatha-Yoga-Pradīpikā (I.22) stipulates that one should press the crossed ankles against the anus. Contemporary manuals explain this posture (*āsana) differently: Sitting with one's legs stretched out in front, one should bend forward. Then one should insert one's arms beneath one's legs and reach up toward the back, locking one's fingers behind the back. Cf. *uttāna-kūrma-āsana*.

kūrma-nādī ("tortoise channel") is mentioned in the *Yoga-Sūtra (III.31) and is explained in the *Yoga-Bhāshya commentary thereon as a structure in the chest. By performing "constraint" (*samyama) on this *nādī*, the *yogin achieves a motionless (mental) state like that of a serpent or guana.

Kūrma-Purāna was originally probably a *Vaishnava work of the fifth century A.D. that was revised several hundred years later in the light of the *Pāshupata tradition. It contains the *Īshvara-Gītā.

kūtastha ("summit-abiding") is used, for instance, in the *Bhagavad-Gītā (VI.8) to designate the perfected *adept and elsewhere (XV.16) to refer to the "imperishable" (*akshara) dimension of existence.

kutīra ("hut") is a *yogin's hermitage. The *Gheranda-Samhitā (V.5ff.) supplies the following details for its construction: One should construct a solitary hut within an enclosed compound in a good location (*desha) in a just, donation-friendly (subhiksha), and conflict-free state. The hut, smeared with cow dung, should be located neither too high nor too low, and it should be free from insects. The compound should include a well or pond. The *Hatha-Yoga-Pradīpikā (I.13) recommends that the hermitage (*matha) should have no windows and only a small door. The *yogin's dwelling is also called *mandira*. See also *āshrama*.

ku-yogin ("bad *yogin") is an unsuccessful practitioner who, according to the *Bhāgavata-Purāna (II.4.14), is unable to attain the *Divine. The *Uddhāva-Gītā (XXIII.29) says of him that he is led astray by the obstacles (*antarāya), other human beings, or even *deities.

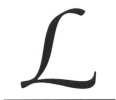

lāghava, lāghutā, or **lāghutva** ("lightness"). The sensation of bodily lightness is one of the by-products of regular and advanced *breath control, especially after rubbing one's sweat (*sveda*) produced by intensive *prānāyāma* into the skin. In the *Gheranda-Samhitā* (I.11), this is the fifth "limb" (*anga*) of the sevenfold path. See also *laghiman*, Levitation, *utthāna*.

laghiman ("levitation") is one of the eight classic paranormal powers (*siddhi*). The *Tattva-Vaishāradī* (III.45) observes that by means of this ability one becomes airborne like the tuft of a reed. The *Mārkandeya-Purāna* (40.31) curiously explains it as "swiftness" (*shīgratva*).

lāghutā. See *lāghava*.

Laghu-Yoga-Vāsishtha was composed by the Kashmiri scholar *Gauda Abhinanda at the beginning of the tenth century A.D., perhaps on the basis of an earlier and no longer extant work. Gauda Abhinanda's composition is generally considered to be an abridgment of the *Yoga-Vāsishtha*, though there are good reasons to assume that the *Laghu* ("Short")-*Yoga-Vāsishtha* is actually an original work that was subsequently cast into the five times larger *Yoga-Vāsishtha* by the same author or another poet-editor. The *Laghu-Yoga-Vāsishtha* comprises six chapters with a total of some six thousand verses. It is presented as the composition of the ancient Sage Vālmīki, the legendary author of the *Rāmāyana*. Vālmīki relates to the seer Bharadvāja a didactic conver-

193

sation that occurred between the God-man *Rāma and the seer *Vashishtha.

As the title of this work indicates, it purports to expound yogic teachings, though its scope is rather more comprehensive, covering not only spiritual and philosophical matters but also cosmology. The general slant of the *Laghu-Yoga-Vāsishtha* is toward the *Yoga of wisdom (*jnāna-yoga). Its metaphysical basis is *Vedāntic nondualism, with a prominent ingredient of *Shaktism. Thus, the supreme *Reality is presented (III.7.1) as possessing all potencies (*shakti). Its aspects are said to be the "power of awareness" (*cit-shakti), the "power of motility" (spanda-shakti), the "power of fluidity" (drava-shakti), and the "power of voidness" (shūnya-shakti).

The ultimate *Reality is pure, omniscient, omnipresent Consciousness (*cit, *citta). It is described (VI.53.24) as follows: "Like the chest of a stone [sculpture], which is void inside and void outside, [the *Absolute] is tranquil, lucid as the vault of the sky, neither visible nor beyond vision."

The phenomenal world is like a dream appearing in the vast expanse of pure Awareness, or *Consciousness. Only the unenlightened being deems it to be external to itself. The human *mind alone creates the illusion of *bondage and the illusion of the process of *liberation. What is to be realized is that ultimately nothing ever happens and that there is simply eternal, objectless *bliss. This extreme idealistic metaphysics has inspired many *Vedānta teachers, including some of the composers of the *Yoga-Upanishads.

laghv-āhāra ("scant diet") is sometimes regarded as one of the component disciplines of self-restraint (*niyama). The *Yoga-Tattva-Upanishad (28) even considers it to be the most important practice of moral discipline (*yama). According to the *Mandala-Brāhmana-Upanishad (I.2.2), a light diet keeps the "defects" (*dosha) in check. See also āhāra, mita-āhāra; cf. atyāhāra.

lajjā ("shame") is occasionally listed among the "defects" (*dosha).

lakshana ("characteristic," "sign"). In the *Yoga-Sūtra (III.13), this word has a technical meaning, signifying an object's specific mode of existence. See also parināma.

lakshya ("perceivable object," "vision"). In *tāraka-yoga, this denotes a meditative visionary state marked by an intense experience of *light. Three variations of this state are distinguished: "inner vision" (*antar-

lakshya), "external vision" (**bahir-lakshya*), and "intermediate vision" (**madhya-lakshya*).

Lakulīsha ("Lord of the Club"), also called Lakuli and Nakulīsha, is the reputed founder of the *Pāshupata sect, whose distinguishing mark is the club (*lakula*) carried by all members. He is remembered to have had four main disciples and to have been seated on an "altar of ashes" when instructing his followers. He lived probably in the first century A.D. and was soon deified.

lalanā-cakra ("carressing wheel") is a psychic center situated in the *head near the uvula. It is also known as *tālu-cakra*. Its curious name is probably explained by the yogic practice of tonguing the *palate or, more specificially, the uvula in order to stimulate the flow of the lunar *nectar. *Lalanā* is also one of the esoteric designations of the *idā-nādī*.

Lallā, a fourteenth-century female *adept of Kashmiri *Shaivism, was a practitioner of *laya-yoga*. In one of her wonderfully poetic sayings she mentions that she was called Lallā (Sanskrit *lalāsa*) because she was ever "desirous" of knowing *Reality.

lambikā-yoga ("Yoga of the hanger"). The *lambikā* ("hanger") is the uvula, which is also called "royal tooth" (**rāja-danta*). This anatomical part carries special significance in *hatha-yoga*. As the *Goraksha-Paddhati* (II.48) explains:

> When the tongue constantly "kisses" the tip of the uvula, [thereby causing] the liquid (*rasa*) to flow—[which may taste] salty, pungent, sour, or like milk, honey, or ghee—this leads to the cure of *diseases, prevents aging, immunity to weapons that are hurled [at one's person]. That [*yogin* who has mastered this practice] will [enjoy] *immortality and the acquisition of the eight "excellences" (**guna*) and obtain the ultimate *perfection.

This technique is part of the *khecarī-mudrā*.

Languor. See *ālasya, styāna, tandrā*.

laulikī ("rolling") is a synonym for *naulī*.

laulya ("fickleness") is, according to the *Hatha-Yoga-Pradīpikā* (I.15), one of the factors detrimental to success in *Yoga. Cf. *dhairya, dhriti*.

Law. See *dharma, sanātana-dharma*.

laya ("dissolution, absorption"). The *Agni-Purāna* (368.1ff.) distinguishes between four types of dissolution: (1) *nitya-laya*, or the "daily death" of millions of beings; (2) *naimittika-laya*, or the "incidental dissolution" of all beings into the *Absolute; (3) *prākrita-laya*, or the "material dissolution" of everything at the end of a world-period, that is, after a cycle of four thousand eons (*yuga*); (4) *ātyantika-laya*, or the "ultimate dissolution" of the individual psyche (*jīva*) into the Absolute.

In *hatha-yoga*, the term *laya* signifies the immersion or absorption of *attention into *Reality by means of the practice of enstasy (*samādhi*). Occasionally, the term *laya* is employed as a synonym for *samādhi*. The *Hatha-Yoga-Pradīpikā* (IV.34) has this relevant stanza: "They say: 'Dissolution, dissolution.' But what is the nature of dissolution? Dissolution is the nonremembering of things due to the nonarising of previous [subliminal] traits (*vāsanā*) [in the condition of *enstasy]."

The same scripture (IV.66) speaks of *Adinātha, the primal God *Shiva, as having taught a crore and a quarter of ways to achieve *laya*. However, it recommends particularly the "cultivation of the [inner] sound" (*nāda-anusandhāna*). By contrast, the *Tejo-Bindu-Upanishad* (I.41) cites *laya* as one of the nine obstacles (*vighna*) of *Yoga. Here the word is probably used in the sense of "inertia."

laya-yoga ("Yoga of [meditative] absorption") is generally used in a broad manner to describe various *Tantric meditation approaches that seek to dissolve the conditional *mind,

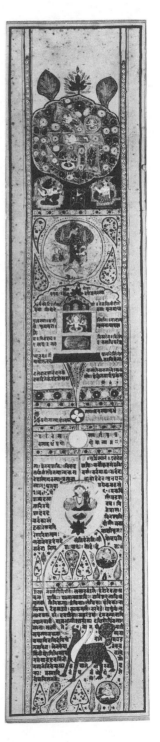

33. The higher psychoenergetic centers (cakra) according to the opening section of a scroll from Kashmir.

often through such means as *breath control and "seals" (*mudrā).
Thus in the *Amaraugha-Prabodha (27f.), for example, laya-yoga is said to
be for the middling practitioner and to consist of the *contemplation of
the *nectar of immortality in one's *body. This involves visualizing God
*Shiva in his brilliant phallic (*linga) form in the *kāma-rūpa at the base
of the spine. After six months, the text assures the reader, one comes
to enjoy powers (*siddhi) and longevity for up to three hundred years.

The *Yoga-Bīja (142) defines laya-yoga as the "identity (aikya) of 'field'
(*kshetra) and 'field knower' is designated as the Yoga of absorption."
The text (143) continues:

> Upon realizing that identity, o Goddess, the mind dissolves. When
> the [condition of] laya-yoga ensues, the life force (pavana) becomes
> stable. Owing to [that condition of] absorption, one reaches *happi-
> ness, the bliss (*ānanda) within oneself, the transcendental state.

Laziness. See ālasya, styāna, tandrā.

Levitation. See ākāsha-gamana, bhū-cara-siddhi, khecaratva, lāghava, mano-
gati, utkrānti, utthāna.

Liberated posture. See mukta-āsana.

Liberation. See apavarga, jīvan-mukti, kaivalya, moksha, mukti, videha-
mukti.

Life force. See prāna.

Light. "Radiance (*prakāsha) alone is eternal," declares the anonymous
author of the *Pāshupata-Brāhmana-Upanishad (II.21), thus reitering an
ancient and worldwide mystical intuition. The *Chāndogya-Upanishad
(III.13.7f.) has this memorable passage:

> Now, the light (*jyotis) that shines beyond the *heavens, upon the
> backs of all, upon the backs of everything, higher than the highest—
> verily, that is the same as this light that is here within the person. It
> is visible . . .
>
> . . . when one perceives [its] warmth in this *body. It is audible when
> one closes one's ears and hears a kind of sound as of a bee, a bull, or
> a blazing fire. One should reverence that visible and audible light. He
> who knows this, he who knows this becomes one beautiful to see,
> one heard of in renown.

The transcendental *Self is luminous, and its experience is vividly described in countless scriptures as being of a blinding light.

Luminosity is in fact a characteristic of many spiritual or inner states. It is an attribute of the life force (*prāna), the various psycho-energetic centers (*cakra), and not least the "serpent power" (*kundalinī-shakti), the great agent of transformation according to *Tantrism. See also tāraka-yoga.

Lightness. See lāghava, Levitation.

līlā ("play"). Some nondualist schools of *Hinduism view the world as a purely spontaneous, arbitrary creation or divine *play. Specifically, līlā refers to the love play of the God-man *Krishna culminating in the nocturnal dance, the *rasa-līlā, in which *Krishna multiplied himself so that each shepherdess (*gopī) thought she alone had his full attention. By contrast, the *dance of God *Shiva, as "king of dance" (*nata-rāja), is one of destruction.

linga ("mark"). In the *Sāmkhya tradition, this term refers "that which has characteristics," namely the human personality, consisting of the higher mind (called *buddhi), the "I-maker" (*ahamkāra), the lower mind (called *manas), the five cognitive senses (*jnāna-indriya) and the five conative senses (*karma-indriya).

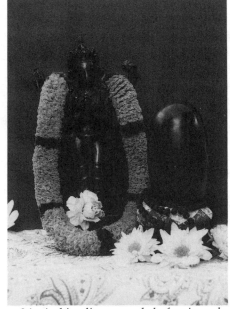

The *Maitrāyanīya-Upanishad (VI.10) applies the term linga to the entire creation extending from the first principle (called *mahat) to the "particulars" (*vishesha). It contrasts this with the linga "without foundation," which is the un-thinkable *Reality itself. In the *Mahābhārata epic (XII.195.15), the linga is the vehicle, or body, of the transmigrating psyche.

34. A shiva-linga, symbol of universal creativity.

The term linga can also denote the phallus or, by extension, the cosmic principle of creativity. The worship of the *Divine through the symbol of a phallus dates back to the *Indus civilization. Early on,

God Shiva became associated with the symbol of the *linga* and its *worship. It is the God's most common emblem. The *Lingāyatas, a branch of *Shaivism, wear a miniature *linga* as an amulet. Metaphysically, the *linga* stands for the unimaginable potency or power of creativity prior to the *creation of the world. In his *Tantra-Āloka* (V.54), the great scholar and adept *Abhinava Gupta explains the word as follows: "This whole [universe] is dissolved (*līnam*) in that, and this whole [universe] is perceived (*gamyate*) as residing within that."

The *Amaraugha-Prabodha* (55) offers this etymological definition: "Where the movable and immovable dissolves by force of *laya*, that is [known as] *linga*."

By the occult law of correspondence "as above, so below," the cosmic *linga* also has its representation within the human *body. Thus the scriptures of *Tantrism and *hatha-yoga* describe experiences involving a radiant *linga* that can be seen in different psychic centers of the body. For instance, the *Brahma-Upanishad* (80) speaks of three types of *linga* that should be made the object of one's *meditation: (1) the *adho-* ("lower") *linga* at the base of the spine; (2) the *shikhin-* ("crest") *linga* at the upper terminal of the central channel (*sushumnā-nādī*); (3) the *jyotir-* ("light") *linga* situated in the psychoenergetic center of the forehead. The *Siddha-Siddhānta-Paddhati* (II.4) mentions a *linga*-shaped flame in the *heart. Cf. *yoni*.

linga-cakra ("phallus wheel"), also known as *linga-sthāna* ("place of the phallus") is a rare synonym for *svādhishthāna-cakra*.

linga-mātra ("pure sign"). In *Classical Yoga, this is the level of cosmic manifestation prior to the emergence of specific *objects. The *Tattva-Vaishāradī* (I.45) also styles this the "great principle" (*mahat-tattva*), and *Vyāsa, in his *Yoga-Bhāshya* (II.19) speaks of it as "mere being" (*sattā-mātra*).

Linga-Purāna is one of the eighteen principal *Purānas. It belongs to the tradition of *Shaivism and discusses *Yoga in many chapters (especially chapters 7–9 and 88) from the perspective of the *Pāshupata school. The text describes the eightfold *path (*ashta-anga-yoga*), and furnishes long lists of obstacles (*vighna*) and omens (*arishta*).

linga-sharīra ("body of characteristics"). According to the *Sāmkhya tradition, this *body consists of the constituent parts of the subtle vehicle called *linga*, with the addition of the sensory potentials (*tanmātra*). This complex is also known as the "subtle body" (*sūkshma-

sharīra) and is contrasted with the "gross body" (*sthūla-sharīra*), the physical organism composed of the material elements (*bhūta*). The gross body in itself is thought to be insentient. It becomes animated when it is linked with the *linga-sharīra*, which is the entity that transmigrates by sheer force of the individual's *karma*. See also *citta-sharīra*, *deha*.

Lingāyata sect. The followers of this cult, which originated in the twelfth century A.D., are also known as Vīra-Shaivas. The founder, or reorganizer, of this moderate religious school within *Shaivisim was Basava or Basavanna (A.D. 1106–1167). The name "Lingāyata" derives from the custom of worshipping *Shiva in the form of the phallus (*linga*), a symbol of creativity. One of the doctrinal innovations of this tradition is the idea of the "six regions" (*shat-sthāla*).

lobha ("greed") is one of the principal "defects" (*dosha*), which must be checked through the constant practice of "nongrasping" (*aparigraha*).

Lock. See *bandha*.

Locust posture. See *shalabha-āsana*.

loka ("realm"). The word, which is derived from the verbal root *ruc/ loc* ("to shine, be bright, visible"), signifies a dimension of cosmic existence. According to *Hindu cosmography, there are seven major realms, each corresponding to a specific state of *consciousness. See also Cosmos.

loka-samgraha ("world gathering"). This compound is found in the *Bhagavad-Gītā* (III.20; 25), where it stands for the ideal of "bringing together," or harmonizing, the world. This goal is proposed as an incentive for righteous or lawful (*dharma*) *action, and it counterbalances the simultaneous demand in *karma-yoga* for "equal-mindedness" (*sama-buddhi*), or the yogic virtue of regarding everything with inspired indifference. See also *sarva-bhūta-hita*, *para-artha-ihā*.

Lotus posture. See *padma-āsana*.

Love. See *bhakti*, *pranidhāna*, *prapatti*.

Lust. See *kāma*.

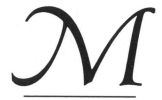

Macrocosm. See *brahma-anda*; cf. Microcosm, *pinda-anda*.

mada ("pride") is sometimes listed as one of the "defects" (**dosha*). This word can also mean "exhilaration" or "intoxication."

mādhu-bhūmika ("he who is on the honey level"). The **Yoga-Bhāshya* (III.51) explains that a **yogin* who has attained to the experience of the "truth-bearing wisdom" (**ritam-bhara-prajnā*) at the highest level of conscious enstasy (**samprajnāta-samādhi*) is known as a *mādhu-bhūmika*. It is this type of practitioner who is tempted by higher beings and who therefore needs to fix his **mind firmly on the goal of "aloneness" (**kaivalya*). This temptation is referred to in the **Yoga-Sūtra* (III.51), which speaks of "high-placed beings" (*sthānin*). Cf. *atikrānta-bhāvanīya, prajnā-jyotis, prathama-kalpika*.

mādhu-vidyā ("honey doctrine") is an ancient teaching expounded in the **Brihad-Āranyaka-Upanishad* (II.5.1ff.). Here honey stands for the nourishing essence of a thing. The underlying idea is that all things participate in the transcendental **Self* (**atman*), which holds together the entire **cosmos. Thus the elements, the sun, lightning, space, and so on have the quality of nutrient honey because of that fundamental **Being. According to the **Tattva-Vaishāradī* (III.54), *mādhu* is the "truth-bearing wisdom" (**ritam-bhara-prajnā*).

mādhurya ("graciousness") is sometimes counted among the practices of moral discipline (**yama*). See also *mārdava*.

201

madhya-lakshya ("middle vision" or "intermediate sign") is one of three types of visionary experience (*lakshya) in *tāraka-yoga. The *Advaya-Tāraka-Upanishad (7) describes it as the experience of different-colored *light leading to the experience of the five types of luminous "ether-space" (*ākāsha). Cf. antar-lakshya, bahir-lakshya.

madhya-mārga ("middle path") is a synonym for *sushumnā-nādī.

Magaradhvāja Yogi 700 is the curious name of a *yogin found on various inscriptions. The figure 700 apparently refers to the number of his disciples. This prominent *adept of *Shavism lived in the twelfth century A.D.

Magic, called abhicāra, indra-jāla, or *māyā in Sanskrit, is the occult art of influencing one's environment through practices and rites that are based on laws other than the causal laws accepted by the rational *mind. The tradition of *Yoga harbors many magical elements, and throughout the centuries the *yogins have not only been celebrated as masters of their own selves but have also been feared as possessors of extraordinary powers. In fact, the word for spiritual perfection and paranormal power is the same in Sanskrit—*siddhi. The tradition of asceticism (*tapas), which is one of the historical tributaries to Yoga, is essentially a form of magic, since it is based on the direct or indirect coercion of invisible beings, often the deities (*deva) themselves. Magical features are especially prominent in the schools of *Tantrism. However, aspirants are frequently warned against the use of magical powers for selfish ends, yet there are also numerous stories of *yogins who have fallen from *grace precisely because they failed to heed such warnings. See also Alchemy, Occultism.

mahā-ātman ("great self"), often written mahātma, refers to a holy person, a "great soul" such as Gandhi. In philosophical contexts, the term stands for the ultimate *Reality.

mahā-bandha ("great lock") is described in the *Hatha-Yoga-Pradīpikā (III.19ff.) thus: One should place the left foot at the perineum (*yoni) and the right foot on the left thigh. After inhaling, one should press the chin firmly against the chest, contract the anal sphincter, and fix the *mind on the central conduit (*sushumnā-nādī) of the *life force. One should retain the *breath for as long as possible and then exhale gently. This procedure is to be repeated with the right foot placed against the perineum (*yoni). Some authorities specify that one should

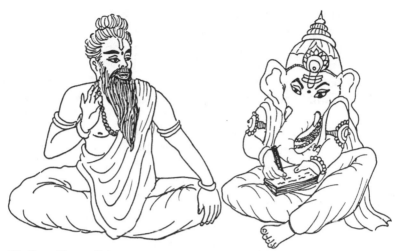

35. *Sage Vyāsa dictating the Mahābhārata epic to God Ganesha, who alone could memorize the sage's words.*

not perform the throat lock (called *kantha-bandha* or **jālandhara-bandha*) but simply block the air flow by performing the "tongue lock" (*jihvā-bandha*). This is done by pressing the tongue against the front teeth. The **Shiva-Samhitā* (IV.21f.) further explains that one should force the **apāna* upward and the **prāna* downward. This technique is thought to invigorate and rejuvenate the *body, strengthen the bones, gladden the *heart, and, most importantly, force the life energy into the central channel (**sushumnā-nādī*), which ultimately awakens the "serpent power" (**kundalinī-shakti*).

Mahābhārata ("Great [Story of] the Bharatas") is one of India's two national epics, the other being the **Rāmāyana*. Even though the *Rāmāyana* has many stories of ascetics (**tapasvin*), it contains virtually no yogic elements. The *Mahābhārata*, however, is replete with references to *Yoga and *Sāmkhya. It is an important document for the schools of *Pre-Classical Yoga. Three didactic passages are of special significance—the **Bhagavad-Gītā*, the **Moksha-Dharma*, and the **Anugītā*.

maha-bhūta ("great element") refers to the five coarse material elements (**bhūta*).

maha-mudrā ("great seal") is explained in the **Gheranda-Samhitā* (III.6f.) as follows: One should press the left heel against the buttocks, while stretching the right leg and catching hold of one's toes. Then one should contract the throat and gaze at the spot between the eyebrows. The practice is repeated with the left leg extended. This technique is said to cure all *diseases, particularly consumption, hemorrhoids, and indigestion. The *Shiva-Samhitā (IV.16) states that one should press the left heel against the perineum (*yoni). In modern texts, this is also known as the "half back-to-front posture" (ardha-pashcima-uttāna-āsana).

The *Goraksha-Paddhati (I.76) defines the mahā-mudrā as the purification (*shodhana) of the entire network of channels (*nādī), the drying up (shoshana) of the liquids (*rasa) of the body. This work also states (I.60) that this technique can transmute the deadliest poison into nectar. The *Hatha-Yoga-Pradīpikā (III.18) claims that this *mudrā awakens the "serpent power" (*kundalinī-shakti). See also nabho-mundra.

mahān or **mahat** ("great one") is a synonym for *buddhi.

Mahānirvāna-Tantra ("Treatise on the Great Extinction") is a widely esteemed *Tantra dating from the eleventh century A.D. It is a comprehensive work and has been called "the most important Hindu Tantra" (Agehananda Bharati, 1965). It contains fourteen chapters that carefully describe the various ritual practices such as the *purification of the location, invocation and worship of one's chosen *deity, *mantra recitation, the left-handed rite of the "five M's" (*panca-ma-kara), and so on. It also contains valuable *kaula lore, which (XIV.179) is considered superior to any other teaching. In XIV.123, this Tantra defines *Yoga as the "union of the psyche (*jīva) with the transcendental *Self," and states that he who has realized the *Absolute transcends both Yoga and worship (*pūjā).

maha-rajas ("great *rajas) is the female form of seminal liquid (*bindu), identified as both menstrual blood and vaginal excretion. It is said to be of red color, which is captured in the word *rajas.

mahārshi ("great seer") is derived from mahā and rishi. It is a title of respect for an *adept.

maha-siddha ("great adept"). Northern *Tantrism knows of eighty-four mahā-siddhas who have realized perfection (*siddhi), or *enlightenment, and who also possess all the various paranormal powers (*siddhi). See also Adept, siddha.

maha-siddhi ("great power") is, according to the *Yoga-Tattva-Upanishad* (76), *liberation itself. See also *siddhi*.

maha-sukha ("great joy") is the supreme *bliss, or perfect delight, that is realized upon *enlightenment. This term is at home particularly in the *Sahajiyā movement, which teaches the ultimate identity of the transcendental *Reality with the immanent reality. Cf. Pleasure.

Mahā-Upanishad is one of the *Samnyāsa-Upanishads, which deal with *renunciation. It defines (V.42) *Yoga as the "pacification of the *mind" and mentions (V.22) that there are seven levels (*bhūmi) of yogic development.

Mahā-Vākya-Upanishad ("Upanishad of the Great Saying") is one of the *Yoga-Upanishads. It consists of only twelve stanzas and recommends the practice of recitation (*japa) of the *hamsa. It states that in order to acquire supreme wisdom (*vijnāna), one must abandon both the "eye of knowledge" (*vidyā-cakshus*), which leads to *liberation, and the "eye of nescience" (*avidyā-cakshus*), which leads to *bondage. The highest *realization is said to have nothing to do with enstasy (*samādhi) or the powers (*siddhi) of *Yoga, or even with the mind's dissolution (*mano-laya). It is simply flawless identity (*aikya*) with the *Absolute.

maha-vedha ("great piercer") is described in the *Hatha-Yoga-Pradīpikā* (III.26ff.) as follows: Practicing the "great lock" (*mahā-bandha), one should inhale and then apply the "throat seal" (*kantha-mudrā*), that is, *jālandhara-bandha. One should repeatedly raise oneself slightly off the ground and allow the buttocks to drop back down. This is thought to force the life energy (*prāna) into the central channel (*sushumnā-nādī). As is clear from the *Shiva-Samhitā* (IV.24), this practice is known as the "piercer" because it forces the concentrated *prāna to pierce through the three "knots" (*granthi). The *Gheranda-Samhitā* (III.21ff.) states: "As a *woman's beauty, youth, and charms are in vain without a man [to admire them], so too are the 'root-lock' (*mūla-bandha) and the 'great lock' (*mahā-bandha) [useless] without the 'great piercer.' "

maha-vrata ("great vow"). According to the *Yoga-Sūtra* (II.31), the "great vow" consists of the five constituent practices of moral discipline (*yama), which are to be observed at all times and under all circumstances.

mahā-yoga ("great Yoga") consists, according to the *Yoga-Shikhā-Upanishad* (I.129f.), of *mantra-yoga, *laya-yoga, *hatha-yoga, and *rāja-yoga. The texts emphasizes the central importance of *breath control when it states (I.138) that what all these approaches have in common is the "joining" (*samyoga) of the in-breath (*prāna) and the out-breath (*apāna). The phrase *mahā-yoga* is also often used synonymously with *samādhi.

mahiman ("magnification") is one of the eight classic paranormal powers (*siddhi). It is the power of infinite expansion. *Vācaspati Mishra, in his *Tattva-Vaishāradī (III.45), explains it as the ability to become as large as an elephant, a mountain, or a whole town, and so on. However, the *Mani-Prabhā (III.44) defines *mahiman* as "pervasiveness" (*vibhūtva*), which suggests that it is not the physical *body that expands but the "subtle body" (*sūkshma-sharīra), or the *mind.

maithunā ("intercourse"), or ritual sex between consecrated male and female initiates, is a central practice of left-hand *Tantrism. The woman, who is known as "seal" (*mudrā), is for the duration of the rite looked upon as the *Goddess or divine *shakti, whereas the male practitioner is God *Shiva. This sacramental intercourse is the climax of the *panca-tattva ceremony. It generally takes place in a circle (*cakra) of initiates with one's *teacher present. He is usually seated together with his consort in the center of the circle.

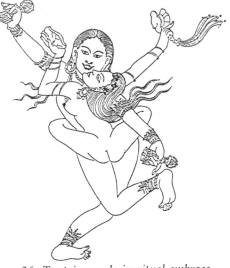

36. *Tantric couple in ritual embrace.*

This is never intended as an occasion for lustful behavior. Rather, the ceremony comes at the end of a prolonged ritual and is essentially a *meditation exercise. Orgasm is generally bypassed through the diffusion of sexual energy throughout the *body. The psychosomatic energy generated through sexual contact is utilized to enhance the initiate's complex visualizations and is transformed into bliss (*ānanda). See also *bindu*, Sexuality.

Maitrāyanīya-Upanishad is a prose scripture belonging to the second or third century B.C. This work, which exists in two recensions and contains numerous interpolations, is the earliest record of a "sixfold Yoga" (*shad-anga-yoga*).

maitrī ("friendliness, friendship") is recognized as a virtue in *Classical Yoga. Together with "compassion" (*karunā*), "gladness" (*muditā*), and "equanimity" (*upekshā*) the projection, or conscious radiation, of friendliness is mentioned in the *Yoga-Sūtra* (I.33) as a means of pacifying the *mind. In *Buddhism, these four virtues are known as the "brahmic stations" (*brahma-vihāra*).

ma-kara ("letter m"). See *panca-ma-kara, panca-tattva*.

makara-āsana ("dolphin posture"). The word *makara* refers to a dangerous marine creature such as a crocodile or shark. However, this posture is widely known in Western *Yoga circles as the dolphin posture. The *Gheranda-Samhitā* (II.4) offer this description: Lying face down with both legs extended and spread-eagled, one should hold the *head with one's hands. According to depictions in modern manuals, the arms form a cradle—hands touching opposite shoulders—in which the forehead is placed. This practice, which is also referred to as the dolphin posture, is said to increase the "bodily *fire," that is, one's metabolism.

mala ("impurity, defilement"). All spiritual traditions are agreed that the ordinary person exists in a state of impurity that prevents the dawning of real wisdom (*jnāna*). The yogic *path can be viewed as a massive attempt at self-purification. Perfect *purity is equated with *liberation. The *Tattva-Vaishāradī* (IV.31) identifies the defilements as the "causes of suffering" (*klesha*) and *karma.

Kashmiri *Shaivism recognizes three fundamental defilements: (1) *ānava-mala*, which is the defilement relating to individuation itself; (2) *māyiya-mala*, or the defilement causing the illusion (*māyā*) that there is an external world populated by a multitude of *objects; (3) *kārma-mala*, or the defilement resulting in motivated *action in that illusory world. All three defilements are coverings surrounding the inherent *light and *bliss of the transcendental *Self. See also *antarāya, dosha, nava-mala*; cf. *shodhana, shuddhi*.

mālā ("garland," "rosary"). Some *yogins use a rosary for their *mantra recitation. Rosaries can be made of a variety of substances, the favorite substance being *rudra-aksha* ("*Rudra's eye")—the dried berries of the tree *Elaeocarpus Ganitrus*. Usually 108 beads are strung together.

manas ("mind") refers generally to the lower mind that deals with organizing the information received from the senses (*indriya). Because of its proximity to sensory functions it is viewed as a sense. In the *Brihad-Āranyaka-Upanishad* (I.5.3), its operational modes are said to be desire (*kāma*), volition (*samkalpa*), doubt (*vicikitsā*), faith (*shraddhā*), lack of faith (*ashraddhā*), resolution (*dhriti*), irresolution (*adhriti*), shame (*hrī*), knowledge (*dhi*), and fear (*bhī*).

The *Yoga scriptures emphasize the volitional and doubting disposition of the *mind. The universal recommendation is that the mind, as the *Shvetāshvatara-Upanishad* (II.9) puts it, should be restrained "like a chariot pulled by unruly horses." The *Laghu-Yoga-Vāsishtha* (VI.9.367), again, compares the mind to a tree that should be cut not merely at the branches but at the root. "The *bliss that arises upon the dissolution of the mind," states the *Maitrāyanīya-Upanishad* (VI.24), "is the Absolute (*brahman)." The same scripture (IV.6) declares that the mind can be either pure or impure, depending on whether or not it is riddled with *desires. According to another stanza (IV.11), when the mind is turned toward sense objects it leads to *bondage, when it is turned away from them, it is the cause of *liberation. The *Hatha-Yoga-Pradīpikā* (IV.26) likens the *manas* to mercury, which is quite unsteady. In verse IV. 29, it is called the "lord" (*nātha) of the senses, whereas the life force (*prāna) is said to be the "lord" of the mind. The connection between the *breath and the mind is one of the great discoveries of Yoga, and much is made of it in *hatha-yoga. See also *buddhi, citta.

manas-cakra ("mind wheel") is an esoteric center of the *body, and is depicted as a white six-petaled lotus in the *head. It is situated above the *ājnā-cakra and is also called *sūrya-mandala* ("solar orb") and *jnāna-netra* ("eye of wisdom"). See also *cakra, jnāna-cakshus*.

mana-unmanī ("mental exaltation"). This phrase is sometimes used in *Tantrism and *hatha-yoga as a synonym for *samādhi ("enstasy"). The *Hatha-Yoga-Pradīpikā* (IV.3) contains this stanza: "When the life force (*prāna) flows in the *sushumnā, the [condition of] *mana-unmanī* is accomplished. Otherwise, the other practices are only an exertion for *yogins." See also *amanaskatā, unmanī*.

mandala ("circle, orb"). In general terms, *mandala* refers to a region, often inside the *body. More specifically, it is a circular arrangement similar to the *yantra* that serves as a tool of *concentration. It contains three principal geometric elements. In the center is the "seed" (*bindu*), representing the point of potentiality of both the *cosmos and the *mind. The surrounding circles represent various levels of existence. They are in turn encompassed by a square with open "gates." Beyond this can be a variety of other elements. In Tibetan *Buddhism, such *mandalas* can be complex pictorial representations. However complicated or simple a *mandala* may be, it always represents consecrated space and is thought to be the body of one's chosen deity (*ishta-devatā*). The *mandala* is used to worship that deity and, through complex visualization practices, to become one with it.

Mandala-Brāhmana-Upanishad is one of the *Yoga-Upanishads. It consists of eighty-nine paragraphs divided into five sections. Sections III–V appear to be an independent text. The teachings of this *Upanishad are linked with the name of *Yājnavalkya. He expounds an eightfold Yoga (*ashta-anga-yoga*), whose component practices differ from *Patanjali's path. Yājnavalkya also speaks of the five "defects" (*dosha*), namely lust (*kāma*), anger (*krodha*), faulty breathing (*nish-vāsa*), fear (*bhaya*), and sleep or drowsiness (*nidrā*). These are conquered by abstention from volition (*samkalpa*), patience (*kshamā*), a scanty diet (*laghv-āhāra*), attentiveness, and the cultivation of the truth. This work also refers to the three visionary experiences (*lakshya*) and the five types of "ether-space" (*ākāsha*) known in *tāraka-yoga. It further mentions three types of gaze (*drishti*) during *meditation. The goal of this *Yoga is "transmindedness" (*amanaskatā*), the condition of "living liberation" (*jīvan-mukti*), also known as "Yoga sleep" (*yoga-nidrā*).

Mandavya is mentioned in the *Tattva-Vaishāradī* (IV.1) as an example of a *yogin* who used potions (*aushadhi*). He is mentioned in many *Purānas, and the *Mahābhārata* (I.107f.) relates an incident in which he was impaled by robbers and kept himself alive through his yogic powers. He was feared for the potency of his curses.

mandira ("dwelling" or "temple"). See *kutīra*.

manduka-āsana ("frog posture"). This posture (*āsana*) is mentioned already in the *Mahābhārata* epic (XII. 292.8). It is inadequately described in the *Gheranda-Samhitā* (II.34) as follows: One should place the (wide apart) knees forward and the feet backward so that the toes touch each other. In other words, the practitioner almost sits on the heels. Cf. *uttāna-manduka-āsana*.

māndukī-mudrā ("frog seal"). According to the *Gheranda-Samhitā* (III.62f.), this practice is done by closing one's mouth and twirling the tongue (like a leaping frog) against the *palate. This stimulates the production of the ambrosial liquid (*amrita*) and prevents *illness and aging. See also *khecarī-mudrā, lambikā-yoga*.

Māndūkya-Kārikā of *Gaudapāda is a verse commentary on the *Māndūkya-Upanishad* of the second or third century B.C. The *Kārikā*, which has a valuable subcommentary by *Shankara, includes an exposition of the "intangible Yoga" (*asparsha-yoga*).

Manikkavācakar (Tamil) is one of the early *Shaiva saints. He lived in the middle of the ninth century A.D. in South India. It appears that at the time of his *renunciation, he was a junior minister of King Varaguna II. His devotional poetry forms the eighth book of the *Tirumurai*, the canon of southern *Shaivism.

manipura-cakra ("wheel of the jeweled city"), also known as *manipuraka*, is the psychoenergetic center (*cakra*) at the *navel. It is generally depicted as a ten-petaled lotus of the color of "rain clouds." According to the *Shat-Cakra-Nirūpana* (19), there is a triangular "region" (*mandala*) of *fire within this *cakra. The center's presiding *adept is *Rudra, the presiding *Goddess is the four-armed, dark-hued Lākinī. The "seed syllable" (*bīja-mantra*) is *ram*, which pertains to the fire element. The *Goraksha-Paddhati* (I.23) fancifully derives the name *mani-pura* from the fact that this is

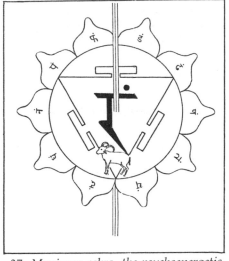

37. *Manipura-cakra, the psychoenergetic center located at the navel.*

also the location of the "bulb" (*kanda*), which is pierced by the central channel (*sushumnā-nādī*) "like a gem by a string."

According to the *Shiva-Samhitā* (V.81), the *yogin who contemplates this esoteric structure not only conquers *disease and *death but also acquires the ability to enter another *body, as well as to make gold, discover medical remedies, and locate hidden treasures. See also *nābhi-cakra*.

Mani-Prabhā ("Jewel Luster") is a sixteenth-century subcommentary on the *Yoga-Bhāshya*, authored by Rāmānanda Sarasvatī.

mano-gati ("mind walk") is the paranormal power (*siddhi*) to go in one's *mind wherever one wishes. See also *ākāsha-gamana*, *khecaratva*.

mano-javitva ("fleetness [as of] the mind") is a paranormal power (*siddhi*) that enables the *adept to move about at the speed of the *mind, that is, instantaneously. It is referred to, for instance, in the *Yoga-Sūtra* (III.48) which states that this ability is acquired in conjunction with complete mastery of the matrix of *Nature.

mano-laya ("dissolution of the mind"). See *laya*.

manomaya-kosha ("sheath composed of mind"). This is one of the five "envelopes" (*kosha*) occluding the *Self. It is otherwise known as the lower mind (*manas*). See also *deha*.

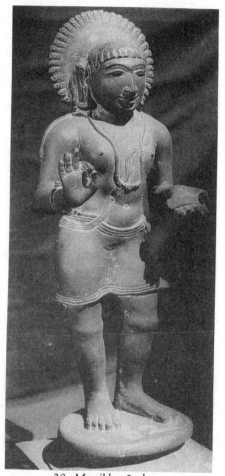

38. Manikkavācakar.

Manthana is mentioned in the *Hatha-Yoga-Pradīpikā* (I.6) as an *adept of *hatha-yoga*. He may be identical with Manthana Bhairava who authored a work on alchemy entitled *Ānanda-Kānda*.

mantra is derived from the verbal root *man* ("to think") and the suffix *tra* suggesting instrumentality. It is thought or intention expressed as *sound. Thus the word *mantra* denotes "prayer," "hymn," "spell," "counsel," and "plan." In yogic contexts, *mantra* stands for numinous phonemes that may or may not have communicable meaning. The **Kula-Arnava-Tantra* (XVII.54) defines it as follows: "A *mantra* is so called because it saves one from all *fear through pondering (**manana*) of the luminous *deity who is of the form of *Reality."

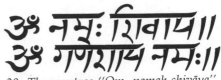

39. The mantras "Om, namah shivāya" and "Om, ganeshāya namah."

However, this is only one of the purposes to which *mantras* are put. They are also frequently employed as simple magical devices to achieve worldly ends.

A *mantra* is a *mantra* by virtue of it having been communicated in an initiatory setting. Thus, even the most famous of all *mantras*, the sacred syllable *om, becomes a *mantra* only when it has been empowered by one's teacher (*guru). Every *mantra* is associated with a particular invisible power, or *deity. Some *mantras*, such as *om*, designate the *Absolute as such.

A *mantra* can consist of a single sound or a string of phonemes that have no apparent meaning. It can also consist of a whole meaningful sentence as in the case of the ancient *gāyatrī-mantra.

Of special significance are the **bīja-* or "seed" *mantras*, which express the quintessence of a *mantra* and of the corresponding *deity. Thus the *bīja-mantra* of *Kālī is *krīm*, of *Shiva *hrīm*, of Mahālakshmī *shrīm*, and so on. See also *nāda, mantra-yoga, shabda.*

Mantra-Mahodadhi ("Ocean of Mantras") is an encyclopedic work on *mantra-yoga, consisting of twenty-five chapters with over 3,300 stanzas. This text was completed in May–June A.D. 1889 by Mahidhara, a renowned commentator on the *Yajur-Veda. He also wrote an auto-commentary called *Naukā* ("Boat").

mantra-shāstra ("teaching on *mantras"), also known as *mantra-vidyā* ("science of *mantras"), is the body of speculations about the numinous potential of human sounds. See also *nāda, shabda.*

mantra-yoga is one of the principal branches of the *Yoga tradition. The **Yoga-Tattva-Upanishad* (21f.) defines it as the recitation (*japa) of various *mantras made up of the "matrices" (*mātrikā), that is, the primary sounds of the Sanskrit alphabet. This discipline, which is said to be suitable for the inferior practitioner who has little insight into spiritual life, should be pursued for twelve years. It gradually leads to wisdom (*jñāna) as well as the classic paranormal powers (*siddhi).

The *Yoga of the recitation of numinous sounds undoubtedly has its roots in the spells of archaic *magic. This is evident from the *Rig-Veda, whose mantras are presented as having magical properties. They were important ingredients of the sacrificial cult. Mantric recitation became an exact and exacting science at the hands of the *brahmins, for the invisible powers have to be worshipped and invoked with precision lest they should turn against the sacrificer.

The practice of mantric recitation is one of the earliest components of *Yoga. Even though mantras retained their original character as magical tools for achieving one's desires in the Yoga tradition, they acquired a new function, namely to aid the *yogin's spiritual maturation. In other words, mantras became instruments of *Self-realization. Mantra-yoga as an independent branch of Yoga is, however, a relatively late development in the long history of Yoga. Its appearance is closely connected with the emergence of *Tantrism. It is treated in numerous scriptures belonging to that cultural movement. There are also a number of works that specifically expound mantra-yoga, notably the encyclopedic *Mantra-Mahodadhi, the *Mantra-Yoga-Samhitā, the Mantra-Mahārnava ("Great Flood of Mantras"), the Mantra-Mukta-Āvali ("Independent Tract on Mantras"), the Mantra-Kaumudī ("Moonlight on Mantras"), and the Tattva-Ānanda-Tarangiṇī ("River of the Bliss of Reality").

According to the *Mantra-Yoga-Samhitā, mantra-yoga has sixteen "limbs" (*anga): (1) *Bhakti, or "devotion," which is threefold—"prescribed devotion" (vaidhi-bhakti) consisting of ceremonial worship, "devotion involving attachment" (rāga-ātmika-bhakti), and "supreme devotion" (para-bhakti); (2) *shuddhi, or "purification," which consists in ritual cleansing of the *body and *mind, the use of a specially consecrated location (*desha) for practice, and facing in the right direction during *recitation; (3) *āsana or "posture"; (4) panca-anga-sevana, or "serving the five limbs," which consists in the daily practice of reading the *Bhagavad-Gītā ("Lord's Song") and the Sahasra-Nāma ("Thousand Names [of the *Divine]"), reciting songs of praise, of protection, and heart opening; (5) *ācara ("conduct"), which is of three kinds, namely "divine" (divya), "left-hand" (*vāma), involving worldly activity, and "right-hand" (*dakshina), involving *renunciation; (6) *dhāranā, or "concentration"; (7) divya-deva-sevana, or "serving the divine space," which consists of sixteen practices that convert a given place into consecrated space (*desha) suitable for mantric *recitation; (8) prāna-kriyā, or "breath ritual," which is the *sacrifice of one's *breath into the *Divine and is accompanied by a number of rites, including the "placing" (*nyāsa*) of the life force (*prāna*) into different parts of the *body; (9) *mudrā*, or "seal," which consists of a variety of hand gestures that focus the mind; (10) *tarpana*, or "satisfaction," which is the practice of offering libations of water to the invisible powers in order to make them favorably disposed; (11) *havana*, or "invocation," which is the calling upon one's chosen deity (*ishta-devatā*) by means of *mantras*; (12) *bali*, "offering," consisting in the giving of gifts of fruit or flowers to one's chosen deity; (13) *yaga*, or "sacrifice," which can be external or internal, the latter being thought superior to the former; (14) *japa*, or "recitation"; (15) *dhyāna*, or "meditation"; (16) *samādhi*, or "enstasy," which is also called the "great condition" (*mahā-bhāva*) in which the *mind dissolves in the *Divine.

It is clear from these practices that *mantra-yoga* is pronouncedly ritualistic, which reflects not only its origins in the sacrificial cult of ancient India but also its *Tantric provenance.

Mantra-Yoga-Samhitā ("Compendium on Mantra-Yoga") is a systematic exposition of *mantra-yoga* comprising 566 stanzas. Its date is unknown, though it can tentatively be assigned to the seventeenth or eighteenth century A.D. The "Yoga of sound" is defined (I.4) thus: "The Yoga that is practiced by means of the support of [the right] disposition (*bhāva*) and sound (*shabda*) and [by means of the support] of the self [composed of] 'name and form' (*nāma-rūpa*), that is called *mantra-yoga*."

This work discusses the qualifications of the teacher (*guru*) and the aspirant (*shishya*), ritual *purification practices, *breath control, projection (*nyāsa*) techniques, various kinds of worship (*pūjā*), and how to determine the right kind of *mantra* for the student by means of a diagram (called *cakra*).

marana-siddhi ("death power") is the paranormal power (*siddhi*), mentioned in the *Kaula-Jnāna-Nirnaya* (IV.14), to kill through mere thought.

mārdava ("gentleness") is sometimes counted among the practices of moral discipline (*yama*). See also *mādhurya*.

mārga ("way"). See *bhakti-mārga*, *nivritti-mārga*, Path, *pravritti-mārga*.

mārga-anurakti ("attachment to the path") is mentioned in the *Mandala-Brāhmana-Upanishad* (I.1.4) as one of the constituent practices of self-restraint (*niyama*). See also *mumukshutva*.

Mārkandeya is a renowned *adept who is mentioned in the *Mahābhārata* epic and in many *Purānas, notably the *Mārkandeya-Purāna*. It is probable that there was more than one sage by this name.

Mārkandeya-Purāna is one of the earliest extant *Purānas. It deals with *Yoga specifically in chapters 36–44, which in the main consist in a long dialogue between *Dattātreya and Alarka. This work prescribes a rather ritualistic life-style for the *yogin*, which in some scriptures of *Post-Classical Yoga is called *kriyā-yoga*.

marman ("joint") refers to a particularly vital spot in the body, reminiscent of acupuncture points. Native Indian medicine knows of 107 such places in the *body, the principal *marman* being the *heart. The *Yoga scriptures generally speak of eighteen *marmans*. Thus the *Shāndilya-Upanishad* (I.8.1f.) names the feet, big toes, ankles, shanks, knees, thighs, anus, penis, *navel, heart, throat, the "well" (*kūpa*) meaning the "throat well" or jugular notch, the palate (*tālu*), *nose, eyes, the middle between the eyebrows (*bhrū-madhya*), forehead, and the *head. According to the *Kshurikā-Upanishad* (14), one should cut through these vital spots by means of the "mind's sharp blade." The underlying practice is to focus *attention and *breath on each *marman* and to free it from tensions so that the life force (*prāna*) can flow freely again.

mātanginī-mudrā ("elephant seal") is described in the *Gheranda-Samhitā* (III.88ff.) thus: Standing up to the neck in water one should draw in the water through both nostrils and expel it again through the mouth. Next, one should suck it up through the mouth and expel it through the *nose. It is said that by regularly repeating this cycle several times one becomes as strong as an elephant.

matha ("hut" or "monastery"). See *āshrama, kutīra*.

mati ("conviction"), which is sometimes regarded as one of the practices of self-restraint (*niyama*), is explained in the *Darshana-Upanishad* (II.11) as "faith" (*shraddhā*) in the *Vedic teachings and avoidance of any doctrines that run counter to the *Vedas.

mātrā ("measure") is a unit of measurement that has traditionally been used to calculate the duration of various exercises, particularly breath control (*prānāyāma*). A *mātrā* is defined in the *Yoga-Cūdāmany-Upanishad* (100) as the time taken by a single breath (*shvāsa*) to occupy the "space" above and below, that is, to fill the lungs. According to the *Yoga-Tattva-Upanishad (40), however, it is the time it takes to snap one's fingers after circling the knee with one's hand. The *Tattva-Vaishāradī (II.50) specifies that the knee must be circled three times to arrive at the correct duration. The *Mārkandeya-Purāna (XXXIX.15) states that a mātrā is the time taken by opening and closing one's eyes.

In earlier works, such as the *Bhagavad-Gītā (II.14), the term mātrā can stand for "matter" or "material *object."

mātrikā-nyāsa ("placing the mothers"). The mātrikās (literally, "little mothers") are the letters of the Sanskrit alphabet, which are the foundation of all *mantras. In depictions of the different "lotuses" (*padma), representing the psychospiritual centers (*cakra) of the *body, the fifty letters of the alphabet are often seen inscribed in the petals. In the ritual of mātrikā-nyāsa, the Sanskrit alphabet is placed in the body of the initiate, thereby empowering him or her with the power of the deity (*devatā). See also nyāsa.

mātsarya ("envy" or "jealousy") is often mentioned as an undesirable character trait that must be overcome. Especially, the practitioner of the left-hand *path (*vāma-marga) of *Tantrism—the "hero" (*vīrya)—must have conquered sexual jealousy, because during the sacred rite of intercourse (*maithunā) his female partner is rarely the same person twice. No *attachment must be formed between the participants of this *Tantric ceremony. A synonym for mātsarya is īrshyā.

matsya-āsana ("fish posture") is described in the *Gheranda-Samhitā (II.21) thus: One should assume the "lotus posture" (*padma-āsana) and then lie back while cradling the *head with one's arms.

Matsyendra ("Lord of Fish"), or Matsyendranātha, who is remembered as one of the eighty-four "great adepts" (*mahā-siddha), probably lived at the beginning of the tenth century A.D. He appears to have been the founder of the Yoginī branch of the *Kaula school of *Tantrism in Assam. In Tibet he is known as Mīnanātha or Luipā (probably a shortened version of Lohipāda ("He Who Hails From the River Lohit in Assam"), and in Nepal he is venerated as the deity Avalokiteshvara. He is traditionally regarded as the first human *teacher of *hatha-yoga and may have been the originator of the *Nātha sect. Matsyendra is said to have had twelve (or twenty-two) disciples, the most famous being *Goraksha. In northern India, there are many legends about him and Goraksha. Matsyendra is credited with the authorship of a number of works, including the old *Kaula-Jnāna-Nirnaya*, which, however, was probably written a century after his time. According to some scholars, *matsyendra* and *goraksha* are titles suggesting specific initiatory levels.

matsyendra-āsana ("Matsyendra's posture") is described in the *Gheranda-Samhitā* (II.22f.) as follows: While sitting one should twist the trunk sideways. One should place the left leg next to the right thigh and the right elbow on the same thigh, holding the chin with the right hand. This position has to be repeated in the other direction. According to the *Hatha-Yoga-Pradīpikā* (I.27), this exercise fans the gastric *fire, cures all *diseases, and awakens the "serpent power" (*kundalinī-shakti*).

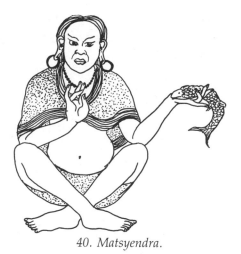

40. Matsyendra.

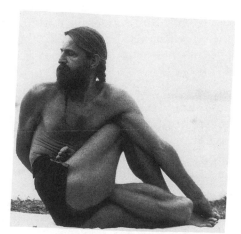

41. Matsyendra-āsana.

mauna ("silence") is the characteristic condition of the *muni, the silent sage. According to the *Bhagavad-Gītā* (XVII.16), *mauna* is an aspect of mental austerity (*tapas*). It is occasionally counted among the constituent practices of moral discipline (*yama) as well as self-restraint (*niyama). The *Yoga-Bhāshya (II.32) distinguishes between *kāshtha-mauna* or "stock-stillness" and *ākāra-mauna* or "formal silence." *Vācaspati Mishra, in his *Tattva-Vaishāradī (II.32), explains the former as the practice of abstaining from signaling one's intentions even by means of gestures, while the latter is simply abstention from speech. In the *Laghu-Yoga-Vāsishtha (IV.5.29), *mauna* is equated with *liberation. However, the *Shiva-Samhitā (V.4) considers it to be one of the possible obstacles (*vighna) on the spiritual *path. Cf. *katthana*.

Mauni, an *adept in the lineage of *Goraksha, is said to have been the *teacher of Vāmanayya, a minister of King Cola who ascended the throne in 1012 A.D.

māyā ("she who measures") is a key concept of the *Vedānta tradition. It is generally translated as "illusion." However, in such early *Yoga and *Sāmkhya scriptures as the *Bhagavad-Gītā (VII.14) and the *Shvetāshvatara-Upanishad (IV.10), the word is used in the sense of "creative power," referring to the three primary constituents (*guna) of *Nature. By the māyā of the "Lord" (*īshvara), states the Gītā (XVIII.61), all beings are whirled about as if they were mounted on a machine.

Only in some radical idealist schools of later *Vedānta did the word acquire the meaning of "illusion" or "phantom existence." For instance, in the *Shiva-Samhitā (I.64), māyā is called the "mother of the universe" (vishva-jananī), the universe being a "play of illusion" (māyā-vilāsitā). More moderate nondualist schools understand maya as "relative existence" rather than "hallucination." It is used in contrast to the absolute *Reality, which is nondual. See also līlā, parināma, sat-kārya-vāda.

mayūra-āsana ("peacock posture") is described in the *Gheranda-Samhitā (II.29f.) thus: Placing one's palms on the ground, one should balance the *body with one's stomach resting on the elbows. Then one should raise one's legs in the air. This is said to stimulate digestion and cure abdominal *diseases.

Medicine. The links between native Indian medicine and *Yoga are manifold. Yoga makes use not only of medical concepts but also has adopted a number of procedures described in the *Āyur-Veda scriptures. Examples are the notion of the different forms of life energy (*prāna), bodily humors (*dhātu), vital areas (*marman), the signs (*arishta) of approaching *death, and *dietary considerations, as well as the use of enemas (*vasti) and sniffing water (*neti). The Yoga tradition has, in turn, influenced the medical authorities both conceptually and technologically. Many *yogins past and present have a background in the healing arts. Thus the members of the *Kānphata order have a considerable reputation in the practice of medicine.

Works that illustrate well the close relationship between Yoga and *Āyur-Veda are the *Mishraka ("Mixture") and the *Sat-Karma-Samgraha, both authored by Cidghanānanda, who probably lived in the eighteenth century. See also Anatomy.

Meditation is the practice of systematically vacating and unifying *con-sciousness. Even though the meditative state is structured differently from the ordinary *waking state, it is nonetheless accompanied by awareness. In fact, it is characterized by an unusual degree of lucidity. See also *dhyāna, jhāna, nididhyāsana*; cf. *samādhi*.

Memory. See *smriti*.

meru is the name of the golden mountain that, according to *Hindu mythology, exists in the center of the earth. It is supposed to be 350,000 miles high and as many miles deep. This mountain serves as the pleasure ground of the *deities of the Hindu pantheon. In *Yoga and *Tantrism, *meru* is a secret term for the central axis of the human *body, the spinal column, and is often also called *meru-danda* ("*meru*-staff"). *Meru* is also the central bead of a rosary (**mala*). See also Cosmos.

Microcosm is known as **pinda-anda* in Sanskrit. This term denotes the human *body, which is born of an egg (*anda*) and which yet contains the entire universe in itself. *Yoga subscribes to the archaic notion that body and *cosmos are structurally homologous. Therefore, the world can be transcended by transcending the body in all its aspects. Cf. Macrocosm.

Meykandar (Tamil) is a famous *adept of the *Shaiva-Siddhānta tra-dition who lived in the mid-thirteenth century A.D. He authored the *Shiva-Jnāna-Bodha* ("Illumination of the Wisdom of *Shiva"), consisting of only twelve verses based on the *Raurava-Āgama*. This is the first Tamil attempt at a systematic exposition of the theological doctrines of Southern *Shaivism. Meykandar had forty-nine disciples.

Mīna is mentioned in the *Hatha-Yoga-Pradīpikā* (I.5) as an early master of *hatha-yoga*. Some traditions identify him with *Matsyendra, and others speak of him as a disciple of *Jālandhari.

Mind. See *buddhi, citta, manas*.

Mishraka ("Mixture") is a work by *Cidghanānanda dealing with *dis-eases due to faults in one's *Yoga practice. See also *Sat-Karma-Samgraha*.

mita-āhāra ("moderate diet") is sometimes considered to be one of the practices of moral discipline (*yama*). The *Hatha-Yoga-Pradīpikā* (I.58) defines it as agreeable and nutritious food that is consumed in order to delight God *Shiva. This work echoes widespread dietary wisdom when it stipulates that one should leave one fourth of the stomach empty. The *Gheranda-Samhitā* (V.16ff.) states: "He who practices *Yoga without moderation in diet incurs various *diseases and obtains no success." See also *āhāra*, *laghv-āhāra*; cf. *atyāhāra*.

Modesty. See *hrī*.

moha ("delusion") is frequently counted among the "defects" (*dosha*). The *Yoga-Vārttika* (II.34) explains it as a mistaken notion, such as the idea that merit accrues from sacrificing animals. The most serious form of *moha* is the self-delusion that one is a limited ego-personality rather than the transcendental *Self.

moksha ("liberation"). In the *Laghu-Yoga-Vāsishtha* (V.9.48), *moksha* is explained as follows: "*Liberation is neither beyond the sky nor in the netherworld, nor on earth. Liberation is said to be the dissolution of the *mind upon the obliteration of all aspirations (*āshā*)." In other words, *liberation is an intrapsychic event, not a locality. It is a shift in *consciousness whereby one transcends all duality. The event of liberation, paradoxically, coincides with the realization that both liberation and *bondage are merely conceptual constructs and hence of no ultimate significance. The *Laghu-Yoga-Vāsishtha* (VI.13.25) puts it this way: "There is neither bondage nor liberation. There is only the *Absolute beyond ill." The same scriptures (VI.13.93) emphatically states: "What is called 'liberation' does not have space, or time, or any other state." See also *apavarga*, *jīvan-mukti*, *kaivalya*, *mukti*, *videha-mukti*.

Moksha-Dharma ("Liberation Doctrine") is a remarkable didactic section in the *Mahābhārata* (XII.168–353), which records teachings of many schools of *Pre-Classical Yoga and *Sāmkhya.

Moon. See *candra*.

Morality is a vital aspect of spiritual life, though it must not be equated with spirituality in general. A moral, or "good" way of life—embodying such values as love, forgiveness, generosity, etc.—is the foundation on which all higher spiritual practice can thrive. Whereas morality prevents the accumulation of further *karmic demerit, or *sin, spiritual practice aims at the transcendence of both good and evil. See also *yama*.

Mrigendra-Tantra is an authoritative scripture of the *Pāshupata tradition which was composed between A.D. 500 and 800. It deals with *Yoga in a special chapter in two apparently independent passages. One passage mentions a yogic *path consisting of the following "limbs" (*anga): *breath control, *sense withdrawal, *concentration, *meditation, "inspection" (*vīkshana), and *enstasy. Yoga itself—as the *angin*, or "possessor of the limbs"—is said to be the eighth component.

mrita-āsana ("corpse posture"), which is also known as *shava-āsana, is described in the *Gheranda-Samhitā (II.19) as follows: One should lie flat on the ground like a corpse. This is said to remedy fatigue and also to quieten an agitated *mind.

mrityu ("death") is sometimes regarded as one of the "defects" (*dosha) of human existence. See also Death, *kāla*.

muditā ("gladness"), or a positive state of *mind, is to be consciously projected. See also *karunā, maitrī, upekshā*.

mudrā ("seal"). This word has a number of different connotations in *Yoga and *Tantrism. Thus, in *hatha-yoga it stands for practices similar to the postures (*āsana). The *Gheranda-Samhitā (III) knows of twenty-five such "seals," which include the "looks" (*bandha) and, curiously, also five concentration practices (*panca-dhārana): *ashvinī-mudrā, *bhujanginī-mudrā, *jālandhara-bandha, *kākī-mudrā, *khecarī-mudrā, *mahā-bandha, *mahā-mudrā, *mahā-vedha, *māndukī-mudrā, *mātangī-mudrā, *mūla-bandha, *nabho-mudrā, *pāshinī-mudrā, *sahajolī-mudrā, *shakti-cālanī-mudrā, *shāmbhavī-mudrā, *tādāgī-mudrā, *uddīyāna-bandha, *vajrolī-mudrā, *viparīta-karanī-mudrā, and *yoni-mudrā, as well as *pārthavī-mudrā, *ambhasī-mudrā, *vāyavī-mudrā, āgneyī-mudrā, and ākāshī-mudrā. All these "seals," the text states, are to be kept secret with great care. They should especially not be taught to a rogue *disciple or one lacking in devotion. These *mudrās* give both "enjoyment" (*bhoga) and "liberation" (*mukti). They have great curative and rejuvenating power and also increase the gastric fire (*jāthara-agni). The *Hatha-Yoga-Pradīpikā (III.8) calls them "divine" (*divya), because they lead to liberation and also produce the classic paranormal abilities (*siddhi) of a liberated being. Another important "seal," which is not named in the *Gheranda-Samhitā, is the *shan-mukhī-mudrā.

The term *mudrā*, moreover, denotes certain hand gestures used during yogic rituals and in the course of the performance of particular postures (**āsana*) and *meditation. In the *Soma-Shāmbhu-Paddhati*, no fewer than thirty-seven hand *mudrās* are described. The best known in yogic circles are **abhaya-mudrā*, *anjali-mudrā* (performed by joining the palms in front of the chest), **cin-mudrā*, **dhyāna-mudrā*, and **jnāna-mudrā*.

In *Tantrism, two further meanings of *mudrā* are current. Here the term can refer to the female participant in the sexual ritual (**maithunā*) as well as to parched grain, one of the five ingredients of the **panca-tattva* rite, which is thought to have aphrodisiacal properties. Finally, the **hatha-yogins* also apply the term *mudrā* to the large earrings worn by members of the **Kānphata* order.

Muktananda, Swami (A.D. 1908–1983) was a great contemporary *adept of **kundalinī-yoga*. A **dis-ciple of Swami Nityananda, he in turn had a large following in India and Western countries, initiating thousands of men and women through direct spiritual transmis-sion (**shakti-pāta*). Among his more prominent American stu-dents was the late "Rudi" (Swami Rudrananda), who taught Swami Chetananda and Franklin Jones (alias Da Free John, alias Da Love-Ananda), who was also initiated by Swami Muktananda himself. Philosophically, Swami Muktan-anda was at home in Kashmiri *Shaivism.

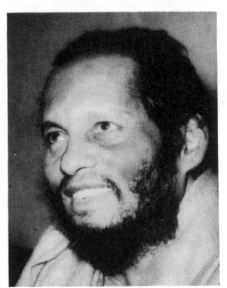

42. *Swami Muktananda.*

mukta-āsana ("liberated posture") is described in the **Gheranda-Samhitā* (II.11): One should place the left heel at the root of the genitals and the right heel above the genitals. The **Yoga-Yājnavalkya* (III.14) gives this alternative: One should place the left ankle above the penis and the right ankle above that.

mukti ("release") is a synonym for *moksha. The *Mārkandeya-Purāna (XXXIX.1) understands it as the operation (*viyoga*) from spiritual *ignorance upon the dawn of true wisdom (**jnāna*) and as one's identity (**aikya*) with the (Absolute and nonidentification with the primary constituents (**guna*) of *Nature. According to the *Shiva-Purāna (IV.41.3), there are four types or degrees of such release: *sālokya-mukti* is release through dwelling in the same space (**loka*) as *God; *sāmnidhya-mukti* is release through proximity to God; *sārūpya-mukti* is release through assuming the same form as God; and *sāyujya-mukti* is release through being perfectly yoked to God. See also *jīvan-mukti, videha-mukti*.

Muktikā-Upanishad is a *Vedānta scripture dating from the late fourteenth century A.D. and consisting of two parts. In the second part, various yogic processes are mentioned.

mūla-bandha ("root lock") is one of the three "locks" (**bandha*) employed in *hatha-yoga. It is described in the *Gheranda-Samhitā (III.14ff.) as follows: One should, with the aid of the left heel placed against the perineum (**yoni*), contract the perineum and carefully press the *navel against the spinal cord. The right heel should be placed against the penis. This technique is said to lead to the mastery of the *breath and bring about the rejuvenation of the *body. According to the *Yoga-Kundaly-Upanishad (I.42ff.), the naturally downward-moving *apāna breath is forced upward by contracting the anal sphincter muscle. The *Hatha-Yoga-Pradīpikā (III.61ff.) notes that the *mūla-bandha* helps the *prāna and *apāna to unite with the *nāda and *bindu. This "lock" is also thought to stimulate the *body's inner *fire and to arouse the dormant "serpent power" (**kundalinī-shakti*). One of the side effects of this practice is the diminution of urine and faeces. The *Tejo-Bindu-Upanishad (I.27) furnishes a symbolic definition, stating that the *mūla-bandha* is that which is the root of all the worlds.

mūlādhāra-cakra ("root-prop wheel") is the lowest of the seven principal psychoenergetic centers (**cakra*) of the *body. Most schools depict this center as a four-petaled lotus situated at the anus or the perineum (**yoni*). The petals are generally described as being of crimson hue. Its "seed syllable" (**bīja-mantra*) is *lam*, which pertains to the *earth element. The center's presiding *adept is Dviranda, and its presiding *Goddess is Dākinī. This center contains the radiant triangle called *kāma-rūpa* ("desire formed") within which is found the golden phallus (*linga*) of *Shiva. This *cakra* is the source of the central channel (*sushumnā-nādī*) of the life force, and the resting place of the "serpent power" (*kundalinī-shakti*). Regular *contemplation of this psychoenergetic center yields, among many other things, the paranormal ability to jump like a frog and, in advanced stages, to actually *levitate.

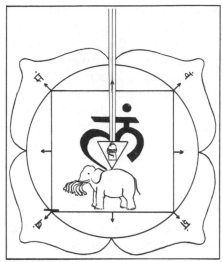

43. *Mūlādhāra-cakra, the psychoenergetic center located at the base of the spine, the seat of the kundalinī-shakti.*

mūla-shodhana ("root cleansing") is one of the four kinds of "washing" (*dhauti*) used in *hatha-yoga. It is described in the *Gheranda-Samhitā* (I.42ff.) thus: So long as the rectum is not properly cleansed, the *apāna* breath does not circulate freely. Hence one should carefully cleanse the rectum with water by means of a stalk of turmeric or one's middle finger. See also *cakrī-karma*.

mumukshutva ("desire for liberation") is a *Vedānta term adopted by some *Yoga authorities. The desire to transcend the ego-personality is an essential prerequisite for spiritual growth. Without it, a person's commitment to the trials of discipline is apt to be weak. On the other hand, however, the desire for *liberation must be free of any neurotic urge to escape the world or oneself. The person aspiring to *liberation is called *mumukshu* as opposed to the "pleasure seeker" (*bubhukshu*). See also *mārga-anurakti*.

muni ("sage") is a word that is etymologically related to *mauna ("silence"). It appears that this designation was originally used in ancient *Vedic times to refer to religious ecstatics outside the circles of orthodox *Brāhmanism. The word is probably related to the Greek term *mania* ("exaltation"). At the time of *Shankara (c. A.D. 800), however, the *muni* was regarded as representing the highest type of spiritual perfection.

In the *Laghu-Yoga-Vāsishtha* (VI.7.3), two types of *muni* are distinguished. The ordinary type is known as *kāshtha-tapasvin* or the "ascetic who stands stock-still." The second, superior type is the *jīvan-mukta,* who, as the name indicates, is *liberated while still embodied. See also *keshin*.

mūrchā ("fainting") can occur during some yogic practices, notably *breath control. According to the *Yoga-Mārtanda* (55), it can be overcome by practicing the *khecarī-mudrā*.

Mūrchā is also the name of one of the eight types of breath retention (*kumbhaka*) described in the *Hatha-Yoga-Pradīpikā*) (II.69): At the end of inhalation, one should firmly practice the "throat lock" (*jālandharabandha*) while exhaling slowly. This is so called because it causes the *mind to swoon into *happiness.

mūrti ("form") usually refers to the visible manifestations of the deities (*devatā*) that are to be worshipped, invoked, or *meditated upon. Often this is an image of the *Divine or one's teacher (*guru*), who is venerated as an embodiment of the transcendental *Reality.

Mysticism. See Yoga.

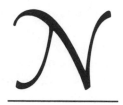

nābhi ("navel") is counted as one of the sensitive areas (**marman*) of the **body.

nābhi-cakra ("navel wheel") is a synonym for **manipura-cakra*. It is the only **cakra* referred to by name in the **Yoga-Sūtra* (III.29), the textbook of **Classical Yoga, which states that by practicing "constraint" (**samyama*) upon this psychoenergetic center, one acquires **knowledge about the body's **anatomy. According to the **Shāndilya-Upanishad* (I.4.6), it is here that the psyche (**jīva*) resides "like a spider in its web."

nābhi-kanda ("navel bulb"). See *kanda*.

nabho-mudrā ("ether/space seal"). The term *nabhas* is a synonym for **ākāsha*. This "seal" (**mudrā*) is described in the **Gheranda-Samhitā* (III.7) as follows: Regardless of the activities one is engaged in, one should always turn the tongue backward against the **palate and restrain one's **breath. This can be called **khecarī-mudrā* in daily life. According to the **Yoga-Cudāmany-Upanishad* (45), however, *nabho-mudrā* is a synonym for **mahā-mudrā*.

nāda ("sound") is a particular kind of sound (**shabda* or **dhvani*). According to the **Yoga-Shikhā-Upanishad* (III.3), it is the second level of manifestation of the "Absolute as sound" (**shabda-brahman*). The *nāda* is the inner sound that becomes audible when the network of psychoenergetic currents (**nādī*) has been duly purified. This sound manifests in a variety of ways. The *Darshana-Upanishad* (VI.36) distinguishes three degrees of it, resembling the sound of a conch, a thunder cloud, and a mountain cataract respectively. The *Nāda-Bindu-Upanishad* (34f.) compares the first degree of sound manifestations to the sound produced by the ocean, a thunder cloud, a kettle drum, or a waterfall. The second degree is said to resemble the sound made by a drum, a big drum, or a bell. The third degree is likened to the sound of a small bell, a bamboo flute, a lute, or a bee. The *Hamsa-Upanishad* (16) speaks of ten modes of the inner sound, the last being called the "sound of the thunder cloud" (*megha-nāda*), which is the only fit focus for *concentration. Certain other phenomena are said to be associated with the different levels of the inner sounds, and they become significant from the fourth level on. In ascending sequence, the phenomena described are as follows: tremor of the *head, the profuse production of the "nectar of immortality" (*amrita*), enjoyment of the ambrosial liquid, the acquisition of secret *knowledge, "higher speech" (*para-vācā*), the ability to make oneself invisible and to see infinitely, and finally identification with the *Absolute. The *Hamsa-Upanishad* (43), furthermore, compares the *nāda* to a snake charmer, since it captivates the fickle mind (*manas*).

The *Hatha-Yoga-Pradīpikā* (III.64) speaks of the union of the *prāna and *apāna with the *nāda* and *bindu. That is to say, through controlled breathing and mental *concentration a conjunction between the out-breath and the in-breath is effected. This occurs in the central channel (*sushumnā-nādī*), and it produces the inner sound. That inner sound, riding on the focused *breath, then proceeds to the *bindu, which is the inaudible aspect of sound, envisioned to exist above the *heart. This work (IV.90ff.) states:

As a bee drinking the nectar cares not for the scent, so the *mind absorbed in the *nāda* does not crave for sense objects.

The sharp hook of the *nāda* effectively curbs the mind, [which is like] a mad elephant, roaming in the garden of the sense objects.

When the mind is bound by the noose of the *nāda* and has discarded [its habitual] restlessness, it reaches full *steadiness, like a bird with clipped wings.

The *nāda* is the snare by which the deer is bound within, and it is the hunter who slays the deer within.

The *nāda* is thought to originate in the center of the spine, which the *Dhyāna-Bindu-Upanishad* (95) calls the "fiddle stick" (*vīnā-danda*). In order to elicit the inner sound more readily, some *yogins* practice what is known as the "six-openings seal" (*shan-mukhī-mudrā*), blocking off the nostrils, eyes, and ears.

The *nāda* is represented in writing as a crescent or semi-circle (*ardha-mātra*) as in the sacred syllable *om*.

nāda-anusandhāna ("cultivation of the [inner] sound"), also called *nāda-upāsana* ("worship through sound"), is of great importance in *hatha-yoga*. According to the *Hatha-Yoga-Pradīpikā* (IV.66), this is the primary means of accomplishing mental absorption (*laya*). This discipline is said to have four stages (*avasthā*).

Nāda-Bindu-Upanishad is one of the *Yoga-Upanishads. This work, consisting of only fifty-three stanzas, expounds a *Vedānta-based *nāda-yoga*. The inner sound (*nāda*) is stated (31ff.) to be the vehicle that will transport the *yogin* beyond the ocean of phenomenal existence; it drowns all external noises and focuses the *mind. The practice of *vaishnavī-mudrā* is recommended. The ultimate goal of this Yoga is *liberation upon the shedding of the physical body.

nāda-sphutatva ("explosion of the [inner] sound") is mentioned in the *Hatha-Yoga-Pradīpikā* (II.78) as one of the signs of *perfection. See also *nāda*.

nāda-yoga is a prominent teaching in the *Yoga-Upanishads. It is indirectly referred to already in the *Maitrāyanīya-Upanishad* (VI.22), which speaks of those who listen to the sound (*shabda*) inside the *heart by placing the thumbs against the ears. The subtle sound that becomes thus audible must not be confused with the thumping of the heart muscle or ringing in the ears.

nādī ("conduit, channel" or "vein, artery") refers both to the blood-carrying veins or arteries and to the channels in or along which the life force (*prāna*) circulates. A more sophisticated interpretation understands the *nādīs* as the flow patterns of the psychosomatic energy. They are also called *hitā* and *sirā*.

Their number is generally affirmed to be 72,000, although, as the *Tri-Shikhi-Brāhmana-Upanishad* (II.76) assures us, they are really countless. The *Shiva-Samhitā* (II.13) claims the existence of 350,000 *nādīs* in all. Some works state that seventy-two *nādīs* are particularly important,

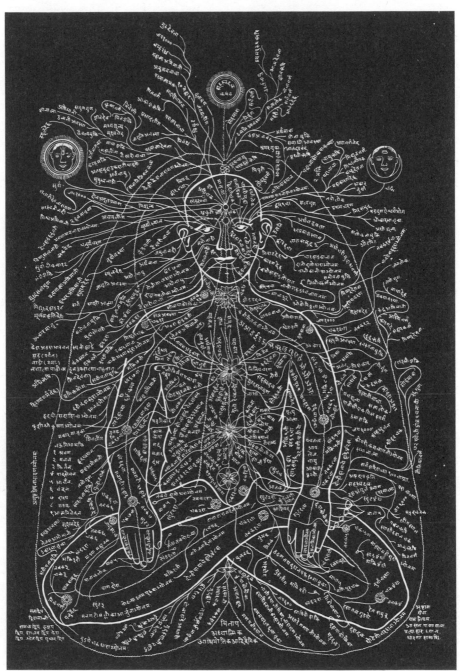

44. *The network of subtle energy conduits (nādī-cakra) that sustain the physical body.*

but most mention only ten, twelve, or fourteen by name. Thus, according to the *Darshana-Upanishad (IV.6ff.), the fourteen major conduits of the life force are: *sushumnā, *idā, *pingalā, *sarasvatī, *pūshā, *varunā, *hasti-jihvā, *yashasvinī, *ālambusā, *kuhū, *vishva-udārā, *payasvinī, *shankhinī, *gāndhārā.

An earlier tradition, recorded in the *Brihad-Āranyaka-Upanishad (IV2.3) and the *Chāndogya-Upanishad (VIII.6.6), speaks of 101 nādīs. The *Katha-Upanishad (VI.16) teaches that one among these 101 channels passes to the crown of the *head and leads to *immortality. This teaching is reiterated in some of the *Yoga-Upanishads. Thus, the *Yoga-Shikhā-Upanishad (VI.5) identifies the nādī extending to the head as para-nādī, which is otherwise known as the *sushumnā-nādī.

Among these multitude of pathways of the *life force, three have special esoteric significance: the central channel, called *sushumnā-nādī, and the two channels that wind around it in helical fashion, which are known as the *idā-nādī and the *pingalā-nādī.

The *Varāha-Upanishad (V.28) describes the twelve main channels as a "multicolored cloth" in the middle of which is the *nābhi-cakra. In the *Shāndilya-Upanishad (I.4.11) and the *Yoga-Yajnavalkya (IV.46), which both acknowledge fourteen principal nādīs, this network of channels is likened to the ashvattha, the sacred fig tree. All the nādīs are said to originate in the "bulb" (*kanda). They are the locus of the psyche (jīva).

The *Laghu-Yoga-Vāsishtha (VI.9.111) states that the nādīs bind the *body like creepers. This, however, is only true so long as they are laden with "impurities" (*mala). In that case, the life force (*prāna) cannot circulate freely in them, and especially it cannot enter the central channel. Hence the *yogin is advised to practice exercises for their *purification. The Shāndilya-Upanishad (I.7.1) promises results after only three months. See also amrita-nādī, nādī-shodhana, rākā-nādī.

nādī-cakra ("wheel of channels") can mean either the entire network of "conduits" (*nādī) of the *life force or the "heart lotus" (hridaya-pundarīka).

nādī-shodhana ("purification of the channels") is an essential prerequisite of advanced breath control (*prānāyāma). The higher breathing practices and techniques for awakening the "serpent power" (*kundalinī-shakti) are dangerous so long as the nādīs have not been thoroughly purified.

According to the *Gheranda-Samhitā (V.36), the purificatory practices are of two basic types, namely samanu and nirmanu. The former is done by means of a "seed" or *bīja-mantra and is really a more advanced *meditation and breathing practice. The latter consists in the six "washing" (*dhauti) practices, which should precede the samanu exercise. For the samanu process, one should assume the "lotus posture" (*padma-āsana), place the teacher (*guru) in one's *heart, and contemplate the "seed" syllable of the wind element, which is yam. This exercise has the following stages: (1) Inhale through the left nostril while repeating the sound yam sixteen times; (2) restrain the *breath for sixty-four repetitions; (3) slowly exhale through the right nostril over a period of thirty-two repetitions; (4) raise the "fire" (*agni) from the region of the *navel toward the *heart; (5) inhale through the right nostril while repeating sixteen times the "seed" syllable of the *fire element, which is ram; (6) retain the breath for sixty-four repetitions; (7) exhale through the left nostril over a period of thirty-two repetitions; (8) contemplate the luminous reflection of the "moon" (*candra) at the tip of the nose, inhale through the left nostril while repeating sixteen times the "seed" syllable tham; (9) retain the breath for sixty-four repetitions while contemplating the "nectar" (*amrita) flowing from the "moon"; (10) exhale through the right nostril while repeating thirty-two times the syllable lam.

According to the *Hatha-Yoga-Pradīpikā (I.39), the nādīs are purified by means of the regular practice of the "adept's posture" (*siddha-āsana), though this scripture (II.7ff.) also recommends a form of alternate breathing. The *Darshana-Upanishad (V.10) stipulates that one should practice alternate breathing while in seclusion three to four times daily for a period of three to four days. See also nādī-shuddhi.

nādī-shuddhi ("purity of the channels") is sometimes used synonymously with *nādī-shodhana, though strictly speaking, it refers to the end state of purity. Among the signs of a purified system of nādīs are bodily lightness (*lāghava), increased glow of the "*fire" in the abdomen, and the manifestation of the inner sound (*nāda). See also cihna.

nāga ("serpent") is one of the secondary types of life force (*prāna). Most texts ascribe to it the function of belching and vomiting. According to the *Siddha-Siddhānta-Paddhati (I.68), it is present in all the limbs and is responsible for motion and discharge.

Nāgojī Bhatta, who is also known as Nāgesha, was one of the great *Hindu scholars of the late sixteenth century A.D. He wrote many original works on *Vedānta and also a larger and a shorter commentary on the *Yoga-Sūtra.

naishkarmya-karman ("trans-action action") is a key concept of *karma-yoga*. First taught in the *Bhagavad-Gītā* (III.4), this doctrine states that a person is not karmically affected by his or her actions if those actions are done in the spirit of *sacrifice. *Naishkarmya-karman* is ego-transcending activity and must be carefully distinguished from mere action (*karman*) and inaction (*akarman*).

Nakulīsha. See Lakulīsha.

nāma-rūpa ("name [and] form") is a *Vedānta phrase that denotes the phenomenal universe, which is a mental construct and hence distinct from *Reality. It is the conventional reality to which Goethe poetically referred as "Schall und Rauch" (sound and smoke). The Ultimate is nameless and formless. See also Name.

Nāmadeva (A.D. 1270–1350) was a contemporary of *Jnānadeva, whose work he continued. Traditional accounts state that in his early life Nāmadeva was a waylayer and that he was brought to his senses by the tears of a *woman whose husband he had killed. After his conversion, he became one of the great spokesmen for the medieval *bhakti movement. He left behind a large number of instructional verses (*abhanga*). See also Ekanātha, Gahinīnātha.

Name. Although most schools of *Hinduism deem the *Divine in itself to be nameless and formless, it has traditionally been worshipped under many names (*nāma*), which are all sacred. In fact, there are compilations known as *Sahasra-Nāma* ("Thousand Names") that are entirely dedicated to listing the many names by which the Divine may be invoked. This is a form of *mantra practice.

Namm, (Tamil), one of the *Ālvārs, is the last and also the most revered of the *Vaishnava poet-saints of South India. He lived probably toward the end of the ninth century A.D. He composed numerous hymns that are part of the *Vaishnava canonical literature and a love poem entitled *Tiru-Virutta*, as well as two other minor works. He has at times been considered as an incarnation (*avatāra*) of God *Vishnu whom he worshipped. His poetry epitomizes the devotional (*bhakti*) approach to *enlightenment.

Nārada. There were probably several individuals by this name, unless we doubt Nārada's historicity altogether, for which there is no stringent reason. A seer Nārada is already mentioned in the *Atharva-Veda*

(V.19.9). He cannot be thought to be identical with the sage who, for instance, figures so prominently in the *Mahābhārata epic and in many of the *Purānas, or with the Nārada who is the author of one of the two extant *Bhakti-Sūtras.

Nārada-Parivrājaka-Upanishad, which was probably composed about A.D. 1200, is the most extensive text of the group of *Samnyāsa-Upanishads. It describes (V.11ff.) six classes of ascetics: kutīcaka, bahūdaka, *hamsa, *parama-hamsa, turiyātīta, and *avadhūta. Only the last two are said to enjoy the "aloneness" (*kaivalya) of the *Self. This work (V.26) decries the value of the disciplines prescribed in *Yoga and *Sāmkhya scriptures, though in chapter VI speaks of the "knower of *Vedānta" (vedānta-vid) as a *yogin. Its Yoga is clearly of the *nondualist variety.

Nāradeva is mentioned in the *Hatha-Yoga-Pradīpikā (I.8) as one of the masters of *hatha-yoga. Nothing is known about him.

nāraka ("pertaining to the human") stands for "hell." References to *hell are found already in the ancient *Rig-Veda (VII.104 etc.), but the first clear picture of what this entails is given in the *Upanishads.

The *Yoga-Bhāshya (III.26), the oldest available commentary on the *Yoga-Sūtra of *Patanjali, reflects popular notions when it speaks of the seven hell realms. These are in ascending order: avīci ("that which is waveless [i.e., static]"), mahā-kāla ("great death/blackness"), ambarīsha ("frying pan"), raurava ("that which pertains to ruru [a demon]"), mahā-raurava ("that which pertains to the great ruru"), kāla-sūtra ("thread of death/blackness"), and andhatāmisra ("thick darkness"). These names are in part explained by the predominant elements that characterize those hellish regions or states of being, namely *earth, *water, *fire, *air, and *ether. In these realms, creatures suffer the consequences of their own misdeeds in other lives. See also Cosmos, pātāla; cf. svarga.

nāraka-dvāra ("gate to hell"). The *Bhagavad-Gītā (XVI.21) speaks of three gates to hell, namely desire (*kāma), anger (*krodha), and greed (*lobha).

Nārāyana ("He Who Is Man's Abode") is one of God *Vishnu's or *Krishna's many names.

Nārāyana Tīrtha was a great *Vedānta scholar who probably lived in the eighteenth century A.D. He wrote two commentaries on the *Yoga-Sūtra, namely the *Sūtra-Artha-Bodhinī and the *Yoga-Siddhānta-Candrikā, in which he interprets *Classical Yoga from a *Vedāntic point of view, drawing especially on the discipline of devotion, or *bhakti-yoga.

nāsa-agra-drishti ("gaze at the tip of the nose") is prescribed for a variety of "postures" (*āsana) and *meditation practices. See also drishti.

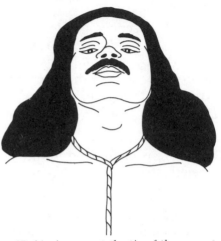

nātha ("lord") is the distinguishing title of *adepts of the *Nātha sect and of members of the *Kānphata order, notably *Matsyendra and *Goraksha.

Nātha sect, or Nāthism, is a teaching lineage within *Shaiva *Tantrism. The origins of Nāthism are obscure. However, it has correctly been described as a particular phase of the *Siddha cult, whose

45. *Yogic gaze at the tip of the nose (nāsa-agra-drishti).*

members aspired to the transubstantiation of the human *body. It was within the Nātha sect that *hatha-yoga came to be developed. Its two most outstanding *adepts are *Matsyendra and his disciple *Goraksha. Northern India knows of a tradition of nine nāthas. Different lists name different individuals. The best known list has the names of Matsyendra-, Goraksha-, *Carpata-, Mangala-, Ghugo-, *Gopi-, Prāna-, Sūrata-, and Cambananātha.

The success of this sect was partly due to the fact that its teachers did not recognize caste barriers, and their teachings were adopted by outcastes and kings alike. In the course of time, the followers of Nāthism became a "casteless" caste of spinners, weavers, and metal workers. See also Kaula sect.

Nāthamuni, who probably lived in the tenth century A.D. in Cola, was the first learned sage of the *Vaishnava tradition of South India. He is said to have been a practitioner of the eightfold *path (*ashta-anga-yoga) and to have often walked about naked, living on food thrown to him. Among the scriptures authored by him is the *Yoga-Rahasya*

This widely traveled teacher had eleven principal disciples. He was the grandfather of *Yamunācārya, *Rāmānuja's teacher.

Nāthism. See Nātha sect.

Nature. See Cosmos, *prakriti*.

naulī, also known as *laulikī* ("rolling"), is described in the *Hatha-Yoga-Pradīpikā* (II.33f.) thus: With the shoulders bent forward one should vigorously rotate the abdominal muscles. This practice, which is one of the "six acts" (*shat-karma*), is said to be the "crown" of *hatha-yoga*, stimulating the gastric *fire and curing all disorders of the bodily *humors.

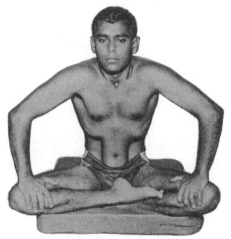

46. Naulī, a curious technique of hatha-yoga.

nava-cakra ("nine wheels"). Some traditions speak of a system of nine psychoenergetic centers (*cakra*), which generally includes the well-known set of seven plus the "palate center" (*tālu-cakra*) and the "ether center" (*ākāsha-* or *vyoma-cakra*), which is part of the *sahasrāra-cakra*.

nava-dvāra ("nine gates") refers to the nine bodily apertures. Thus, the *Mahābhārata* epic (XII.203.35) speaks of the *body as the "virtuous city with nine gates." This notion was already current in ancient *Vedic times. In *Yoga, these nine openings are to be shut "like a tortoise withdraws its limbs," as the *Yoga-Tattva-Upanishad* (141) puts it. See also *dvāra*.

nava-kārana ("nine causes"). According to an abstruse philosophical doctrine expounded in the *Yoga-Bhāshya* (II.28), there are nine types of cause: (1) *utpatti-kārana*, or "generative cause" (e.g., the *mind as the cause of mental processes); (2) *sthiti-kārana*, or "permanent cause" (e.g., the mind whose permanence alone can fulfill the *Self's innate purposiveness); (3) *abhivyakti-kārana*, or "cause of manifestation" (e.g., the Self's continuous apperception of all mental processes creates, for instance, the experience of color); (4) *vikāra-kārana*, or "modifying cause" (e.g., fire is the cause that modifies the food to be cooked); (5) *pratyaya-kārana*, or "cause of presentation" (e.g., the notion of smoke is the cause of the notion of fire); (6) *prāpti-kārana*, or "cause of attainment" (e.g., the performance of *Yoga is the cause of *liberation); (7) *viyoga-kārana*, or "cause of disunion" (e.g., the performance of Yoga is the cause of the Self's disjunction from the impure psyche); (8) *anyatva-kārana*, or "cause of otherness" (e.g., a goldsmith is the cause of the gold's transformation into jewelry); (9) *dhriti-kārana*, or "cause of sustenance" (e.g., the *body is the cause that sustains the senses). See also Causation.

nava-mala ("nine blemishes") is a synonym used in the *Yoga-Bhāshya* (I.3) for the "obstacles" (*antarāya*). See also *mala*.

Nava-Shakti-Shatka ("eight [stanzas] on the Nine Powers") is a short work of two folios ascribed to *Goraksha.

Navel. See *nābhi*.

neti is one of the "six acts" (*shat-karma*) of *hatha-yoga*. According to the *Gheranda-Samhitā* (I.49), this practice is performed by inserting a fine thread nine inches in length into one nostril and pulling it out through the mouth. This is thought to cure disorders of phlegm (*kapha*), improve one's vision, and facilitate the practice of *khecarī-mudrā*. Modern *yogins* use a thin rubber thread (*sūtra*). This practice is also called *sūtra-neti* and

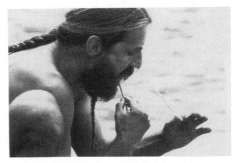

47. Netī, cleansing of the sinuses by means of a rubber thread (sūtra) or water (jala).

distinguished from *jala-neti*, which involves pouring water (*jala*) into one nostril at a time.

neti-neti (composed of *na iti*, "not thus") is a well-known *Upanishadic response to the inquiring student who desires a positive description of the transcendental *Self. Whatever can be said of *Reality is not ultimately true. Descriptions are merely pointers to that which is beyond all mental constructs.

nididhyāsana (derived from the desiderative of the verbal root *dhyai*, "to meditate, contemplate") is a *Vedānta term for, and is similarly defined to, *dhyāna.

nidrā ("sleep") is widely considered one of the great enemies of *Yoga practice and is hence often listed among the "defects" (*dosha). Already the *Mahābhārata (XII.209.1) states that one should abandon it. Elsewhere (XII.263.46) this work lists sleep among such defects as "desire" (*kama), "anger" (*krodha), "greed" (*lobha), and "fear" (*bhaya).

In *Classical Yoga, *sleep is considered to be one of the five "fluctuations" (*vritti) of *consciousness. *Patanjali, in his *Yoga-Sūtra (I.10), defines it as that mental state that is based on the experience (*pratyaya) of the nonoccurrence of other mental phenomena. This means it is a kind of rudimentary awareness. That sleep is not simply the absence of conscious activity is, according to the *Yoga-Bhāshya (I.10), demonstrated by the fact that when one wakes up, one remembers "I have slept well." The *Yoga-Sūtra (I.38) also states that insights derived from sleep can be made a topic of *meditation. A variety of yogic techniques can be used to combat sleep, including *breath control, particularly the *sīt-karī-prānāyāma, and the *khecarī-mudrā. See also Dream, *sushupti*, *svapna*, *yoga-nidrā*.

nidrā-jaya ("conquest of sleep") is listed in the *Siddha-Siddhānta-Paddhati (II.32) as one of the practices of moral discipline (*yama).

nihsangatā ("noncontact, nonattachment") is mentioned in the *Siddha-Siddhānta-Paddhati (II.33) as one of the practices of self-restraint (*niyama). Socializing is typically felt to be detrimental to the *yogin's inner work. The reason for this is that contact with others tends to reinforce *attachment. See also *sanga*.

nirānanda-samāpatti ("coinciding beyond bliss") is a level of enstatic realization—*samādhi—postulated by *Vācaspati Mishra in his *Tattva-Vaishāradī (I.41). It follows upon *sa-ānanda-samāpatti. This stage of the enstatic experience is, however, explicitly denied by *Vijnāna Bhikshu in his *Yoga-Vārttika (I.41).

Niranjana is mentioned in the *Hatha-Yoga-Pradīpikā (I.7) as an *adept of *hatha-yoga. No biographical information is available on him.

nirāsmita-samāpatti ("coinciding beyond 'I-am-ness' ") is proposed by *Vācaspati Mishra in his *Tattva-Vaishāradī (I.41) as the stage following upon *sa-asmitā-samāpatti. It is a form of conscious enstasy (*samprajnāta-samādhi). However, the weighty authority of *Vijnāna Bhikshu, as expressed in his *Yoga-Vārttika (I.41), goes against accepting this enstatic coincidence as a legitimate level in the mystical scale.

nirbīja-samādhi ("seedless enstasy") is *Patanjali's term for that supreme state of *consciousness resulting from the total "restriction" (*nirodha) of all conscious processes. This *enstatic condition is called "seedless" in the *Yoga-Sūtra (I.51) because it transcends the "causes of affliction" (*klesha) in their latent form as "subliminal activators" (*samskāra). According to the *Yoga-Bhāshya (I.18), however, it is to be explained as lacking any objective prop (*ālambana) on which *attention could be fastened. This state is also called supraconscious enstasy (*asamprajnāta-samādhi), but, more accurately, represents the final phase of that elevated enstatic state, namely the *dharma-megha-samādhi.

nirguna ("unqualified") applies to the transcendental *Reality, which eternally abides beyond the qualities (*guna), or primary constituents, of *Nature. The manifest world, by contrast, is said to be "qualified" or saguna.

nirlipta ("nondefilement") is, according to the *Gheranda-Samhitā (I.9), the seventh aspect of the "sevenfold discipline" (*sapta-sādhana). See also shauca.

nirmāna-citta ("created consciousness"). This term is traditionally interpreted in the sense of "artificially created mind." However, it seems to have a more philosophical meaning in the *Yoga-Sūtra (IV.4) where it stands for the "individualized consciousness" that evolves out of the principle (*tattva) of "pure I-am-ness" (*asmitā-mātra). See also citta.

nirmāna-kāya ("created body"). This term is well known in Mahāyāna *Buddhism, where it refers to the earthly *body of the *Buddha. In *Yoga, however, a magical ability (*siddhi) is intended, as is clear from the following stanza of the *Mahābhārata epic (XII.289.26): "O, Bull of Bharata, having obtained power (*bala), the Yoga [follower] should fashion for himself many thousands [of bodies], and he should roam the earth with all of them." The *Tattva-Vaishāradī (III.18) mentions the *adept Avatya as an example of a master who, by means of his yogic powers, created an "artificial" body for himself.

nirodha ("restriction"). In *Classical Yoga, four levels of restricting *consciousness are recognized: (1) *vritti-nirodha*, or "restriction of the fluctuations (*vritti*)," which is achieved by means of meditation (*dhyāna*); (2) *pratyaya-nirodha*, or "restriction of presented ideas (*pratyaya*)," which is accomplished on the level of conscious enstasy (*samprajnāta-samādhi*); (3) *samskāra-nirodha*, or "restriction of subliminal activators (*samskāra*)," which occurs on the level of supraconscious enstasy (*asamprajnāta-samādhi*); (4) *sarva-nirodha*, or "complete restriction," which coincides with the realization of the "cloud of *dharma enstasy" (*dharma-megha-samādhi*).

The term *nirodha* is also sometimes used as a synonym for *kumbhaka*, or breath retention.

nirvāna ("extinction") is a term that is generally associated with *Buddhism, where it refers to the "nonblowing," or cessation, of all *desire—a condition that is synonymous with *enlightenment. However, the term is also employed in some schools of *Yoga. Thus, for instance, already the *Bhagavad-Gītā (II.72) speaks of the *yogin's "extinction in the Absolute" (*brahma-nirvāna*). The *Gita* (VI.19) also has this pertinent stanza: " 'As a lamp standing in a windstill [place] flickers not'—that simile is recalled [when] a *yogin with yoked attention (*citta*) practices the union (*yoga*) of the self [with the transcendental *Self]."

nirvāna-cakra ("wheel of extinction") is a synonym for *sahasrāra-cakra*. The specific location of this psychoenergetic center (*cakra*) is at the upper termination point of the central channel (*sushumnā-nādī*), which is also known as the "brahmic fissure" (*brahma-randhra*).

nirvicāra-samāpatti ("suprareflexive coincidence") is one of the forms of conscious enstasy (*samprajnāta-samādhi*) in *Classical Yoga. This *enstatic state is devoid of the cognitive elements, called "reflexion (*vicāra*), that characterize the condition of "reflexive coincidence" (*savicāra-samāpatti*). It thus corresponds to *nirvitarka-samāpatti* on a higher level. See also *samādhi, samāpatti*.

nirvicāra-vaishāradya ("suprareflexive lucidity") is the culmination of *nirvicāra-samāpatti* and, according to the *Yoga-Sūtra* (I.47), is coterminous with the state of perfect clarity of the inner being known as *adhyātma-prasāda*.

nirvikalpa-samādhi ("formless enstasy") is the *Vedānta equivalent of the supraconscious enstasy (*asamprajnāta-samādhi) in *Classical Yoga. As the *Laghu-Yoga-Vāsishtha (V.10.81) puts it, this state obliterates all the subconscious traits (*vāsanā), leading to *liberation. According to the *Mandala-Brāhmana-Upanishad (V.2), the experience of this *enstatic condition reduces urine, feces, and sleep. See also samādhi; cf. savikalpa-samādhi.

nirvitarka-samāpatti ("supracogitative coincidence") is one of the forms of conscious enstasy (*samprajnāta-samādhi) in which all "cogitation" (*vitarka) has ceased. It follows upon the *enstatic state of "cogitative coincidence" (*savitarka-samāpatti) and is analogous to *nirvicāra-samāpatti. See also samādhi, samāpatti.

nishadana ("seat") is a rare synonym for *āsana ("posture").

nishcaya ("determination") is, according to the *Hatha-Yoga-Pradīpikā I.16), one of the factors conducive to success in *Yoga.

nishkarma-karman. See naishkarmya-karman.

nishpatty-avasthā ("state of maturity") is the fourth and final stage (*avasthā) of the yogic *path. The term nishpatti means "maturity" or "ripeness." The *Varāha-Upanishad (V.75) states that on this level of spiritual accomplishment the *yogin reaps, by means of the "Yoga of spontaneity" (sahaja-yoga), the fruit of "liberation while alive" (*jīvan-mukti). The *Shiva-Samhitā (III.66) notes that spiritual maturity is reached through gradual practice. The *Hatha-Yoga-Pradīpikā (IV.76f.) has these stanzas:

> Having pierced "Rudra's knot" (*rudra-granthi) [situated in the *ājnā-cakra], the *life force reaches the seat of the All [i.e., of the Lord]. Then a flutelike sound or the sound of a lute is heard.

> When the *mind has "become unified" (ekī-bhūta), which is called *rāja-yoga, the *yogin becomes equal to the Lord (*īshvara) in that he is able to create and destroy [whole worlds].

nishvāsa ("[faulty] breathing") is one of the "defects" (*dosha) mentioned in the *Mandala-Brāhmana-Upanishad (II.1). This presumably refers to the shallow, irregular breathing of the ordinary person, which must be corrected through breath control (*prānāyāma). Cf. shvāsa.

Nityanātha is mentioned in the *Hatha-Yoga-Pradīpikā* (I.7) as a master of *hatha-yoga*. He may be identical with the author of a work on *alchemy entitled *Rasa-Ratna-Ākāra*.

nivritti-mārga ("path of cessation"), as opposed to the "path of activity" (*pravritti-mārga*), stands for the spiritual orientation of the *yogin*, who has renounced the world.

Nivrittinātha was the elder brother and teacher of the famous Marathi poet-yogin *Jnānadeva.

niyama ("restraint") is the second "limb" (*anga*) of the eightfold path (*ashta-anga-yoga*), as taught by *Patanjali. According to his *Yoga-Sūtra* (II.32), it has five constituent practices, namely purity (*shauca*), contentment (*samtosha*), asceticism (*tapas*), study (*svādhyāya*), and devotion to the Lord (*īshvara-pranidhāna*). In the *Tri-Shikhi-Brāhmana-Upanishad* (II.29), *niyama* is defined as one's "continuous attachment to the supreme *Reality." This scripture also mentions that *niyama* encompasses the following ten practices: asceticism (*tapas*), contentment (*samtushti*), "affirmation" (*āstikya*) of the *Vedic heritage or of the existence of the *Divine, liberality (*dāna*), adoration (*ārādhana*), "listening to [the scriptures of] *Vedānta" (*vedānta-*shravana*), modesty (*hrī*), conviction (*mati*), recitation (*japa*), and vow (*vrāta*).

The *Uddhāva-Gītā* (XIV.34) furnishes a list of twelve practices, namely bodily and mental purity (*shauca*), which are counted separately, recitation (*japa*), asceticism (*tapas*), sacrifice (*homa*), faith (*shraddhā*), hospitality (*atithya*), worship (*arcanā*), pilgrimage (*tīrtha-atana*), exertion for the good of others (*para-artha-iha*), contentment (*tushti*), and service to one's teacher (*ācārya-sevana*). The *Linga-Purāna* (I.8.29f.) additionally mentions "control over the penis" (*upastha-nigraha*) and fasting (*upavāsa*), bathing (*snāna*), and silence (*mauna*). The *Siddha-Siddhānta-Paddhati* (II.33) adds to the above: living in solitude (*ekānta-vāsa*), noncontact (*nihsangatā*), indifference (*audāsinya*), dispassion (*vairāgya*), and "following the teacher's footsteps" (*guru-carana-avarūdhatva*). Cf. *yama*.

Nonviolence. See *ahimsā*; cf. *himsā*.

nriti ("dance"). Restraint of the life force in the lowest psychoenergetic center of the *body, the *mūlādhāra-cakra*, sometimes leads to spontaneous dancing. See also Dance.

nyāsa ("casting, placing"). In the *Yoga-Sūtra* (III.25), this term is used synonymously with *samyama. It is the focusing of *attention to the point where subject and object merge. In other contexts, especially in *Tantrism, *nyāsa* refers to a variety of rites that are designed to gradually assimilate the *body into the body of one's chosen deity (*ishta-devatā*) or one's *teacher by touching specific parts of the body and reciting empowering *mantras. These rites are usually preceded by the "purification of the elements" (*bhūta-shuddhi*).

The first step in the *nyāsa* ritual is the infusion of the life (*jīva*) of the *deity into one's *body, a process that is called *jīva-nyāsa*. This is followed by "placing" the fifty letters of the Sanskrit alphabet into one's body, which is known as *mātrikā-nyāsa*. Then the practitioner salutes various deities associated with different parts of the body, which is known as *rishi-nyāsa*. Next comes the "placing of the six limbs" (*shad-anga-nyāsa*), which consists of "placing the limbs" (*anga-nyāsa*) and "placing the hands" (*kara-nyāsa*). The former rite is done by touching various places on the *head while reciting specific *mantras. The latter rite consists in assigning *mantras to the various parts of one's hands. Thus, *nyāsa* is an esoteric means of distributing psychospiritual power (*shakti) in the *body and thereby creating a new inner and outer reality for oneself.

Nyāya is one of the six classical systems (*darshana) of *Hinduism. The Nyāya tradition seeks to ascertain truth by means of correct logical procedures or "rules" (*nyāya*). The origins of this school of thought are as yet little known, though there appears to have been a historical connection to the *Yoga tradition. The founder of this school was Gautama, who probably lived during the early post-Christian era and is credited with the authorship of the *Nyāya-Sūtra*.

O

Obedience. See *guru-shushrūshā.*

Object. Whether the world of objects is viewed to be real, as in *Classical Yoga, or illusory, as in most schools of *Vedānta, all traditions of *Hinduism concur that the universe of forms is inferior to the formless *Reality. The reason for this is that forms inevitably undergo change (*parināma), whereas the Formless is eternally stable. For the human being, change implies varying degrees of suffering (*duhkha), and hence only the realization of the unchanging *Being promises abiding *happiness. She also *artha, lakshya, vishaya.*

Observances, moral. See Morality, *yama.*

Obstacles. See *upasarga, vighna;* see also *dosha.*

Occultism. Even the most intellectually sophisticated schools of *Yoga contain elements of *magic or occultism. One may be tempted to view these features as simply being dysfunctional remnants of an earlier, uninformed age. However, any attempt to demythologize Yoga is doomed to failure, because it would involve the obliteration of vital aspects of this ancient tradition.

The new discipline of *parapsychology has so far been too busy defending itself against the consensus opinion of the scientific establishment to proceed much beyond statistical experiments of no ultimate conclusiveness. No overarching model has yet been formulated that could accommodate and satisfactorily interpret all known facts,

243

whether tested or alleged. Until such a model is available, a more appropriate orientation would be to adopt a stance of epistemological humility toward matters that are not immediately intelligible from within the framework of "objective" science. We can, after all, place a certain faith in the fact that Yoga looks back on a much longer *history of experimentation than modern science, and in an area that hitherto science has almost completely ignored—namely the area of our species' higher psychospiritual capacities. See also *siddhi*.

Offering, sacrificial. See *bali*, *dāna*, *karma-yoga*, *pushpa*.

ojas. Derived from the verbal root *vaj* meaning "to be strong," *ojas* denotes "force, strength, vitality." In *Āyur-Veda it is the quintessence of the constituents (*dhātu*) of the *body. Some modern interpreters deem it to be albumen or glycogen, but *yogins* assure us that it is rather a subtle force that is distributed over the entire body and nourishes it incessantly. *Ojas* is the vital principle that is contained or stored in the seven *dhātus*.

The greatest concentration of *ojas* is found in semen (*bindu*, *shukra*), which explains why all traditions recommend, if not total abstention, at least stringent sexual economy. The underlying idea is that the conservation of semen increases the *ojas* store and thus enhances not only one's *health but also the quality of one's *consciousness. See also *brahmacarya*.

om. The sacred monosyllable *om* is the oldest and most venerated of all *Hindu *mantras*, and is also employed in *Buddhism. It is also called the "root"—or *mūla-mantra* and often precedes other *mantras*. The *om*-sound symbolizes the *Divine. The *Maitrāyanīya-Upanishad* (VI.22) refers to it as the sound of the soundless *Absolute. It is by

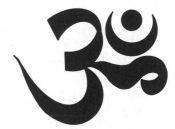

48. *The sacred syllable om.*

means of this numinous sound that the *yogin* focuses his *attention to the point where he can transcend the finite *consciousness in its entirety. The above *Upanishad (VI.24) likens the *body to a bow, the syllable *om* to an arrow, the focused *mind to the arrow's tip, and the ultimate Mystery as the target. This scripture also observes: "Just as a spider climbing up by means of its threads finds open space, so indeed the meditator climbs up by means of *om* and finds autonomy (*svātantrya*)."

The *Māndūkya-Upanishad*, which is entirely dedicated to an analysis of the theology and esotericism of the monosyllable *om*, opens with the following passage:

> *Om!* This syllable (**akshara*) is this whole world. Its further explanation is:
>
> The past, the present, and the future—everything is but the sound *om*.
>
> And whatever else that transcends triple time—that, too, is but the sound *om*.

This same scripture explains that *om* is composed of four parts or "measures" (**mātrā*), namely *a, u, m*, and the *anusvara* represented by a dot placed above the letter *m*, which signifies a nasal humming. These four parts are compared to the four states of consciousness— waking, dreaming, sleeping, and the "fourth" (**turīya*), which is the transcendental *Self beyond the *mind. See also *bindu, caturtha, hamsamantra, nāda, pranava*.

Omens. See *arishta, cihna*.

Omniscience. See *sarva-jnātva*.

One-pointedness. See *ekāgratā*.

Ontology. This philosophical discipline is concerned with *Being and its categories. *Hindu philosophy, including *Yoga, is largely grounded on the ontological conceptions developed in the influential *Sāmkhya tradition. See also *tattva*.

Order. See *dharma*.

oshadhi. See *aushadhi*.

P

pada-artha-bhāvanā-bhūmi ("level of the realization of the essence"). The phrase *pada-artha* means "thing [corresponding to] the word (*pada*)." It signifies the ultlimate *Reality. This realization is one of the seven levels of wisdom (*sapta-jnāna-bhūmi*). It is explained in the *Varāha-Upanishad (IV.2.9) as the "apperception" (*avabodhana*) of the ultimate Reality following the prolonged focusing of the *mind upon that Reality.

Pada-Candrikā ("Moonlight on the Words [of *Patanjali]"). See *Yoga-Sūtra-Artha-Candrikā*.

pada-sevana ("service at the feet [of *God]") is one of the "limbs" of the *Yoga of devotion (*bhakti-yoga*). This is part of the ritual worship of the *Divine installed in the shrine as an image (*mūrti*) or as a symbol, such as the phallus (*linga*).

padma ("lotus") is a synonym for *cakra.

padma-āsana ("lotus posture"), also called *kamala-āsana*, is described in the *Gheranda-Samhitā (II.8) as follows: Placing the right foot on the left thigh and the left foot on the right thigh, one should cross the hands behind the back and catch hold of one's big toes. The chin should be placed on the chest and the *gaze should be fixed on the tip of the nose (*nāsa-agra*). This posture (*āsana*) is said to cure all *diseases. The *Hatha-Yoga-Pradīpikā (I.45f.) gives an alternative version: One should place the feet, soles up, on the opposite thighs and place the hands, palms up, between the thighs. Both versions are commonly recommended for the practice of breath control (*prāṇāyāma*).

Pādukā-Pancaka ("Five [Verses on] the Footstool") is a work of only seven stanzas describing the *meditation on the five esoteric loci of *kundalinī-yoga*, namely the twelve-petaled lotus at the *heart, the triangle in its pericarp, the region of the *nāda and *bindu, the "jewel seat" (*mani-pītha*) within it, the *hamsa below that seat, and the triangle above it.

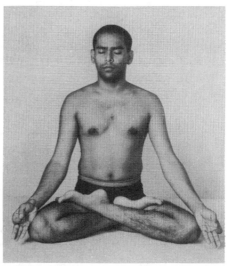

49. Padma-āsana, a favorite meditation posture.

Pain. See *duhkha*; cf. Pleasure.

pakva ("ripe, mature"). In *hatha-yoga*, the ordinary *body is thought to be "immature" or "unbaked" (*apakva*). The purpose of the various practices of this *Yoga is to strengthen the body and help it ripen into a "divine body" (*divya-deha*).

Palate is an important esoteric location (*desha*) of the *body. See also *tālu*.

panca-ākāsha ("five ether/spaces"). See *ākāsha*.

panca-anga-sevana ("serving the five limbs") is a constituent practice of *mantra-yoga*. The five "limbs" (*anga*) of one's chosen deity (*ishta-devatā*) are said to be the daily ritual reading of the *Bhagavad-Gītā and the *Sahasra-Nāma* ("Thousand Names [of *God]"), singing songs of praise, reciting formulates of protection, and the opening of one's *heart.

panca-avasthā ("five states"). See *avasthā*.

panca-bhūta ("five elements"). See *bhūta*.

panca-dasha-anga-yoga ("fifteenfold Yoga"). The *Tejo-Bindu-Upanishad* (I.15ff.) teaches a yogic *path consisting of the following fifteen "limbs" (*anga): (1) moral discipline (*yama); (2) self-restraint (*niyama); (3) "abandonment" (*tyāga); (4) silence (*mauna); (5) "place" (*desha); (6) "time" (*kāla); (7) posture (*āsana); (8) "root lock" (*mūla-bandha); (9) "bodily equilibrium" (deha-samya); (10) steadiness of vision (drik-sthiti); (11) "breath restraint" (prāna-samyamana), which is the same as *prānāyāma; (12) sense withdrawal (*pratyāhāra); (13) concentration (*dhāranā); (14) "meditation on the *Self" (ātma-dhyāna); and (15) enstasy (*samādhi). Most of these practices are interpreted symbolically rather than literally. Cf. *ashta-anga-yoga, sapta-sādhana, shad-anga-yoga*.

panca-dhāranā ("five concentrations") refers to the *Tantric and *hatha-yoga practice of concentration (*dhāranā) on the five material elements (*bhūta). This can be done by focusing either on the symbols of these elements or on their associated deities (*devatā). Thus, according to the *Tri-Shikhi-Brāhmana-Upanishad (II.133ff.), the *earth element is to be visualized as a yellow square, the *water element as a silvery crescent, the *fire element as a red flame, the *air element as a smoke-colored sacrificial altar, and the *ether element as lustrous deep black space. Their presiding *deities are Aniruddha, *Nārāyana, Pradyumna, Samkarshana, and Vasudeva respectively. In each case, *concentration must be accompanied by breath retention (*kumbhaka). The concentration on the earth element is supposed to be two hours in duration, with each subsequent concentration lasting two hours more than the preceding one.

The *Yoga-Tattva-Upanishad (69ff.) explains that one should retain the *breath in the bodily region (*sthāna) governed by each of the five elements. The five elemental regions of the *body are as follows: (1) prithivī-sthāna ("earth area"), extending from the soles of the feet to the knees; (2) apam-sthāna ("water area"), extending from the knees to the hips; (3) vahni-sthāna ("fire area"), extending from the hips to the *navel; (4) vāyu-sthāna ("wind area"), extending from the navel to the *nose; (5) ākāsha-sthāna ("ether area"), extending from the nose to the top of the *head.

These five types of *concentration, which may have been practiced already at the time of the *Shvetāshvatara-Upanishad (II.13), are listed in the *Gheranda-Samhitā (III.68ff.) as "seals" (*mudrā) and are respectively called *pārthivī-, *āmbhasī-, *āgneyī-, *vāyavī-, and *ākāshī-dhāranā-mudrā. They lead to bodily firmness and, in addition, each concentration is said to yield certain paranormal powers (*siddhi).

panca-ma-kara ("five *m*-letters"), also known as *panca-tattva*, stands for the five core practices of the left-hand *Tantric ritual, which all have names starting with the letter *m*. These are *madya* ("wine"), *māmsa* ("flesh"), *matsya* ("fish"), *mudrā* ("parched grain"), and *maithunā* ("intercourse"). The consumption of wine, meat, fish, and parched grain is thought to stimulate the sexual drive, and *maithunā*, as the crowning practice of this ritual, is the means of employing the accumulated sexual energy for the arousal of the "serpent power" (*kundalinī-shakti*).

Pāncarātra ("five nights") is a pronouncedly monotheistic *Hindu tradition that worships God Vasudeva, or *Vishnu, and is as old as *Buddhism. Originally a non-*Vedic religious culture, the Pāncarātra tradition, whose followers called themselves *Bhāgavatas, gave rise to *Vaishnavism. Apart from its emphasis on monotheistic worship, it also introduced into *Hinduism the idea of temples and images, and challenged the existing caste system by its ideal of equality among people. The name *pānca-rātra* is obscure but suggests the kind of syncretism that characterizes this tradition.

There are said to be 108 "compilations" (*samhitā*) of the Pāncarātra tradition, though in effect over 200 titles are known. These works ideally treat of four topics, namely wisdom (*jnāna*), *Yoga, cultic activity (*kriyā*), such as the construction of temples or the creation of images of the *Divine, and ritual conduct (*caryā*).

Pancashikha, a renowned authority of the *Sāmkhya tradition, may have flourished in the first century A.D. References to him are found in a number of works on *Yoga, including the *Yoga-Bhāshya*.

panca-tattva ("five substances") is a synonym for *panca-ma-kara*.

panca-vyoman ("five ether/spaces"). See *ākāsha*.

pandita ("pundit, scholar"). The *Bhagavad-Gītā* (IV.19) describes the true pundit as one whose doings are devoid of desire (*kāma*) and motive (*samkalpa*), that is, who is a genuine practitioner of *karma-yoga*. See also *grantha*, *shāstra*.

pāpa ("sin" or "evil"). The concepts of sin and evil played an important role already in the moral life of the ancient *Vedic people. The *Rig-Veda* contains many *prayers for the forgiveness of sin. The Vedic seers (*rishi*) accepted sin as part of the human condition. Sin is the inevitable by-product of the experience of separation between I and you. Only the *breath, which is frequently equated in the *Rig-Veda* with the *Self (*ātman*), is not overcome by evil. Hence, attunement to the Self is the only means of combatting sin and evil.

The *Vedic understanding of sin also informs later *Hindu thought. Thus, the *Bhagavad-Gītā* (III.36f.) has the following exchange between the God-man *Krishna and his disciple *Arjuna:

> Now, by what is this man impelled to commit evil, even unwittingly, o Vrshneya [i.e., *Krishna]? As though constrained by force?
>
> It is desire (*kāma*), it is *anger born of the dynamic quality (*rajo-*guna*), all-devouring and greatly evil—know this as the enemy here [on earth].

*Desire, then, is at the root of all evil. But desire is itself rooted in the ego-sense (*ahamkāra*), the illusion that one is divorced from the rest of existence. Only *wisdom, or gnosis (*jnāna*), can move a person beyond sin. For, through wisdom one is made whole. As (*Krishna explains in the *Bhagavad-Gītā* (IV.36ff.):

> Even if you were the most evil of all evildoers, you will cross all crooked [streams of life] with the raft of wisdom.
>
> As a kindles fire reduces its fuel to ashes, o Arjuna, so does the fire of wisdom reduce all actions to ashes.
>
> For, nothing here [on earth] purifies like wisdom; and this [a person] perfected in *Yoga will find of himself in time within himself.

Already in the pre-Christian ethical literature (*dharma-shāstra*), sin is said to be atoned by means of strenuous *breath control, as a high form of austerity (*tapas*). This idea is repeated in many later *Yoga texts. Controlled breathing is a form of self-sacrifice, the application of *wisdom. See also *adharma, dosha, kilbisha, pātaka*; cf. *dharma, punya*.

para-anta-jnāna ("knowledge of the end [of one's life]") is, according to the *Yoga-Sūtra* (III.22), acquired from omens (*arishta*) or by practicing enstatic "constraint" (*samyama*) in regard to one's *karma. See also Death.

para-arthatva ("other-purposiveness"). In the *Yoga-Sūtra* (III.35), this term is used to express the notion that *Nature exists solely for the purposes of the *Self, which, by contrast, has no purpose beyond itself. The two primary purposes of Nature are to serve either the worldly enjoyment (*bhoga*) or the liberation (*moksha*) of the Self.

para-artha-ihā ("exertion for the weal of others") is listed in the *Uddhāva-Gītā* (XIV.34) among the practices of self-restraint (*niyama*). See also *loka-samgraha*.

para-brahman ("supreme Absolute") is the unqualified ultimate *Reality about which nothing can be said. See also Absolute, *brahman*; cf. *shabda-brahman*.

para-citta-jnāna ("knowledge of another mind") is one of the paranormal powers (*siddhi*). According to the *Yoga-Sūtra* (III.19), it is acquired by "direct perception" (*sākshātkārana*) of the contents of another person's *consciousness. See also Mind.

para-deha-pravesha ("entering another body"), also called *para-kāya-pravesha* (or *-āvesha*), is an important yogic power (*siddhi*) claimed for many *adepts. It results from intense *contemplation on the *ājnā-, the *anāhata-, or the *mūlādhāra-cakra. The *Laghu-Yoga-Vāsishtha* (VI.9.117) mentions that this can be accomplished by means of exhalation (*recaka*), when the steadied life force (*prāna*) is kept at a distance of twelve digits from the face. This, however, presupposes an awakened "serpent power" (*kundalinī-shakti*). A well-known story, told in the *Shankara-Dig-Vijaya*, relates how *Shankara entered the corpse of a king in order to experience the pleasures of his harem so that he, Shankara, a renouncer with no knowledge of *sexuality, might win an intellectual tournament.

According to the *Kaula-Jnāna-Nirnaya* (XX.8), this ability extends to animal bodies. Thus, in the *Mahābhārata* epic (XII.260.5–262.45), there is the story of Syūmarashmi, who entered the *body of a cow in order to converse with the sage *Kapila. This paranormal ability has sometimes been equated with the phenomenon of "astral projection," though more appears to be involved.

parama-anu ("superatom"). In the *Yoga-Sūtra* (I.40), this phrase simply means the "most minute." However, *Vyāsa, in his *Yoga-Bhāshya* (I.43), borrows the *Vaisheshika idea that everything consists of atoms (*anu*). He thus regards objects as "conglomerations of atoms" (*anu-pracaya*). In his comments on this passage, *Vācaspati Mishra introduces the concept of *parama-anu* or "superatoms," which he seems to use interchangeably with *anu*.

parama-ātman ("supreme Self") is the transcendental *Self, as opposed to the psyche (*jīva) or "living self" (*jīva-ātman).

parama-hamsa ("supreme swan") signifies the *adept who enjoys *liberation, or *enlightenment. See also *avadhūta, hamsa*.

parama-īshvarī ("supreme Goddess") is a synonym for *kundalinī*.

parampara ("[from] one [to] another") refers to the chain of oral transmission and *empowerment from teacher (*guru) to disciple (*shishya). It is traditionally considered to be very auspicious and important to be a member of such a teaching lineage, though there have always been *adepts who became *enlightened without the benefit of a human teacher. See also *dīkshā*.

Paranormal powers. See Parapsychology, *siddhi, vibhūti*.

Paranormal perception. See *divya-shrotra, divya-desha, divya-darshana, pratibhā*.

Parapsychology. Claims of paranormal abilities and occurrences are a "universal constant" of the world's psychospiritual traditions. The literature of *Yoga is replete with references to numerous major and minor "powers" (*siddhi) that the *yogin is thought to acquire in the course of his spiritual discipline. Almost an entire chapter of the *Yoga-Sūtra, the classical work on Yoga philosophy and practice, is dedicated to paranormal abilities and the techniques by which they can be acquired. The method recommended by *Patanjali is known as "constraint" (*samyama), which is the combined practice of *concentration, *meditation, and *enstasy with regard to the same *object of contemplation. This method is said to yield a special kind of knowledge, and it is recognized as a form of valid cognition (*pramāna) by most other schools of *Hindu philosophy. It is also known as *yogi-pratyaksha* or "*yogin's* perception."

There is probably no psychic phenomenon known today that is not mentioned somewhere in the vast spiritual literature of India, but the most spectacular claims revolve around the doctrine of the eight major paranormal powers of *mahā-siddhis*, also known as "lordly powers" (*aishvarya): *animan, *mahiman, *lāghiman, *prāpti, *prākāmya, *vashitva, *īshītritva, and *kāma-avasāyitva. These are said to be by-products of an *adept's highest spiritual realization. Most *Hindu authorities understand these major paranormal powers literally, but some interpret them symbolically, and a few regard them as pertaining only to the "subtle body" (*sūkshma-sharīra). While we must remain alert to the ever-present readiness of the human *mind to delude itself and engage in fantasies, modern paraspychology has amassed enough evidence for the existence of paranormal phenomena. Therefore, today *some* of the claims of *Yoga and other similar spiritual traditions seem no longer implausible. See also Psychology.

para-sharīra-āvesha ("entering another body") is a synonym for *para-deha-pravesha*.

para-vairāgya ("superior renunciation"). In *Classical Yoga, this phrase refers to the higher form of dispassion (*vairāgya) and is defined in the *Yoga-Sūtra* (I.16) as the "nonthirsting for the primary constituents" (*guna-vaitrishnya) of *Nature. It is a final "No" to the world in its entirety. Unlike ordinary dispassion, this superior form is realizable only after experiencing the enstatic condition (*samādhi). It results from the "vision of the Self" (*purusha-khyāti). In the *Mani-Prabhā* (I.51) it is paraphrased as "eagerness for the so-called *dharma-megha[samādhi]."

paricāya-avasthā ("accumulation state") is the third of four stages (*avasthā) of yogic development. The *Hatha-Yoga-Pradīpikā* (IV.74f.) describes it as follows: One hears a sound like that of a drum in the "ether/space" of the *ājnā-cakra. Then the life force (*prāna) reaches the "great void" (*mahā-shūnya*), which is the seat of all powers (*siddhi). When one has transcended "mind(-generated) bliss" (*citta-ānanda*), there arises "spontaneous bliss" (*sahaja-ānanda), whereupon one becomes free from *pain, aging, *disease, *hunger, and somnolence (*ni-drā). According to the *Shiva-Samhitā* (III.60), this stage is characterized by the life force entering into the central channel (*sushumnā-nādī). This is accompanied by the awakening of the "serpent power" (*kundalinī-shakti).

paridhāna ("putting around") is a secret process, referred to in the *Hatha-Yoga-Pradīpikā* (III.112), by which the "serpent power" (*kundalinī-shakti) can be awakened. This practice may be the same as *naulī.

parināma ("transformation") is a key term in the philosophy of *Patanjali. It denotes serial change. According to the *Yoga-Sūtra* (III.13), transformation is of three basic types: (1) *dharma-parināma*, or the change in the form of a substance; (2) *lakshana-parināma*, or the change implicit in the fact that time (*kāla) consists of past, present, and future; (3) avasthā-parināma, or the qualitative change due to the effects of time (i.e., aging), as when an earthen vessel breaks and turns to dust. Patanjali seeks to apply these insights to *consciousness and its transmutation through the techniques of *Yoga. Patanjali's philosophy of change disallows permanency to the phenomena of *Nature. Only the transcendental Self (*purusha) is considered to enjoy "immutability" (aparināmitva). See also Evolution.

pārthavī-dhāranā-mudrā ("earthy concentration seal"), which is also called adho-dhāranā, is one of the five *concentration techniques described in the *Gheranda-Samhitā (III). It consists in focusing *mind and *life force on the *earth element held at the *heart for a period of 150 minutes. This is said to cause steadiness (stambha) and bring one in control over the earth itself. See also dhāranā, mudrā, panca-dhāranā.

parvan ("joint"). *Patanjali distinguishes between four levels (parvan) ("unof manifestation of *Nature: *vishesha ("particularized"), *avishesha ("unparticularized"), *linga-mātra ("differentiated"), and *alinga ("undifferentiated").

paryanka ("couch") is a posture (*āsana) mentioned, for instance, in the *Yoga-Bhāshya (II.46). According to *Vācaspati Mishra's commentary on this passage, it is executed by holding the knees with one's arms while reclining. Modern manuals describe this posture differently: Starting out in the "hero posture" (*vīra-āsana), one should then arch backward until the *head rests on the ground. The arms are supposed to cradle the head.

pashcima-tāna-āsana ("back extension posture"), which is also known as *ugra-āsana, is described in the *Tri-Shikhi-Brāhmana-Upanishad (II.51) as follows: Seated with the legs stretched out in front, one should bend forward until one can grasp the big toes with one's hands and the head comes to rest

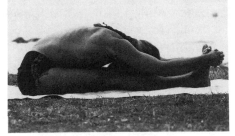

50. Pashcima-tana-āsana.

on one's knees. As the *Yoga-Cūdāmany-Upanishad (49) observes, this is really a "lock" (*bandha) because of the constriction in the abdominal area achieved by this posture. The *Shiva-Samhitā (III.92) states that this is also called *ugra-āsana. See also āsana.

pashcima-uttāna-āsana ("back stretching posture") is a common synonym for *pashcima-tāna-āsana*.

pāshinī-mudrā ("bird-catcher seal") is described in the *Gheranda-Samhitā* (III.65) thus; One should place one's legs around the back of the neck, holding them firmly like a noose (*pasha*). This not only gives strength (*bala*) and vigor (*pushti*) but also awakens the "serpent power" (*kundalinī-shakti*).

pashu ("animal"). The *Shiva-Purāna* (VII.1.5.61) describes all beings—from the Creator-God *Brahma down to the least creature—as animals bound by a noose (*pasha*), whose fodder is *pain and *pleasure.

Pāshupata is the earliest and most influential sect of *Shaivism, whose members worship God *Shiva as *Pashupati. The founder of this sect is *Lakulīsha. The main scripture of this tradition is the *Pāshupata-Sūtra* attributed to Lakulīsha, which deals with *Yoga in its fifth chapter. It has an extensive treatment of the moral disciplines (*yama*) and the practices of self-restraint (*niyama*), and it recommends detachment from all past, present, and future things and attachment to the *Divine. Its yogic *path, which is highly ritualistic, must be distinguished from the *pāshupata-yoga* described in the *Purānas, which is more akin to the *Classical Yoga of *Patanjali. The *Pāshupata-Sūtra*, discovered only in the 1930s, has a valuable commentary by Kaundinya entitled *Panca-Artha-Bhāshya* ("Discussion on the Five Topics [of Pāshupata Philosophy]"). Another important work of the Pāshupata sect, which was most prominent in Gujarat, is Haradatta's ninth-century *Gana-Kārikā* consisting of merely eight verses. This text is often wrongly attributed to Bhāsarvajna, who wrote the commentary *Ratna-Tīkā* on it.

Pāshupata-Brāhmana-Upanishad is one of the *Yoga-Upanishads. It consists of a total of seventy-eight verses distributed over two sections. It presents a symbolic sacrificial philosophy exalting the inner *sacrifice. It recommends a form of *nāda-yoga*, or *Yoga of sound, in which the *mind is to be applied to the *hamsa. The specific approach put forward in this scripture (II.6) is called *hamsa-arka-pranava-dhyāna* or "meditation on the humming sound [i.e., *om] of the radiant 'swan.' " It enjoins (II.21) silence (*mauna*) on the grounds that *light (*prakāsha*) alone exists. This text further states (II.31) that the person who knows the *Self is neither *liberated nor unliberated, since such ideas pertain only to those who are still bound. For the same reason, prohibitions about food (*anna*) are said not to apply to the Self-realized *adept who is both food and the eater of food (in the spirit of the ancient *Taittirīya-Upanishad).

pāshupata-yoga is the collective name given to a variety of *Shaiva teachings that belong to the period after *Patanjali. The yogic doctrines are expounded in such scriptures as the *Shiva-, the *Linga-, and the *Kūrma-Purāna. Their avowed goal is union with God *Shiva.

Pashupati ("Lord of Beasts") is one of the names of God *Shiva. During the excavations at Mohenjo Daro, one of the big cities of the *Indus civilization, a terracotta seal was discovered that depicts a figure seated cross-legged upon a platform and wearing a two-horned headdress, adorned with jewelry, and endowed with what appears to be an erect phallus (*linga) and surrounded by various animals. This figure has frequently been thought to be the earliest representation of Pashupati, though this interpretation has not remained unchallenged.

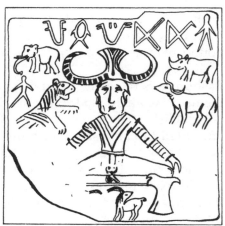

54. Shiva Pashupati, "Lord of Beast," drawn after a terracotta seal from the Indus civilization.

Passion. See kāma, rāga, rajas, rati.

pātāla ("nether region"). According to the *Yoga-Bhāshya (III.26), there are seven nether regions above the seven hells (*nāraka). These are respectively known as mahātāla, rasa-tāla, atāla, sutāla, vitāla, tāla-atāla, and pātāla—the word tāla meaning "plane." See also Cosmos.

pātaka ("sin") stands for sin (*pāpa) that is so serious that it deprives one of one's caste membership, which means one's livelihood. According to the *Yoga-Cūdāmany-Upanishad (108), the practice of *breath control can expiate even such cardinal sin.

pātanjala-darshana ("Patanjali's view") is the native *Hindu term for what modern scholars call *Classical Yoga.

Pātanjala-Rahasya ("Patanjali's Secret") is a short subcommentary on the *Tattva-Vaishāradī* that offers many concise definitions and quotations from other works. Its author is Rāghavānanda Sarasvatī, who probably lived in the nineteenth century A.D.

Pātanjala-Sūtra. See *Yoga-Sūtra*.

Pātanjala-Yoga-Sūtra differs from the well-known work of *Patanjali. This text, which comprises 501 aphorisms, was dictated by the blind pundit Dhanraj of Benares to Bhagavan Das in 1910.

Patanjali. There have been several prominent men named Patanjali in the history of *Hindu thought. The famous grammarian by that name, who wrote a learned commentary on Pānini's *Ashta-Adhyāyī* ("Eight Lessons [in Grammar]"), lived some time in the second century B.C. He is different from Patanjali the author of the *Nidāna-Sūtra* ("Aphorisms on Origin"), an important work for the study of the *Vedic ritual literature. Both are very probably different from their namesake who composed the *Yoga-Sūtra*, although native Indian tradition maintains that the grammarian and the Yoga writer are identical. From internal evidence of the *Yoga-Sūtra* and general historical considerations, Patanjali the Yoga authority may have lived in the second century A.D.

Virtually nothing is known about him. According to *Hindu tradition, he was an incarnation of *Ananta, or Shesha, the thousand-headed ruler of the serpent race. Ananta, desiring to teach *Yoga on earth, is said to have

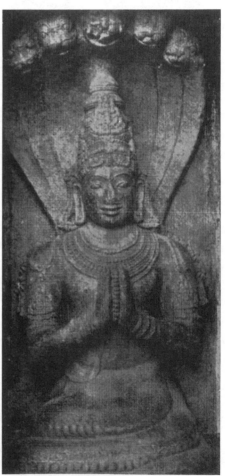

52. *Patanjali, surrounded by serpents who are the guardians of esoteric lore.*

fallen (*pat*) from *heaven onto the palm (*anjali*) of a virtuous woman, named Gonikā. He was clearly an *adept of Yoga with a penchant for philosophy. Often wrongly regarded as the "father of Yoga," Patanjali's great contribution was to have compiled and systematized existing knowledge and given Yoga a philosophical shape that allowed it to compete with other contemporary schools of thought. See also Hiranyagarbha.

Patanjali-Carita ("Patanjali's Life") is an eighteenth-century narrative by Rāmabhadra Dīkshita that speaks of the sage *Patanjali as the author of the *Yoga-Sūtra and a medical treatise of uncertain title.

Path. Spiritual life is almost universally represented as a path that leads from a state of spiritual ignorance (*avidyā) to *wisdom or *enlightenment. Only in some radical schools, such as the *sahaja movement, is this metaphor rejected. See also *mārga*, *sādhana*.

Patience. See *kshamā*, *kshānti*, *titikshā*.

paurusha ("manliness, valor"). This is an important notion in the *Yoga-Vāsishtha (II.4.10ff.), where manly *effort is placed above *fate. Without effort, suffering (*duhkha) cannot be overcome. As this work (II.7.31) affirms: One must not depend on destiny. Cf. Grace.

pavana ("wind") is a synonym for *prāna and *vāyu*.

Pavana-Vijaya ("Conquest of the Wind") is a fairly recent work on *breath control, consisting of 349 stanzas distributed over nine chapters.

pāyasvinī-nādī ("watery current") is a channel (*nādī) of the life force (*prāna) that is situated between the *pūshā- and the *sarasvatī-nādī and that extends to the right ear.

Peacock posture. See *mayūra-āsana*.

Perception. See *drishti*, *grahana*, *pratyaksha*, *sākshātkāra*.

Perfection. See *siddhi*.

Perfection of the body. See *kāya-sampat*

Perspiration. See *sveda*.

phala ("fruit") refers to the moral reward, or *karmic payoff, of one's *actions. According to the *Bhagavad-Gītā (XVIII.12), this fruition is threefold: (1) *anishta* ("undesirable"), or as *Shankara explains in his *Gītā* commentary, leading to a future existence in *hell; (2) *ishta* ("desirable"), or leading to a future existence in some heavenly realm; (3) *mishra* ("mixed"), or, presumably, leading to a future human existence.

The practice of *karma-yoga*, as taught in the *Bhagavad-Gītā*, consists principally in the inward *renunciation of the fruit of one's deeds. As this scripture (II.47) puts it: "In action alone is your 'rightful interest' (*adhikāra*), never in its fruit. Let not your motive be the fruit of action, nor let your attachment be to inaction (*akarman*)."

A related concept is *vipāka* ("fruition").

Phallus. See *linga*.

Phlegm. See *kapha, shleshma*.

pinda ("lump") is the term used in many *hatha-yoga works to denote the human *body. The *Siddha-Siddhānta-Paddhati (I) speaks of six *pindas, the physical body, which is called "embryonic body" (*garbha-pinda*) being the coarsest manifestation. See also *deha, kosha, sharīra*.

pinda-anda ("lump egg") denotes the human *body as an exact replica of the *macrocosm. Thus, according to the *Siddha-Siddhānta-Paddhati (III.2ff.), the entire *cosmos is faithfully reflected in the body. For instance, the mythological "tortoise" that upholds the universe resides at the sole of the feet, the different nether regions (*pātāla*) are at the toes, the knees, and the thighs. The realms of the earth world (*bhū-loka*) are to be found in various parts of the trunk, while the heavenly realms are located in the head. See also Microcosm.

pingalā-nādī ("tawny current") is one of three primary channels of the life force (*prāna*). It is situated to the right of the central conduit (*sushumnā-nādī*) and terminates in the right nostril according to most scriptures, though the *Shiva-Samhitā (II.26) has it end in the left nostril. It is associated with the sun (*sūrya*) and is responsible for heating the *body. It corresponds on the physical level to the sympathetic nervous system. Cf. *idā-nādī*.

pītha ("seat") is sometimes used synonymously for *āsana*. The term can also refer to a sacred site, such as a temple, or a special locus of spiritual energy (*shakti*) within the *body, corresponding to a *cakra. For instance, the *Laghu-Yoga-Vāsishtha (VI.2.100f.) speaks of the thirty-six *tīrthas in the body where *God should be worshipped.

pitri-yāna ("way of the ancestors"). The *pitris* are one's distant ancestors, whereas the word *preta* refers to a recently departed ancestor. Because, according to *Hindu eschatology, *death does not imply the final annihilation of a being, the ancestors are thought to inhabit the nether regions (*pātāla) or, if they were evildoers, the realms of hell (*nāraka). The pious *Hindu remembers his ancestors in daily rites and feeds them through sacrificial offerings. However, ever since the time of the earliest *Upanishads, the "way of the ancestors" has been described as a way of "return" (*āvritti*), that is, *rebirth. In the *Bhagavad-Gītā (VIII.25), it is known as the "dark course" (*krishna-gati*). The ancestral destiny is contrasted with the "way of the gods" (*deva-yāna). See also *ātivāhika-deha*.

pitta ("gall") is one of the three humors (*dhātu). It is associated with the following qualities: fat, hot, pungent, and liquid. Some works recommend *bhastrikā-prānāyāma for the removel of excess gall. See also *kapha*, *vāta*.

pīyūsha ("milk, cream") is a synonym for *amrita.

plāvinī ("floater") is one of the eight types of breath retention (*kumbhaka) taught in *hatha-yoga. The *Hatha-Yoga-Pradīpikā (II.70) describes it as follows: By generously inhaling and filling the abdomen (i.e., the lower half of the lungs) with air, one can float on water as easily as a lotus. See also *prānāyāma*.

Play. From the vantage point of *enlightenment, or *liberation, conditional existence appears inconsequential (*alpa*), and the individual's struggle for continuity seems even absurd. Everything in *Nature's orbit is bound to change and, ultimately, disintegrate. The *ego's desperate bid for survival is doomed to be frustrated, and no lasting *happiness can be found even in the highest dimensions of the multilevel *cosmos. Yet, this *fait accompli* does not disturb the enlightened *adept, who has realized the permanent *Reality, the *Self, beyond the phenomenal world of constant change. On the contrary, because of his realization of the innate bliss (*ānanda), he is able to reengage life with all its absurdities: Knowing that the *body and the *mind are destined to die, together with all their dreams and hopes, he places no great store in them, but meets all experiences as a play (*līlā) of the *Divine. Play is an appropriate metaphor for the world process, since it is utterly spontaneous, inconsequential, and beyond anyone's control. This notion is particularly at home in the schools of non-dualism, or *Advaita-Vedānta: The world and its countless events are the sport of the singular Reality. See also Dance.

Pleasure. Ordinary life revolves around the maximization of pleasure (*sukha) and the minimization of pain (*duhkha). While it is clearly desirable to avoid *pain, the *Yoga authorities also enjoin that one should overcome pleasure. Like pain, pleasure has a binding effect on the *mind. It calls for its repetition and in due course leads to addiction. The Yoga masters propose an ideal that is quite different from the "pleasure principle." They claim that we find ultimate fulfillment only in the personal realization of the transcendental *Reality, which is inherently blissful (*ānanda).

Plough posture. See *hala-āsana*.

Post-Classical Yoga encompasses many different schools and yogic traditions that flourished after the time of *Patanjali, the originator of *Classical Yoga. Post-Classical Yoga includes the teachings of the *Yoga-Upanishads, *Tantrism, and *hatha-yoga. In contrast to the dualistic metaphysics espoused by Patanjali, these later teachings are based on the kind of nondualist (*advaita*) philosophy that also characterizes *Pre-Classical Yoga.

Posture. See *āsana, bandha, mudrā*.

Powers. See *bala*, Parapsychology, *siddhi, vibhūti*.

Prabhudeva is mentioned in the *Hatha-Yoga-Pradīpikā* (I.8) as one of the masters of *hatha-yoga*. No biographical information about him is available.

Practice. See *abhyāsa*.

pradhāna ("foundation") is a term common to *Yoga and *Sāmkhya, which denotes the transcendental matrix of *Nature as apart from the multiple monads of *Consciousness, or Selves (*purusha). In the *Tattva-

Vaishāradī (II.23), the term is explained as "that by which the host of evolutes (**vikāra*) is brought forth (*pradhīyate*)."

pradhāna-jaya ("mastery over the foundation [of *Nature]") is mentioned in the *Yoga-Sūtra (III.48) as one of the fruits of practicing "constraint" (**samyama*) upon the perceptual process (**grahana*). This paranormal power (**siddhi*) makes the *yogin a master of the entire *cosmos. It is also called **aishvarya*. *Vācaspati Mishra, in his **Tattva-Vaishāradī* (III.18), observes that an *adept with this power is able to create thousands of bodies for himself and to freely roam through *heaven and earth.

Pradīpikā. See *Hatha-Yoga-Pradīpikā, Yoga-Anushāsana-Sūtra-Vritti, Yoga-Pradīpikā*.

Prahlāda, who is mentioned already in the *Bhagavad-Gītā (X.30), was an *adept of the early *Vaishnava tradition. Legend has it that his father Hiranyakashipu ordered Prahlāda to be killed because he was enraged by his son's devotion (**bhakti*) to God *Krishna. In later times, Prahlāda came to be associated with the myth of God *Vishnu's incarnation as Nara-Simha ("Man-Lion"). He is a prominent figure in the *Bhāgavata-Purāna.

prajalpa ("talkativeness") is, according to the **Hatha-Yoga-Pradīpikā* (I.15), one of the factors by which *Yoga is foiled. Cf. *mauna*.

prajnā ("wisdom, knowledge"), a synonym for **jnāna*. It stands for insight leading to *liberation or even for the essence of *liberation itself. In the *Mahābhārata (XII.173.2), *wisdom is extolled as the highest virtue: "Wisdom is the foundation of beings. Wisdom is deemed the highest acquisition. Wisdom is the greatest good in the world. Wisdom is deemed *heaven by the virtuous."

According to the *Yoga-Sūtra (I.49), *prajnā* is gnosis obtained in the enstatic condition (**samādhi*) and is quite distinct from *knowledge gained by *inference or from *tradition. It is based on "direct perception" (**sākshātkāra*). On the highest level, this superknowledge is designated as being "truth-bearing" (**ritam-bhara*).

prajnā-āloka ("luster of wisdom") results, according to the *Yoga-Sūtra (III.5), from one's mastery of the practice of enstatic "constraint" (**samyama*).

prajnā-jyotis ("he who has wisdom's light") is a type of *yogin who, according to the *Yoga-Bhāshya (III.51), has subjugated the *elements and *senses and who can preserve his spiritual accomplishments and build upon them to achieve *liberation. Cf. atikrānta-bhāvanīya, mādhu-bhūmika, prathama-kalpika.

prākāmya ("wish fulfillment") is one of the great paranormal powers (*siddhi). The *Yoga-Bhāshya (III.45) explains it as the "nonobstruction of one's will." As *Vyāsa elucidates, this power enables the *yogin, for instance, to dive into solid earth as if it were liquid.

prakāsha ("brightness, luminosity"). See Light.

prakriti ("creatrix") is the *Yoga and *Sāmkhya term for *Nature, or creation. Although the word prakriti does not appear prior to the *Bhagavad-Gītā (III.39) and the *Shvetāshvatara-Upanishad (IV.10), which belong to the same era, the underlying concept was known much earlier and was often termed *avyakta ("unmanifest").

The designation prakriti was originally also used for the eight principal evolutes of *Nature, namely the unmanifest (*avyakta) dimension, which *Patanjali calls *alinga, the higher mind (*buddhi), the *I-maker" (*ahamkāra), and the five elements (*bhūta). In the *Bhagavad-Gītā (VII.4.), *Krishna speaks of these eight divisions (*tattva) as his "lower nature," whereas his "higher nature" is the "life principle" (*jīva-bhūta), the Self (*purusha).

*Hinduism views *Nature as a multilevel hierarchical organization extending from the visible realm composed of the five *elements to the transcendental "foundation" (*pradhāna), or "root-Nature" (mūla-prakriti). The visible dimension is designated as "coarse" (*sthūla), and all the other, hidden dimensions are called "subtle" (*sūkshma). The *Sāmkhya tradition has developed the most sophisticated model explaining the gradual evolution (*parināma) from the transcendental core of Nature to the manifest realm accessible to the five senses (*indriya). This model has been adopted and adapted by most of the *Yoga and *Vedānta schools. In its various forms, it serves as a kind of map for the *yogin who seeks to proceed, in *consciousness, from the external to the internal and then to the transcendental dimension of Nature and, at last, beyond Nature's orbit to the supraconscious Self.

According to the metaphysics of *Classical Yoga and *Sāmkhya, *Nature in all its aspects is utterly insentient. Only the transcendental Self, the *purusha, enjoys *Consciousness. Whereas the Self is perfectly and eternally immobile, a pure witness (*sākshin), Nature is inherently in motion. Its dynamics is due to the interplay of its three types of "primary constituent" (*guna), namely *sattva, *rajas, and *tamas. In combination, they weave the entire pattern of cosmic existence, from high to low. The *gunas* underlie all material *and* psychic realities. The *mind and the *ego are counted among the material phenomena, which are illumined by the transcendental static Consciousness, or *cit.

The relationship between this supposedly insentient Nature and the exclusively sentient *Self has proved a philosophical stumbling block. In the *Mahābhārata epic (XII.303.14ff.), this relationship is compared to the relationship between fly and fig, fish and water, fire and fire basin. Later thinkers wrestled with the epistemological question of how a radically transcendent Self-monad could possibly experience anything.

In *Classical Yoga, *Nature is also called the "visible" (*drishya), whereas the *Self is known as the "seer" (*drashtri) or the "power of seeing" (*drik-shakti). The relationship between these two ultimate principles is said to be one of "preestablished harmony" (*yogyatā). In the commentarial literature on the *Yoga-Sūtra, this fit between *prakriti* and *purusha) is explained by the doctrine of "reflection" (*pratibimba): The "*light" of the transcendental Self is mirrored in the highest, or most subtle, aspect of Nature, namely the *sattva. When the *sattva* of *consciousness is as pure as the transcendental Self, the condition of "aloneness" (*kaivalya), or *liberation, obtains.

prakriti-laya ("absorption into *Nature") is mentioned in the *Yoga-Sūtra (I.19) as the *destiny of those who fail to transcend the "notion of becoming" (*bhava-pratyaya*) and achieve a kind of pseudoliberation in a disembodied (*videha*) state at the core of Nature. This describes the condition of the *deities who, compared to human beings, live immeasurably long lives but who are nevertheless doomed to die. As *Vyāsa explains in his commentary on the above aphorism of *Patanjali, the pressure of the rudimentary *consciousness of the *prakriti-layas* sooner or later forces them to experience renewed *embodiment in one or the other realm of Nature. Genuine *liberation, which transcends Nature completely, is forever. See also *laya*.

pralaya ("dissolution") is the disappearance of the material universe at the end of its cycle of manifestation. *Hindu cosmo-mythologists have calculated this duration to be 2.16 billion years. This is thought to be the length of a single waking day, or *kalpa, in the life of the Creator-God *Brahma. During his sleep, which has the same duration, only the subtle dimensions of the universe, inhabited by the *deities and sages, exists. When Brahma awakens from his sleep, the *cosmos is newly created. Upon completing his hundredth year, Brahma himself dies, and the entire universe, with all its coarse and subtle dimensions, dissolves into the *Divine. This moment is known as the "great dissolution" (mahā-pralaya). See also yuga.

pramāda ("heedlessness"), or inattention, is one of the obstacles (*antarāya) mentioned in the *Yoga-Sūtra (I.30). *Vyāsa, in his *Yoga-Bhāshya (I.30), defines it as the lack of cultivation of the means to enstasy (*samādhi). In the *Yoga-Kundaly-Upanishad (I.59), the synonym pramattatā is employed, which is said to be one of the ten obstructions (*vighna).

pramāna ("measure," "standard"). In *Classical Yoga, pramāna stands for "valid cognition." Like all the other schools of *Hinduism, *Yoga does not bypass the important philosophical issue of the possibility and scope of *knowledge. Thus, *Patanjali recognizes three sources of valid cognition, namely perception, (*pratyaksha), inference (*anumāna), and testimony (*āgama).

prāna ("life"). The word prāna (literally, "breathing forth") is found already in the *Rig-Veda (X.90.13), where it stands for the "breath" of the macranthropos, the cosmic *purusha, and for the *breath of life in general. Early on, it came to be equated with the Absolute (*brahman) as the transcendental source of all life. In secular contexts, prāna denotes "air." However, in the sacred scriptures of *Hinduism, prāna almost invariably signifies the universal life force, which is a vibrant psychophysical energy similar to the pneuma of the ancient Greeks. The *Yoga-Vāsishtha (III.13.31) defines prāna as the "vibratory power" (spanda-shakti) that underlies all manifestation.

Later writers distinguish between the universal or "primary life force" (*mukhya-prāna) and the life force as it enlivens the individual being. The individuated prāna, which is also identified with the psyche (*jīva, *hamsa), is said to reside at the *heart. Its color is red. However, in the *Tri-Shikhi-Brāhmana-Upanishad (II.79ff.), the prāna is said to circulate in the mouth, the *nose, the *heart, the *navel, and the big toes and to be responsible for the assimilation of *food. According to the *Yoga-Yājnavalkya (IV.58f.), it is situated in the middle of the abdomen and has the function of separating water, solid food, and the "essence" (*rasa).

The individuated type of prāna has from the earliest times been thought to have five aspects: (1) prāna, or the ascending *breath issuing from the *navel or the *heart and including both inhalation and exhalation; (2) *apāna, or the breath associated with the lower half of the trunk; (3) *vyāna, or the diffuse breath circulating in all the limbs; (4) *udāna, or the "up-breath" held responsible for eructation, speech, and the ascent of *attention in higher states of *consciousness; (5) *samāna, or the breath localized in the abdominal region where it is connected with the digestive processes. Prāna and *apāna also frequently stand for inhalation and exhalation respectively. Common synonyms for prāna are marut, *vāta, *vāyu, and pavana.

In the period following *Shankara—early ninth century A.D.—the authorities of *Yoga and *Vedānta often added a set of five "secondary breaths" (upaprāna) comprising the following: *nāga ("serpent"); *kūrma ("tortoise"); *kri-kara ("kri-maker"); *deva-datta ("God-given"); and *dhanam-jaya ("conquest of wealth").

These ten types of life force are generally thought to circulate in, or along, 72,000 "channels" (*nādī) that feed all the organs of the *body. Already in the ancient *Taittirīya-Upanishad (II), this intricately patterned life energy is conceived as forming a distinct field, which is called *prāna-maya-kosha.

In the *Chāndogya-Upanishad (II.13.6), the five principal *breaths are referred to as the "gate keepers to the heavenly world," which suggests an esoteric understanding of the close relationship between breath and *consciousness, which led to the invention of the various techniques of breath control (*prānāyāma). See also svara.

prāna-dhāranā ("concentration of the life force") is the technique of projecting the life force (*prāna) into specific parts of the *body in order to restore a particular organ to *health. This practice, which is mentioned in the *Tri-Shikhi-Brāhmana-Upanishad (II.109), is said to conquer all illnesses (*roga) and fatigue (klama).

prāna-maya-kosha ("sheath composed of the life force") is one of the five "sheaths" (*kosha) covering the innate luminosity of the transcendental *Self. Some modern occultists equate this field with the aura.

prāna-rodha or **prāna-samrodha** ("restraint of the life force") is a synonym for *prānāyāma. Complete restraint of the life force (prāna) is also known as prāna-jaya ("conquest of the life force"). *It is usually gauged by the *yogin's capacity to hold his *breath for prolonged periods of time. In order to demonstrate this extraordinary ability, some yogins have let themselves be buried for several hours and even days at a time in allegedly airtight containers underground.

präna-samyama ("constraint of the life force") is a synonym of *pränäyäma*. According to the *Brihad-Yogi-Yäjnavalkya-Samhitä* (IX.35), it is the fourth "limb" (*anga*) of *Yoga, whereas the *Tejo-Bindu-Upanishad* (I.31) lists it as the eleventh "limb" of its "fifteenfold Yoga" (*pancadasha-anga-yoga*). The *Tri-Shikhi-Brähmana-Upanishad* (II.30) gives it a symbolic meaning, defining it as the conviction that the world is false (*mithyä*).

präna-spanda ("quiver of the life force"). According to the *Laghu-Yoga-Väsishtha* (V.9.78), when the ever-dynamic life force (*präna*) is stopped, the movements of the *mind are likewise arrested. See also *spanda*.

pranava ("humming") is the esoteric designation of the sacred syllable *om*, which is recited with a nasalized hum. According to the *Yoga-Sütra* (I.28), the *pranava* should be recited and its inner meaning should be contemplated for the cultivation of "inward-mindedness" (*pratyak-cetana*). Since it is the primary *mantra*, it is also known as "primal seed" (*ädi-bïja*). The *Shiva-Puräna* (I.17.4) offers the following imaginative etymology: *pra* from *prakriti* ("Nature") and *nava* ("boat"), because the *pranava* is the boat by which the *yogin* can cross the ocean of existence and reach the shore of the *Absolute. See also *bïja, bindu, japa, näda*.

pränäyäma ("breath control") is the fourth "limb" (*anga*) of the eight-fold *path taught by *Patanjali in the early post-Christian centuries. The word *pränäyäma* is composed of *präna* ("breath") and *äyäma* ("extension"), which hints at the principal objective of breath control, namely the phase of retention (*kumbhaka*). Prolonging the duration of the withheld *breath is thought to prolong life itself. *Pränäyäma* is recognized as one of the chief means of rejuvenating and indeed immortalizing the *body. However, the ultimate purpose of *pränäyäma* is to control the movement of the *mind. As the *Yoga-Shikhä-Upanishad* (I.61) states, the life force cannot be controlled by mere speculation, talk, the snare of books, contrivances, spells, or medications. It must be checked through the practice of *pränäyäma*. The *yogin* who attempts to practice *Yoga without controlling the breath is compared (I.62f.) to a person who wants to cross the ocean in an unbaked earthen vessel, which only invites trouble.

Pränäyäma is the main technique of *hatha-yoga* by which the "serpent power" (*kundalinï-shakti*) is forced to enter the central channel (*sushumnä-nädï*) and begin its ascension to the *head. The scriptures of *hatha-yoga* know of eight kinds of *breath control, which are also called "retentions" (*kumbhaka): *sūrya-bedha or -bedhana ("sun-piercing"); *ujjayī ("victorious")' *sīt-karī ("sīt-maker"); *shītalī ("cooling"); *bhastrikā ("bellows"); *bhrāmarī ("humming"); *mūrchā ("swooning"); and *plāvinī ("floater"). In place of the sīt-karī and plāvanī forms of breath control, the *Gheranda-Samhitā (V.46) mentions *sahita ("combined") and *kevalī ("absolute") prāṇāyāma instead.

Breath control has three phases, namely inhalation (*pūraka), retention (*kumbhaka), and exhalation (*recaka). In addition, the *Hatha-Yoga-Pradīpikā (II.72) distinguishes between *sahita- and *kevala-kumbhaka. Whereas the former practice involves deliberate inhalation and exhalation, the kevala-kumbhaka is breath retention on the spot.

Before prāṇāyāma can be started, the aspirant must engage various purificatory practices (called *dhauti). Some of the types of prāṇāyāma also serve this purpose. Upon mastery of *breath control, the *yogin is fit to proceed to the higher stages of *Yoga. The *Gheranda-Samhitā (V.1) mentions four essential prerequisites for the practice of prāṇāyāma. These are *sthāna, or right place; *kāla, or right time; *mita-āhāra, or moderate diet; and *nādī-shuddhi, or purity of the channels (*nādī) through which the *life force circulates. The *Shiva-Samhitā (III.37) recommends that prāṇāyāma should not be practiced shortly after a meal or when one is hungry. It also states that one should take some milk and butter before starting. However, these restrictions do not apply to a practitioner who is accomplished.

The *Hatha-Yoga-Pradīpikā (II.15) advises caution in performing breath control: "Just as a lion, an elephant, or a tiger is tamed gradually, so should the *life-force be controlled; else it will kill the practitioner."

Properly executed, however, prāṇāyāma has great curative value, and the texts mention hiccup, cough, asthma, and pain in *head, ears, and eyes among the *diseases that can effectively be healed through breath control. Prāṇāyāma is also said to reduce one's feces, urine, and phlegm (*kapha). Furthermore, it strengthens and invigorates the body-mind and even is claimed to have a rejuvenating effect.

The practice of prāṇāyāma is associated with a variety of psychosomatic phenomena. The *Shiva-Samhitā (III.40ff.) mentions four stages in this process. In the first stage, perspiration (*sveda) is caused, and the sweat should be massaged into the limbs. In the second stage, the *yogin experiences trembling (*kampa). In the third stage, he begins to jump "like a frog." In the fourth stage, he experiences great lightness (*lāghutā) and is able to walk on air. See also shīt-krama.

pranidhāna ("devotion," "dedication") is one's whole-hearted application to the spiritual process. See also *īshvara-pranidhāna*.

prapatti ("resignation," "surrender") is a key concept of the *Pānca-rātra or *Vaishnava tradition. It represents unconditional surrender to the *Divine in which the devotee (*bhakta*) drops all concern even about *liberation, instead trusting entirely the mercy of *God. This attitude of radical devotion (*bhakti*) is epitomized in the final admonition of the God-man *Krishna in the *Bhagavad-Gītā* (XVIII.66): "Relinquishing all teachings (*dharma*), come to me alone for shelter. I will deliver you from all *sin. Do not grieve!"

The practitioner cultivating *prapatti* starts from the recognition of his or her own insignificance and helplessness. Gradually, the devotee grows more deeply attached to the *Divine until his or her self-effacement leads to perfect ecstatic oblivion in *God.

Some scriptures, like the *Yati-Indra-Mata-Dīpikā* (VII.28), regard *prapatti* as an alternative to the arduous discipline of the "sevenfold discipline" (*sapta-sādhana*) and the eightfold *path (*ashta-anga-yoga*). The devotee has to surrender himself to the *Divine only once to be assured of *God's saving grace (*prasāda*). There is no evidence that *Rāmānuja, the great medieval proponent of devotion (*bhakti*), taught this total surrender to the will of God. Yet, some 150 years after Rāmānuja's death, his followers split into two groups, known respectively as the "Southern" and the "Northern" school, in Tamil *tengalai* and *vadagalai*. The former explain *prapatti* as sheer receptivity to the grace of God, whereas the latter believe that the devotee must take certain positive steps to deserve that *grace, including the recitation of sacred *mantras*. Throughout his writings, Rāmānuja emphasized the importance of meditation (*dhyāna*, *upāsana*) on the Divine. Cf. Effort, *paurusha*.

prāpti ("attainment") is one of the classic paranormal powers (*siddhi*), which is the *adept's ability to expand infinitely. The *Yoga-Bhāshya* (III.45) seriously suggests that the *yogin who enjoys this power can touch the moon with his finger tips.

prārabdha-karman ("started action") is *karma, or *destiny, in progress.

prasāda can mean "clarity" and "tranquility" as well as "grace". *Prasāda*, in the sense of "clarity" or "serenity," is sometimes listed among the practices of moral discipline (*yama*). According to the *Bhagavad-Gītā* (XVII.16), *prasāda* is an aspect of austerity (*tapas*). In another stanza from this work (II.64), serenity is said to be the gift of the *yogin who has brought his self (or *ego) under control. Through serenity, he becomes free from all sorrow (*duhkha). This is also the contention of the *Mahābhārata epic (XII.238.10), which states that through "mental tranquility" (citta-prasāda), one leaves behind both the auspicious (shubha) and the inauspicious (ashubha). In the *Yoga-Sūtra (I.47), the "clarity of the inner being" (adhyātma-prasāda) is said to result from the "suprareflexive lucidity" (*nirvicāra-vaishāradya), a high-level *enstatic experience. Thus, prasāda is sometimes regarded as one of the "signs" (*cihna). In aphorism I.23, *Patanjali recommends the practice of projecting the sentiments of friendship (*maitrī), compassion (*karunā), gladness (*muditā), and equanimity (*upekshā) for the cultivation of the "pacification" (prasādana) of *consciousness.

It is easy to see why the word prasāda should also have acquired the meaning of "grace," since mental tranquility is a precondition for one's entrance into higher states of *consciousness. This event is often experienced as being given "from above," that is, as an act of *grace. Thus, the *Linga-Purāna (I.7.4) affirms: "Through grace, wisdom (*jnāna) is born; through wisdom, *Yoga comes about. By means of Yoga, *liberation is procured. Thence through grace, everything [is accomplished]."

This position is maintained already in the ancient *Katha-Upanishad (II.23), which has this verse: "This *Self is not to be attained through instruction, nor by the intellect, nor by much learning. It is to be attained only by the one whom it chooses. To such a one that Self reveals its own person (tanu)."

The same view is expressed by *Shankara, arguably the finest philosopher of *Hinduism, in his learned commentary on the Brahma-Sūtra (I.1.4): "The knowledge of the Absolute (*brahman) is not dependent on human activity. What then? Just like *knowledge of an *object that is an object of *perception and of other means of knowledge, this [knowledge of the Absolute] also depends solely on that [transcendental] Object." See also anugraha, kripā; cf. Effort.

prasamkhyāna ("elevation") is a high-level *enstatic state, consisting in the "vision of discernment" (*viveka-khyāti). The *yogin must be "nonusurious" (akusīda) toward this experience so that he may realize the "cloud of dharma enstasy" (*dharma-megha-samādhi). According to the *Yoga-Bhāshya (I.2), however, it is another name for the dharma-megha-samādhi. In another passage (II.2), the same work states that it is the fire of prasamkhyāna that burns the "causes of affliction" (*klesha) rendering them sterile. *Shankara, in his *Vivarana (II.4), interprets the term as "perfect vision" (samyag-darshana).

prashvāsa ("breathing forth") is listed by *Patanjali in his *Yoga-Sūtra (I.31) as one of the symptoms accompanying the obstacles (*antarāya), and has here probably the meaning of "faulty breathing." Elsewhere (II.49), however, the term occurs in the sense of "exhalation." See also shvāsa; cf. nishvāsa.

prasveda ("sweat," "sweating"). See sveda.

prathama-kalpika ("he who is of the first form") is the neophyte in the first stage of yogic practice for whom, as the *Yoga-Bhāshya (III.51) puts it, the *light is just dawning. Cf. atikrānta-bhāvanīya, mādhu-bhū-mika, prajñā-jyotis.

pratibhā ("shining forth") is explanined in the *Yoga-Bhāshya (III.33) as "a preliminary form of the knowledge born of discernment (*viveka), just as the light at dawn [heralds] the sun." *Vyāsa also calls this the "deliverer" (*tāraka). The *Yoga-Sūtra (III.36) mentions "flashes of illumination" (pratibhā) in regard to hearing, sensing, sight, taste, and smell. According to the *Yoga-Bhāshya (III.36), these are the "super-senses" (atīndriya) possessed by the *adept. *Patanjali states in his aphorism III.37 that these phenomena are powers (*siddhi) in the *waking state but *obstacles in attaining enstasy (*samādhi). Already the *Mahābhārata (XII.232.22) advises that these "flashes of illumination" arising from one's spiritual practice should be ignored. In another passage of the same work (XII.266.7), we read: "The 'knower of the truth' (tattva-vid) [should conquer] sleep (*nidrā) and pratibhā through the practice of wisdom (*jnāna)." See also divya-cakshus, divya-samvid, divya-shrotra.

pratibima ("reflection"). This is an important epistemological concept of *Classical Yoga. It is an attempt to explain how the transcendental *Self, which is thought to be eternally distinct from *Nature and thus from the human body-mind, can possibly apperceive mental states. While the second-century *Yoga-Sūtra makes no reference to pratibimba at all, the *Yoga-Bhāshya (IV.23) mentions the term once and understands it as the "reflection" of the *object in *consciousness. The *Tattva-Vaishāradī (II.17), written several hundred years later, makes a distinction between *bimba, or the mirroring of the object in consciousness, and pratibimba or the reflection of that content of consciousness to the transcendental *Self. However, the *Vaishāradī* frequently also uses both terms interchangeably. According to *Vācaspati Mishra, consciousness is like a mirror (*darpana*) in which the Self's awareness (*caitanya*) is reflected. This idea is found fully developed in the *Yoga-Vārttika* (I.4) by the *Vedānta philosopher *Vijnāna Bhikshu. He speaks of a "mutual reflection" (*parasparam pratibimbam*).

pratipaksha-bhāvanā ("cultivation of the opposite") is a method suggested by *Patanjali in his *Yoga-Sūtra* (II.33) to combat negative mental states characterized by him as "unwholesome deliberations" (*vitarka*). At the simplest level, this could consist in the mere recollection of the opposite of whatever negative or undersirable intentions or thoughts are assailing one's *mind. But it is easy to see how this could be developed into a full-fledged *contemplation. Thus, the *Yoga-Bhāshya* (II.33) advises the practitioner who is troubled by harmful thoughts to ponder as follows:

> Boiled by the terrifying coals of existence (*samsāra*), I take my refuge in the precepts of *Yoga by bestowing fearlessness of all creatures. Having cast off [all] "unwholesome deliberations," I betake myself to them again like a dog: As a dog [devours] his vomit, so do I betake myself to [that which I have] cast off.

pratiprasava ("counterflow") is a technical term of *Classical Yoga that stands for the "involution" of the primary constituents (*guna*) of *Nature. *Prasava* signifies the "streaming forth" of the ultimate building blocks of Nature into the multiple forms of the universe in all its dimensions. *Pratiprasava*, on the other hand, denotes the process of dissolution of those forms *relative to* the *microcosm of the *adept who is about to win liberation (*kaivalya*). In *Classical Yoga, which subscribes to the ideal of "disembodied liberation" (*videha-mukti*), this coincides with the psychophysical *death of the individual.

pratīti ("conviction," "faith"). The *Yoga-Shikhā-Upanishad* (I.132) declares that when *faith is merged with *recitation of one's *mantra, this becomes *hatha-yoga. See also *shraddhā*.

Pratyābhijna school is the most prominent school of the northern Indian branch of *Shaivism. Founded by Vasugupta (A.D. 770–830), the "discoverer" of the *Shiva-Sūtra, this school gets its name from its central tenet, namely that the individual being is able to "re-cognize" himself or herself as *Shiva, the *Absolute. This notion was first philosophically elaborated by Somānanda, a disciple of Vasugupta, in his *Shiva-Drishti* ("View on Shiva"). The most popular textbook expouding this philosophy, which is still in use among Kashmiri pundits today, is the *Pratyābhijna-Hridaya* ("Heart of Recognition") by Kshemarāja, a pupil of the renowned *adept *Abhinava Gupta.

*Yoga played a significant role among the Pratyābhijna adherents. In fact, the *Shiva-Sūtra* can be considered a manual of Yoga similar to the *Yoga-Sūtra*. Vasugupta and his commentators emphasizes the importance of *grace, as manifested in the "descent of the power" (*shakti-pāta*), proper initiation (*dīkshā*), and "illumined knowledge" (*bodha-jnāna*). The yogic technology employed in this school is close to that of early *hatha-yoga*.

pratyāhāra ("withdrawal"), or sensory inhibition, is the fifth "limb" (*anga*) of the eightfold *path (*ashta-anga-yoga*) of *Patanjali. In the *Yoga-Sūtra* (II.54), *pratyāhāra* is defined as the imitation of the nature of *consciousness by the *senses insofar as they disunite themselves from their respective objects. This is said to result in the supreme "obedience" (*vashyatā*) of the senses, which is the ability to "switch off" and produce a state of extreme inward-mindedness at will. *Vyāsa, in his *Yoga-Bhāshya* (II.54), give the following simile: "As when the queen bee flies up and the bees swarm after her, and when she settles down and they also settle down: similarly, the senses are controlled when consciousness (*citta*), is controlled."

The *Maitrāyanīya-Upanishad* (VI.25) compares *pratyāhāra* to the retraction of our sensory awareness in *sleep. However, this comparison is somewhat unfortunate, because *pratyāhāra* is a completely voluntary process and does not lead to a state of diminished awareness but one of intensified *consciousness. The *Yoga-Cūdāmany-Upanishad* (121) likens this process to the sun withdrawing its luster in the third quarter of the day. The *Shāndilya-Upanishad* (I.8.1) offers a symbolic interpretation of *pratyāhāra*: Everything that is seen should be looked upon as the *Self. This scripture also defines it as the mental performance of the prescribed daily rites, and as the holding of the breath (*vāyu*) in the eighteen sensitive places (*marman-sthāna*) in the sequence.

A favorite image for describing this process is expressed, for instance, in the *Goraksha-Paddhati* (II.24): "As the tortoise retracts its limbs into the middle of the *body, so the *yogin* should withdraw the *senses into himself."

This scripture (II.25ff.) continues as follows:

Knowing that whatever he hears, [be it] pleasant or unpleasant, is the
*Self: the Yoga knower withdraws [his senses].

Knowing that whatever scent he smells with the nose is the Self: the
Yoga knower withdraws.

Knowing that whatever he sees with the eye, [be it] pure or impure,
is the Self: the Yoga knower withdraws.

Knowing that whatever he senses with the skin, tangible or intangible,
is the Self: the Yoga knower withdraws.

Knowing that whatever he tastes with the tongue, [be it] salty or not
salty, is the Self: the Yoga knower withdraws.

According to the *Tejo-Bindu-Upanishad (I.34), pratyāhāra is the
twelfth "limb" of the "fifteen-limbed Yoga" (*panca-dasha-anga-yoga). It
is defined here as the "plesant consciousness" (citta-ranjaka) that beholds the *Self in all things. This is in contrast to most other definitions
that suggest a state of acute inwardness. Thus, the *Tri-Shikhi-
Brāhmana-Upanishad (II.30) defines pratyāhāra as the condition of the
"inward-facing" (antar-mukhin) consciousness. Elsewhere (130), the
same text speaks of it as the withdrawal of the *life force from different
places in the *body. See also indriya-jaya.

pratyaksha ("perception") means literally "having before one's eyes
(aksha)." In *Classical Yoga, this is one of the three means of valid
cognition (*pramāna), the other two being inference (*anumāna) and
tradition (*āgama). The *Mahābhārata epic (XII.211.26), which is representative of *Pre-Classical Yoga, states that perception is the foundation
of the other two epistemological means. Elsewhere (XII.289.7) in this
work, pratyaksha is used to contrast *Yoga with the more theory-
dependent approach of the *Sāmkhya tradition, which is characterized
as resting upon the ascertainment of the *knowledge taught in the
books (shāstra-vinishcaya).
    Pratyaksha also figures as the sixth "limb" of the "sevenfold disci-
pline" (*sapta-sādhana) and in this connection is defined, in the *Gheranda-Samhitā (I.11), as the perception of the *Self, resulting from
meditation (*dhyāna). More commonly, this higher spiritual perception
is called *sākshātkāra to emphasize the fact that *Self-realization is not
*knowledge based on any sensory input but "direct perception." Cf.
viparyaya.

pratyaya can mean "cause" and "notion," or "idea." In the *Yoga-Sūtra*, this term very probably has the meaning of "idea" throughout, although the classical commentators interpret some of its occurrences in the sense of "cause." The word denotes any content of *conscious-ness and is thus more comprehensive than either the five types of mental "fluctuation" (*vritti*) or the higher intuitions (*prajnā*) of enstasy (*samādhi*). Both these mental phenomena are in fact "presented ideas" (*pratyaya*), which are continuously apperceived by the transcendental *Self.

pravritti ("activity") is that mental disposition which is due to the influence of *rajas* and, according to the *Tattva-Vaishāradī* (I.2), consists in such states as distress and grief (*shoka*). In the *Yoga-Sūtra* (I.35), the term also refers to a special mental phenomenon that, in the *Yoga-Bhāshya* (III.25), is explained as a kind of "divine perception" (*divya-samvid*), or what we might call heightened sensory awareness. As Vyāsa points out, such paranormal phenomena are useful insofar as they dispel the aspirant's doubts (*samshaya*).

pravritti-mārga ("path of activity"), as opposed to the "path of ces-sation" (*nivritti-mārga*), is the orientation of the person who does not renounce the world, which consequently leads to rebirth after rebirth (*punar-janman*) punctuated by repeated *deaths (*punar-mrityu*).

prayāna-kāla ("time of departure") is the moment of *death, which is very important in *Yoga. See also *anta-kāla*

prayāsa ("overexertion"). According to the *Hatha-Yoga-Pradīpikā* (I.15), this is one of the factors that impede *progress in Yoga. See also Effort, *vighna*.

prayatna ("effort") is, according to the *Yoga-Tattva-Upanishad* (81), an essential prerequisite for success in *Yoga. As the *Bhagavad-Gītā* (VI.45) affirms, this *effort may have to be kept up over many lifetimes until *perfection is reached. In the *Yoga-Sūtra* (II.47), however, *prayatna* stands for "tension," which must be released for the accurate perfor-mance of the postures (*āsana*). See also *paurusha*, *yatna*; cf. Grace.

Prayer. Many of the hymns (*sūkta*) of the ancient *Rig-Veda* are prayers that combine praise with petition. In some contexts, the *Vedic Sanskrit word *brahman* means as much as "prayerful meditation." Later it came to stand for the ultimate *Reality to which the seers (*rishi*) aspired.

Prayer is intimately connected with the worship of the *Divine as a personal force. Thus, it is a prominent element in the theistic schools of *Vaishnavism and *Shaivism, notably *bhakti-yoga. The purer the prayer, or the least amount of self-will it expresses, the more it approximates mediation (*dhyāna), which is the absorption of the individual *consciousness into the transcendental Consciousness (*cit).

Pre-Classical Yoga is a broad historical category that refers to the numerous *Yoga teachings found in such scriptures as the *Katha-, Maitrāyanīya-, and *Shvetāshvatara-Upanishad as well as the *Mahābhārata, especially the *Bhagavad-Gītā, the *Moksha-Dharma, and the *Anugītā sections of that epic. The metaphysics of Pre-Classical Yoga is essentially *Vedāntic. Cf. Classical Yoga, Epic Yoga, Post-Classical Yoga.

preta ("departed [spirit]") is the postmortem entity of a recently deceased person. The *Yoga-Vāsishtha (III.55.27.ff) states that the pretas experience themselves in a new *body created out of the *offerings of their living relatives. Later they meet the messengers of *Yama, the God of Death. The virtuous souls get snatched away in heavenly carriages, whereas the sinners have to walk through snow and dangerous forests. Upon arrival in the world of Yama, they are judged and then transported either to *heaven or to *hell. After a period of time in either realm, they reincarnate. See also deva-yāna, pitri-yāna.

Pride. See abhimāna, dambha, darpa, mada, smaya.

Prithivī ("earth") is one of the five material elements (*bhūta) that compose the densest level of the *cosmos. See also tattva.

Prithu was an ancient *Vedic emperor of Ayodhya (Audh) and a great sage who is remembered in many *Purānas, especially the Vāyu-Purāna. He appears to have been closely connected with the *Vrātya brotherhoods from whom he learned the secret *knowledge about the syllable *om. According to the *Bhāgavata-Purāna (IV.23), he was initiated into *Yoga by *Sanatkumāra.

prīti ("satisfaction") is sometimes counted among the principles of moral discipline (*yama). See also samtosha, tushti.

Progress. Most esoteric traditions depict spiritual life as a winding *path that, step by step, brings the practitioner (*yogin, *sādhaka) closer to the summit, which is *liberation. A few schools understand liberation as a sudden, spontaneous event, but even then some form of preparation or discipline is thought to be necessary. Those who view spiritual life as a graduated process of increasing self-understanding or self-surrender often distinguish between distinct states (*avasthā) or stages (*bhūmi) of maturation. The texts differ in their assessment of how quickly certain stages can be reached. For instance, the *Amrita-Nāda-Upanishad (*28f.) proposes the following sequence: After three months, wisdom (*jnāna) dawns; after four months, the deities (*deva) can be seen; after five months, the resplendent principle called virāj becomes visible; after six months "aloneness" (*kaivalya), or *liberation, is attained. This optimistic view is not shared, for example, by the anonymous author of the *Yoga-Tattva-Upanishad (21), who states that *wisdom is gained after twelve years of practicing *mantra-yoga, though he concedes that the "purification of the channels" (*nādī-shuddhi) can be accomplished within three months.

Since most *Yoga authorities believe that *liberation is, in the final analysis, a matter of *grace that descends on the well-prepared practitioner, these computations must not be taken too seriously. Presumably, their purpose is to encourage the aspirant. Spiritual progress depends very much on the individual—his or her dedication to the process of *self-transcendence and *karmic (genetic, psychomental) strengths and liabilities.

Psychology. While the aspects and phenomena of the ordinary *consciousness are analyzed in unparalleled detail in *Buddhism, *Hindu Yoga has developed a comprehensive phenomenology of extraordinary states of *consciousness, called *samādhi, for which there is no equivalent even in modern psychology. The notion of the transcendental *Self as "witness" (*drashtri, *sākshin), especially deserves our close attention.

*Yoga psychology is therapy, or healing—in the broadest sense of the word. However, whereas modern psychotherapy has grown out of the clinical treatment of cases that *medicine was unable to help, Yoga has from the beginning been a system of spiritual catharsis and transformation intended to restore the individual to primordial wholeness rather than mere physical or mental *health. The *yogins have always endeavored to transcend the ordinary *consciousness, with its sense of self-dividedness and *suffering, and to realize the undiminishable *bliss of the Self (*purusha, *ātman). In the course of their spiritual disciplines—comprising both bodily and mental techniques—they inevitably encountered the habitual patterns of the psyche, which tend toward conventional modes of motivation and perception. Long before

Sigmund Freud, they discovered the reality of the subconscious. Thus, the authorities of *Classical Yoga speak of the "subliminal activators" (*samskāra) that combine into "traits" (*vāsanā) through which the conventional (i.e., unenlightened) personality system is maintained.

The purpose of *Yoga is nothing less than the complete transmutation of the subconscious *mind through the transcendence of the ego-mechanism, called "I-maker" (*ahamkāra) or "I-am-ness" (*asmitā). This goal, which coincides with *enlightenment, or *liberation, is alien to the worldview of modern psychology and psychotherapy. Nevertheless, humanistic psychology, which was ushered in by Abraham Maslow, and especially transpersonal psychology are more sympathetic toward the yogic ideal of *Self-realization and also appreciate that the enstatic states (*samādhi) are, as the *yogins claim, suprawakeful rather than unconscious. See also Feeling, Hypnosis, Parapsychology, Unconsciousness.

pūjā ("worship") is to *Tantrism what the sacrifice (*yajna) is to mainstream *Vedic religion, or *Brāhmanism. It signifies primarily, though not exclusively, the daily worship of one's "chosen deity" (*ishta-devatā). It involves the following ritual components: (1) *āsana, or the "seat" of the image of the *deity; (2) svāgata, or bidding welcome to the deity; (3) pādya, or water for the washing of the deity's feet; (4) arghya, or the offering of unboiled rice, flowers, etc.; (5) āchamana, or water for sipping, which is offered to the deity twice; (6) mādhu-parka, or honey, milk, or ghee; (7) *snāna, or water for bathing; (8) vasana, or cloth; (9) ābharana, or jewels for beautifying the image (*mūrti) of the deity; (10) gandha, or scents and sandal paste; (11) *pushpa, or flowers; (12) dhūpa, or incense; (13) dīpa, or light; (14) naivedya, or food; (15) vandana or namaskāra, which is worshipful praise. The ceremony also includes the use of *mantra recitation, *breath control, and *meditation.

pūjana ("worship", "reverence"). The *Bhāgavata-Purāna (XVII.14) calls the reverence of *deities, *teachers, sages, and "twice-born" (dvija) members of *Hindu society (that is, brahmins, warriors, and merchants) "physical austerity (*tapas)." See also guru-pūjā, īshvara-pūjana.

Pūjyapāda is mentioned in the *Hatha-Yoga-Pradīpikā (I.7) as an *adept of *hatha-yoga. No information about him is available.

punar-janman ("rebirth"). The idea that a person has more than one lifetime is common to most schools of Indian thought. This notion first emerged with the oldest *Upanishads where it was treated as a secret teaching. Thus, the *Chāndogya-Upanishad (V.10.7) has this passage:

> Thus, those whose conduct here [on earth] is pleasing quickly enter a pleasing womb—the womb of a brahmin [woman], the womb of a [woman of the] warrior [estate], or the womb of a merchant [woman]. But those whose conduct here [on earth] stinks quickly enter a stinking womb—the womb of a dog, the womb of a swine, or the womb of an outcaste.

The notion of *punar-janman* is associated with the idea, first expressed in the *Brihad-Āranyaka-Upanishad (IV.4.5), that the quality of one's being is determined by the quality of one's *actions, so that the doer of good deeds becomes good, whereas the doer of *evil becomes evil. The doctrine of reembodiment extends this idea beyond the orbit of the present lifetime. The connecting link between different *embodiments is *karma.

The ultimate purpose of *Yoga is to escape this never-ending cycle of births and *deaths, to put a stop to the generation and fruition of *karma* and to awaken, or reawaken, to one's identity as the transcendental Self (*ātman, *purusha).

punya ("merit") is the "fruit" of *actions or volitions (*samkalpa) that are morally good, that is, in keeping with the cosmic order (*rita, *dharma). Cf. *pāpa*.

Pupil. See *shishya*.

pūraka ("inhalation") is one of the three phases of breath control (*prānāyāma). The *Brihad-Yogi-Yājnavalkya-Samhitā (VIII.19) defines it as that restriction of the *breath that fills all the "channels" (*nādī). This implies that inhalation is more than the intake of air. It is the attraction into the *body of the universal life force (*prāna). Cf. *kumbhaka, recaka*.

Purāna ("Ancient [Stories]") is a type of popular encyclopedia that, at least theoretically, deals with five topics: the original *creation of the world, the world's re-creation after its destruction, the great *world ages, the genealogy of *deities and sages, and dynastic history. Eighteen major works of this genre, called *mahā-purāna*, are known, which include the *Mārkandeya-, *Vishnu-, *Bhāgavata-, *Kūrma-, *Linga-, and the *Agni-Purāna. Most of these Purānas were composed in the post-Christian era. However, in some instances they draw on traditions that flourished as far back as the *Vedic age.

The yogic teachings in the Purānas belong to *Post-Classical Yoga and are thus broadly nondualist (advaita). They generally make use of the formulations of *Patanjali but tend more toward ritualism. Especially the later Purānas show *Tantric influence.

purashcarana ("preparatory ritual"). In *Tantrism, this is the practice of reciting a *mantra a large number of times in order to activate it in one's *consciousness. This ritual is combined with other practices, such as dietary restrictions and the use of consecrated space.

Purification. See dhauti, shauca, shodhana.

Purity, or shuddhi, is a notion that is central to all spiritual traditions. The transcendental *Reality is commonly conceived as being perfectly pure, in stark contrast with the human *mind, or *consciousness, which is tainted by the mechanism of the *ego. The spiritual *path consists in the progressive *purification of the body-mind until it is cleansed of all "defects" (*dosha) and becomes capable of flawlessly reflecting the *light of the *Divine, or *Self. In *Yoga and *Sāmkhya, this process is understood as the gradual emergence of the *sattva aspect of *Nature.

pūrna ("full, whole") is an ancient *Vedic designation for the *Absolute. The *Yoga-Shikhā-Upanishad (I.19), one of the *Yoga-Upanishads, speaks of the "fullness" (pūrnatva) of the Absolute, which allows it to be both divided (sakala) and impartite (nishkala). The much older Kaushītaki-Upanishad (IV.*) observes that by worshipping that plenum, one becomes filled with "splendor" (yashas) and "*brahmic luster" (brahma-varcasa).

purusha ("male") is the *Yoga and *Sāmkhya term for the transcendental *Self, or pure spirit, which is called *ātman in the *Vedānta tradition. The *Brihad-Āranyaka-Upanishad (I.4.1) furnishes the following fanciful etymology: "Because he, being prior (pūrva) to everthing, consumed (aushat) all *evils, he is [called] purusha." The Go-Patha ("Cow Path")-Brāhmana (I.1.39), a pre-Christian work, explains the word purusha as "he who rests in the castle" (puri-shaya), the "castle" being the *body. This is also the explanation of the *Linga-Purāna (I.28.5), a medieval scripture. More likely than either etymology is the derivation of *purusha* from *pū* "male" and *vrisha* "bull."

The *purusha*, as the transcendental *Consciousness, is the "witness" (*sākshin) of all psychomental experiences. In the *Yoga-Sūtra (I.3), the *Self is called the "seer" (*drastri). *Shankara, in his *Vivarana (I.3), names it the "cognizer" (*boddhri) of "cognitions" (*buddhi). In *Epic Yoga, it is widely referred to as the "knower" (*jna*) or the "field knower" (*kshetra-jna), the "field" being *Nature in the form of the individual *body and *mind.

In *Classical Yoga, the *purusha*, which is styled the "power of Awareness" (*citi-shakti), is conceived as being absolutely distinct from Nature (*prakriti), which lacks all *awareness. Yet, what we call *consciousness is due to the curious correlation (*samyoga) between the *purusha* and *prakriti*. That correlation is to be undermined through the processes of *Yoga, until the *Self shines forth in its original splendor.

The *Katha-Upanishad (V.3) also refers to the *purusha* as the "dwarf" (*vāmana) who dwells in the middle of the *body, that is, at the *heart. This work (IV.12) also states that the *purusha*, in its association with the body-mind, is "thumb sized." In its transcendental status, however, the *purusha* is infinite. This dual nature of the *Self—in its bound and liberated form—has led to the question of whether there are many transcendental Selves or, as the *Vedanta tradition postulates, only a single Self (*ātman). The *Mahābhārata epic (XII.338.2) states that both *Yoga and *Sāmkhya proclaim the existence of multiple *purushas* in the world but that these many *purushas* all have their origin in the single Self, which is eternal, immutable, and incommensurable. That Self is described in the same section as being both the "seer" (*drashtri) and the "seen" (*drashtavya). This view is characteristic of the schools of *Epic or *Pre-classical Yoga. It is, however, not the stance of *Classical Yoga.

Thus, the *Yoga-Bhāshya (I.24) clearly announces that there are numerous *purushas* who enjoy the condition of *liberation. They are called *kevalins, as in *Jainism. Nevertheless, the *Tattva-Vaishāradī (I.41) emphasizes that there is no distinction between these many Selves. Logic dictates that if there is more than one ominpresent and omnitemporal being, they must all coincide in eternity. This argument has escaped both *Patanjali, the author of the textbook on *Classical Yoga, and *Īshvara Krishna, the founder of *Classical Sāmkhya.

purusha-artha ("human purpose"). According to *Hinduism, there are four goals to which people can dedicate themselves: (1) *artha*, or material welfare, prosperity; (2) *kāma*, or pleasure, that is, the quest for physical comfort, emotional well-being, and intellectual delights; (3) *dharma, or virtue, justice—a moral way of life; (4) *moksha, or *liberation. *Yoga is concerned with assisting in the realization of liberation, as the summum bonum of human life. The Marathi *adept *Jnānadeva postulated a fifth goal of human endeavor—love or devotion (*bhakti) to the *Divine.

purusha-khyāti ("vision of the Self") is the essence of the supraconscious enstasy (*asamprajnāta-samādhi). See also ātma-darshana.

purusha-uttama ("supreme male"), also written purushottama, is a *Vaishnava theological term for the *Divine. According to the *Bhagavad-Gītā (XV.18), the purusha-uttama is beyond the kshara-purusha ("mobile self"), which is the individual psyche, and the *akshara-purusha ("immobile Self"), which is the transcendental spirit, or the Self upon *liberation, also known as the principle that is "summit abiding" (*kūtastha).

puryashtaka ("eightfold city") consists, according to the *Laghu-Yoga-Vāsishtha (VI.5.5f), of the "I-maker" (*ahamkāra), the lower mind (*manas), the higher mind (*buddhi), and the five senses (*indriya). This is also called the "subtle body" (*sūkshma-sharīra).

pūshā-nādī ("nourishing current") is one of the "channels" (*nādī) of the life force (*prāna) that is generally thought to be situated to the rear of the *pingalā-nādī and to terminate in the right eye or ear, though sometimes the left eye is specified.

pushpa ("flower [offering]") is part of the *Tantric ritual. According to the *Kaula-Jnāna-Nirnaya (III.24), this should be a mental act consisting of such spiritual practices as nonharming (*ahimsā), sense restraint (*indriya-nigraha), patience (*kshamā), and meditation (*dhyāna).

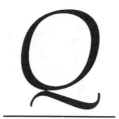

Qualifications, spiritual. See *adhikāra*.

Qualities of Nature. *Yoga and *Sāmkhya cosmology pictures the *cosmos as made up of many levels of existence—from the "coarse" (*sthūla*) material realm to the "subtle" (*sūkshma*) psychic realms, to the unmanifest (*avyakta*) dimension of Nature (*prakriti*). The "stuff" of which all these levels and their respective phenomena are composed are the three types of "qualities" (*guna*). Everything participates in their interplay. Only the transcendental *Reality, or *Self, is eternally beyond these primary constituents of *prakriti*, and hence is said to be *nirguna*.

Quality. See *dharma*.

Quietude. See *shānti*.

R

Rādhā, the divine spouse of *Krishna, is to this day the symbol spiritual womanhood for *Hindus. For the pious followers of *Vaishnaivism, Rādhā has served for centuries as the great ideal of the passionate woman whose love is so full and deep that it transcends the mere carnal and touches the spiritual core of her own and her lover's being. The spiritual love story between the shepherdess (*gopī) and the God-man *Krishna is very touchingly told in the *Bhāgavata-Purāna and, in more openly erotic fashion, in the *Gītā-Govinda.

rāga ("passion," "attachment"). In *Classical Yoga, rāga is one of the five "causes of affliction" (*klesha) and is defined in the *Yoga-Sūtra (II.7) as one's dwelling upon the pleasurable. It is often paired up with *dvesha, meaning "repulsion" or "hatred." The *Bhagavad-Gītā (III.34) calls these the two "waylayers" (paripanthin). See also kāma, rajas, rati.

rāja-danta ("royal tooth") is the estoeric designation of the uvula, which plays an important role in the practice of the *khecarī-mudrā. By stimulating the uvula, the "nectar" (*amrita) is said to flow more profusely. See also lambikā-yoga.

Rāja-Mārtanda ("Royal Sun-Bird"), also called Bhoja-Vritti, is a commentary by King *Bhoja on the *Yoga-Bhāshya. While largely concurring with the interpretations of the *Tattva-Vaishāradī, Bhoja occasionally offers original exegetical observations.

284

rajas is derived from the verbal root *raj/ranj* meaning "to be colored, affected, excited, charmed." This term has several important meanings. Firstly, it designates one of the three primary constituents (**guna*) of **Nature. Rajas is the dynamic principle, whose aspects are listed in the **Maitrāyanī-Upanishad* (III.5) as follows: "thirst" (**trishnā*), affection (**sneha*), passion (**rāga*), greed (**lobha*), violence (**himsā*), lust (**rati*), (false) vision (**drishti*), contradictoriness (*vyāvritatva*), jealousy (**īrshyā*), desire (**kāma*), instability (*asthiratva*), fickleness (*cāncalatva*), possessiveness (*jihīrshā*), material acquisitiveness (*artha-uparjana*), nepotism (*mitra-anugrahana*), dependence on one's environment (*parigraha-avalamba*), "repulsion from undesirable sense objects" (*anishteshu indriya-artheshu dvishti*), and "fondness for desirable [sense objects]" (*ishteshu abhishvanga*).

Secondly, *rajas* denotes the mental or emotional disposition of **passion and as such counts as one of the "defects" (**dosha*). The **Bhagavad-Gītā* (XIV.7) describes it as being of the nature of attraction (**rāga*), springing from "thirst" (**trishnā*) and attachment (**sanga*). It is also said to produce **bondage through one's clinging to **action.

A third connotation of *rajas* is "blood," and in this sense is used to refer to the female "semen," or vaginal secretion. In **Tantrism and some schools of **hatha-yoga, this *rajas* fluid is sucked up through the penis by means of the **vajrolī-mudrā.

Rajas also stands for the female principle, or **shakti*, in general. Thus, the **Yoga-Shikhā-Upanishad* (I.136) states: "In the middle of the perineum (**yoni*), the great place, dwells the well-concealed *rajas*, the principle of the **Goddess, resembling the *japa* and *bandhuka* [flowers]."

See also *mahā-rajas*, *retas*; cf. *bindu*.

rāja-yoga ("royal Yoga") most commonly refers to the **yoga-darshana*, or **Classical Yoga, as pithily expounded in **Patanjali's **Yoga-Sūtra*. It is often contrasted with **hatha-yoga, in which case *rāja-yoga* stands for the higher spiritual practices, whereas *hatha-yoga* is seen as a preparatory discipline. This distinction came into vogue in about the eleventh century A.D. as part of an attempt to integrate the more **meditative, renunciate approach of the eightfold **path (**ashta-anga-yoga*) with the new body-positive teachings of **Tantric *hatha-yoga*.

The **Hatha-Yoga-Pradīpikā* (III.126), which seeks to build a bridge between these two approaches of **Yoga, affirms: "Without *rāja-yoga*, the 'earth' (**prithivī*) is inauspicious. Without *rāja-yoga*, the 'night' (*nishā*) [is inauspicious]. Without *rāja-yoga*, even the different 'seals' (**mudrā*) [are inauspicious]."

This couplet contains a subtle pun on the word *rāja*, which suggests the sovereign's rule, the moon (*rajā*), and the king's (*rāja*) seal. The **Jyotsnā* commentary on this medieval text understands the words "earth" and "night" symbolically. It takes the former to stand for the quality of stability (**sthairya*) of the yogic postures (**āsana*) and the latter for the absence of the flow of the *life force in the practice of breath retention (**kumbhaka*).

The **Yoga-Shikhā-Upanishad* (I.137) explains *rāja-yoga* as the union (**yoga*) between **rajas* and **retas*, or the male and female creative principles. By practicing this union, we are told, the **yogin* "shines" (*rājate*).

rāja-yogin is a practitioner of **raja-yoga*.

rākā-nādī ("full-moon channel") is a current of the *life force mentioned in the **Yoga-Shikhā-Upanishad* (V.24). It is said to fill the *nose with rheum and to cause sneezing after sipping water. See also *nādī*.

Rāma or **Rāmacandra**, prince of the ancient kingdom of Kosala, may have lived in the eighth century B.C. He is the celebrated hero of the **Rāmāyana* epic and in the *Vaishnava tradition is worshipped as one of the incarnations or "descents" (**avatāra*) of God *Vishnu. Rāma, as the name suggests, is generally described as having been of dark color, and is frequently depicted as carrying a bow and arrow. His wife *Sita is the personification of marital *devotion.

Ramakrishna (A.D. 1836–1886), son of a poor Bengali brahmin, is widely recognized as one of the greatest spiritual geniuses of modern *Hinduism. He had his first spiritual experience at the age of six or seven. Throughout his life, he worshipped the Goddess *Kālī and at one point was initiated into *Tantric practice. Subsequently, his teacher Tota Puri instructed him in *Advaita-Vedānta and the practice of "formless enstasy" (**nirvikalpa-samādhi*), which Ramakrishna succeeded in accomplishing in a single day. He lived the life of a renunciate and temple priest at the Kali temple of Dak-

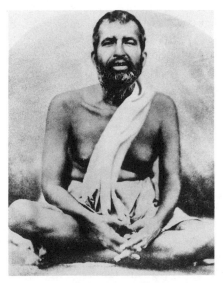

54. *Ramakrishna.*

shineshvar near Calcutta. Yet, Ramakrishna was married, though the marriage was never consummated. His wife, Sarada Devi, was to him the *Goddess incarnate, and she looked upon her husband as her spiritual teacher (*guru). Ramakrishna, a "fool of God" who was oriented more toward mystical experiences than learning, submitted himself to various religious disciplines—including Christianity and Islam—and became convinced that all *paths lead to the same end—*God-realization. Ramakrishna had numerous disciples, among them the world-renowned Swami *Vivekananda.

Rāmānuja was born in South India in A.D. 1017 and is said to have died in A.D. 1137. He was the founder of the Vishishta-Advaita ("Qualified Nondualism") school of *Vedānta and the leading theologian and philosopher of the medieval *bhakti movement. A zealous proponent of *Vaishnavism, Rāmānuja converted numerous people to his religion and reportedly counted among his followers seven hundred ascetics as well as twelve thousand monks and three hundred nuns. His keen intellect and missionary enthusiasm made him the chief opponent of *Shankara's philosophy. Rāmānuja wrote brilliant commentaries on the *Brahma-Sūtra*, the *Bhagavad-Gītā*, and the major *Upanishads, which all occasioned a vast commentarial literature.

Rāmānuja taught that the *Absolute is not merely impersonal and unqualified but includes in its being the phenomenal world. He regarded the changeable world as the body of the *Divine and rejected the idealist notion that the universe is unreal (*mithyā) or illusory (*māyā). *God, whom Ramanuja calls the "Lord" (*īshvara), is the foundation of everything. His existence cannot be inferred but must be accepted on the basis of revelation. Even though everything is dependent on God, there is also free will. A creature can turn toward or away from God. Those who turn to the *Divine with devotion (*bhakti) receive God's favor (*prasāda). For Rāmānuja, *bhakti* is not a state of emotional effusiveness but one of wisdom (*jnāna). See also *prapatti*.

Rāmāyana ("Life of Rāma") of Vālmīki is one of India's two national epics, the other being the *Mahābhārata*. The *Rāmāyana*, a tragic love story, was probably composed a little before the beginning of the Christian era. It has served countless generations as a repository of folk wisdom. In its present form, the epic consists of seven chapters with a total of c. 24,000 stanzas. The hero of the *Rāmāyana* is the God-man *Rāma. The world of this epic is that of asceticism (*tapas) rather than *Yoga.

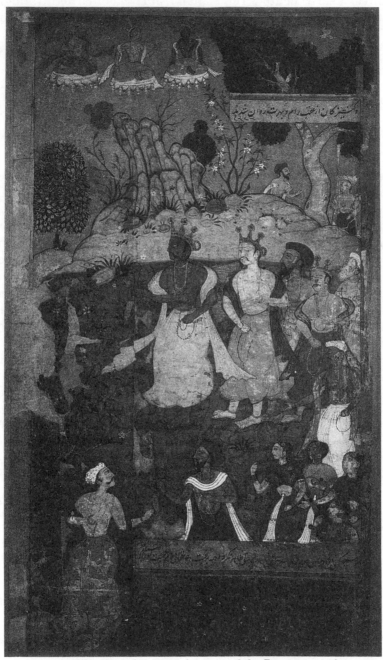

55. Illuminated manuscript page of the Rāmāyana epic.

Ramdas, Swami (A.D. 1884–1963) was a revered modern saint who taught a form of simple *japa-yoga*, the *Yoga of the constant *recitation of the name "Ram" (Sanskrit: Rāma). He renounced the world in 1922 and six years later founded the Ananda Ashram. He is the author of several books.

rasa ("essence") has several connotations. Firstly, in the sense of "taste," it is associated with the tongue and the *water element and thus is one of the functions of the cognitive senses (*indriya-jnāna*). By extension, *rasa* is one's "taste" for the objective world, which, as the *Bhagavad-Gītā* (II.59) observes, lingers even after one abstains from "feeding" on the world. However, this subconscious relish—which is equivalent to the notion of *vāsanā*—disappears when the transcendental *Reality is "seen."

Secondly, *rasa* is the "essence" of pure *bliss in the highest state of devotional surrender to the *Divine. It is the culmination of *bhakti-yoga*. Thirdly, in *alchemy, *rasa* refers to mercury. Fourthly, in yogic alchemy, it stands for the "nectar of immortality" (*amrita*), the great life-giving elixir, hidden in the *body. According to the *Goraksha-Paddhati* (II.48), the *rasa* can be made to flow copiously by "kissing," that is, stimulating the uvula (*rāja-danta*) with the tongue. At first it tastes salty, pungent, and sour, but as the body becomes purified, it tastes like milk, honey, and ghee.

Finally, *rasa* stands for bodily liquid in general and the humors (*dosha*) in particular. Their "drying up" (*shoshana*) is effected by means of the "great seal" (*mahā-mudrā*).

rasāyana ("conduct of mercury"). See Alchemy.

rati is "love passion," as experienced by *Rādhā in relation to the God-man *Krishna. *Rati* is aesthetic *pleasure and its refined distillate of spiritual delight, *the* basic emotion of the erotic spirituality of the *Bhāgavata religion. Thus, the *Krishna followers made a virtue out of what in other, more body-negative schools is viewed as a vice. See also *bhakti*.

ravi ("sun") is a synonym for *sūrya*. Cf. *candra*.

Reality. See Divine, God, *tattva*.

Reason. Even though most schools of *Hinduism place great store in revelation (*shruti*) and faith (*shraddhā*), it is readily apparent from the available literature that the Indians did not indulge in amorphous irrationalism. The theological/philosophical masterpieces, for instance, of *Shankara, *Rāmānuja, and *Vijñāna Bhikshu, compare in their acuity, learning, and lucidity with the great works of Aristotle, St. Augustine, and Thomas of Aquinas.

The *Hindu authorities have not shunned reason and intellect but merely determined and delimited their function and usefulness. They clearly understood that *Reality lies beyond reason, beyond the mind (*manas*), even beyond illumined reason or wisdom (*buddhi*). Therefore, they have used rational arguments to show the limits inherent in reason and to point out a practical, experiential way by which one's innate desire for truth can be fulfilled—the demanding spiritual paths of *self-transcendence and self-transformation to the point of *Self-realization, or *enlightenment. See also *tarka*.

Rebirth. See *punar-janman*.

recaka ("exhalation"), which is also called *reca* and *recya*, is one of three phases of breath control (*prānāyāma*). It is the expulsion, or outward flow, of the life force (*prana*). Cf. *kumbhaka, pūraka*.

Renunciation. See Abandonment, *samnyāsa, tyāga*.

Respiration. See Breath, *prāna, shvāsa*.

retas ("semen") is a synonym for *bindu*. According to the *Goraksha-Paddhati* (II.49), when the *body is filled with the "nectar of immortality" (*amrita*), the *retas* rises. This rising of the semen is a psychosomatic process that is only inadequately characterized as sublimination. It involves higher states of *consciousness. See also *ūrdhva-retas*; cf. *rajas*.

Revelation. See *shruti*; cf. Reason.

Ribhu was a *Vaishnava sage who is referred to and quoted in some of the later *Upanishads. His nondualist teaching is also spoken of in the *Vishnu-Purāna* (II).

Rig-Veda ("Hymn Knowledge") is the oldest of the four *Vedic collections (*samhitā*), dating as far back as 1550 B.C. It comprises ten chapters (called *mandala*) with a total of 1,028 hymns (*sūkta*, *mantra*). This work is the fountainhead of *Brāhmanism. The word *yoga* and its verbal root *yuj* occur frequently in the *Rig-Veda* and generally have the meaning of "yoke" or "discipline," though there is no trace yet of *Yoga proper. See also History, Indus civilization, Pre-Classical Yoga.

riju-kāya ("erect body") is, according to the *Bhāgavata-Purāna* (III.28.8), one of the characteristics of correct posture (*āsana*). The *Yoga-Tattva-Upanishad* (36) treats it as a requirement for the practice of *breath control.

Rishabha is remembered in the *Bhāgavata-Purāna* (V.5.28ff.) as an *adept who besmeared himself with his own excreta but still emitted a sweet fragrance. In the *Shiva-Purāna* (III.4.35), he is introduced as an incarnation of God *Shiva.

rishi ("seer") is the title of the *Vedic bard who "sees" the hymn (*sūkta*, *mantra*) before composing it. *Rishi* and *mahārshi* (*mahā* + *rishi*, "great seer") are honorific titles that are bestowed on saintly folk even today. A female seer is known as *rishikā*. See also *keshin*, *muni*.

rita ("truth" or "order") is a synonym for *satya. It is one of the key concepts of *Vedic times and expresses the universal harmony—both cosmic and moral. See also *dharma*.

ritambhara-prajnā ("truth-bearing wisdom") is, as mentioned in the *Yoga-Sūtra* (I.48), discovered by the *yogin* at the culmination of the "ultrareflexive enstasy" (*nirvicāra-samādhi*). This special *knowledge is said to be "truth bearing" because it discloses the contemplated *object as it is, without any mental distortions.

Ritual, Ritualism. *Yoga has always been connected with some form of religious or magical ritualism. However, certain schools are more ritualistic than others and include rites (*kriyā*) as a significant aspect of their spiritual discipline. In particular, the yogic teachings mentioned in the *Purānas and *Tantras are pronouncedly ritualistic in their orientation. By contrast, the literature of *Classical Yoga, which inclines more toward the philosophical end of the spectrum, is relatively free of the ritual component.

roga ("illness"). For the *Yoga authorities, illness or disease (*vyādhi*) confirms the fundamental insight of *Patanjali that "everything is suffering" (*sarvam duhkham*). As the *Mahābhārata* epic (XII.318.3) puts it: "Bodily and mental illnesses pierce the *body like sharp-pointed arrows shot by a skilled archer."

Although *Yoga is first and foremost a spiritual discipline leading to *self-transcendence and *Self-realization, health (*ārogya*) is valued, and some of the yogic practices clearly have prophylactic and therapeutic value. Especially many techniques of *hatha-yoga* are directly concerned with creating a "divine body" (*divya-deha*) that is immune to disease.

According to the *Hatha-Yoga-Pradīpikā* (II.16f.), *breath control can cure all illnesses but when improperly practiced will cause all sorts of maladies, including asthma, coughs, hiccups, and pain in the *head. Similar claims are made for certain cleansing practices (*dhauti*), "locks" (*bandha*), "seals" (*mudrā*), and even postures (*āsana*). Faulty yogic discipline can produce illnesses of its own. These are discussed together with their remedies in such works as the *Sat-Karma-Samgraha* and the *Mishraka*. See also Medicine.

Rosary. See *mālā*.

Rudra ("Howler"). In *Vedic times, Rudra was an independent *deity but later on became assimilated into God *Shiva. In the *Shiva-Purāna* (VII.1.32.36), the name is explained as "He Who Quells Misery (*rud*)." Rudra appears to have been one of the deities invoked by the *Vrātya brotherhoods. See also *deva*.

rudra is a rare synonym for *prāna* or *vāyu*.

rudra-aksha ("Rudra's eye") is the "third eye" in the middle of the forehead, signifying the *ājnā-cakra*. See also *mālā*.

rudra-granthi ("Rudra's knot") is one of the three "knots" (*granthi*) that block the flow of the *life force through the central channel (*sushumnā-nādī*) of the *body. It is located at the *ājnā-cakra* in the *head.

rūpa ("form") is a multipurpose word. It can denote the *body, physical beauty, a visible thing, or a psychic phenomenon, or "sign" (*cihna*). The last-mentioned meaning is found, for instance, in the *Mahābhārata* (XII.228.18f.), which mentions the following visionary signs that can occur during *meditation: smoke, water, fire, an appearance "like a yellow garment," a phenomenon of the color of wool. The *Shvetāsh-vatara-Upanishad* (II.11) lists phenomena resembling fog, smoke, sun, fire, wind, firefly, lightning, crystal, and the moon, which are said to be preliminary to the ultimate realization of *enlightenment.

S

sa-ānanda-samāpatti ("coinciding with bliss") is one of the subforms of conscious enstasy (*samprajnāta-samādhi*) mentioned by *Vācaspati Mishra in his *Tattva-Vaishāradī* (I.44). It consists in the experience of bliss (*ānanda*) as a result of practicing "constraint" (*samyama*) with regard to the sense organs (*indriya*). See also *samādhi*; cf. *nirānanda-samāpatti*.

sa-asmitā-samāpatti ("coinciding with I-am-ness") is, according to the *Tattva-Vaishāradī* (I.44), a subform of conscious enstasy (*samprajnāta-samādhi*). It is the enstatic experience of the sense of being present without any other mental content. See also *samādhi*; cf. *nirasmitā-samāpatti*.

sabīja-samādhi ("enstasy with seed"). In *Classical Yoga, this is the technical name for various types of conscious enstasy (*samprajnāta-samādhi*). According to the *Yoga-Bhāshya* (I.46), the "seed" (*bīja*) is the *object of *concentration. However, as *Vijnāna Bhikshu notes in his *Yoga-Vārttika* (I.46), the objects themselves are the seeds of *suffering. See also *samādhi*; cf. *nirbīja-samādhi*.

sac-cid-ānanda ("existence, consciousness, bliss") are the three essential aspects of the *Absolute, as taught in *Vedānta. However, these are not qualities, for the Absolute is unqualified (*nirguna*) and impartite (*akala*). Thus, *bliss is not a state of *mind but the condition that remains when all psychomental phenomena, including the experience of *joy, have been transcended. Likewise, "existence" (*sat*, changed to *sac* for euphonic reasons) is not a particular form of existence but *Being. And "consciousness" (*cit*, changed to *cid* also for euphonic reasons) is not individuated conscious but pure Awareness.

Sacrifice. The notion of sacrifice (**yajna*) is central to *Hinduism. The early *Vedic religion has rightly been characterized as one of sacrificial ritualism. During the period of the *Brāhmanas, this was developed into a full-fledged sacrificial mysticism, which served as a bridge to the "inner sacrifice" of the *Upanishads and later *Yoga. If the external sacrifice, involving a variety of *rituals, was the way to *heaven for the Vedic people, the sacrifice of the *self, or *ego, is the way to *liberation for the *Yogin*. Cf. *pūjā, pūjana*.

sādhaka ("accomplisher") is the *Tantric designation for the male spiritual practitioner, or *yogin*. According to the *Shiva-Samhitā* (V.10), there are four types of practitioner, depending on their enthusiasm and commitment to the spiritual process: (1) The *mridu-sādhaka* ("soft practitioner") lacks zeal, is dull witted, sickly, greedy, attached to his wife, fickle, timid, ill, cruel, dependent on others, and given to evil deliberations; he finds fault with his *teacher and is a miracle monger (*bahu-āshin*). Such an individual is said to be fit for *mantra-yoga* and may succeed after twelve years of diligent application. (2) The *madhya-sādhaka* ("middling practitioner") is even-minded, patient, desirous of virtue, soft-spoken, and moderate in all undertakings. He is suited for *laya-yoga*. (3) The *adhimātra-sādhaka* ("ardent practitioner") is fit for *hatha-yoga* and may obtain success after six years of practice; he is steady-minded, disciplined, self-reliant, energetic, compassionate, patient, honest, courageous, mature, filled with *faith; he also has high expectations, worships his teacher's feet, and is constantly engaged in *Yoga practices. (4) The *adhimātratama-sādhaka* ("most ardent practitioner"), who qualifies for any type of Yoga and meets with success after only three years of practice, is highly energetic, zealous, agreeable, valiant, informed about the teachings (**shāstra*), eager to practice, not deluded, not confused, in the prime of his youth, moderate in his *diet, with his *senses under control, fearless, clean, skillful, charitable, a support to all people, competent, firm, wise, content with his lot, forbearing, good-natured, virtuous, well-spoken, and free from major *illnesses; he can also keep his endeavors secret, has faith in the teachings, worships his teacher and the *deities, avoids public gatherings, and practices all forms of Yoga. Cf. *sādhikā*.

sādhana or **sādhanā** ("means of realization") is the spiritual *path, especially of *Tantrism, which leads to perfection (*siddhi). Although all authorities of *Yoga subscribe to the view that we are inherently free, they also concur that in order to realize that native *freedom we must cultivate self-knowledge and an attitude of *dispassion. In other words, we must live from a disposition that is analogous to our inherent freedom, or *enlightenment. This process of "imitation" of the *Divine is the very essence of the spiritual *path. See also *ashta-anga-yoga, sapta-sādhana, shad-anga-yoga, yoga-kritya.*

sādhikā is the *Tantric designation for the female spiritual practitioner, or *yoginī. Cf. *sādhaka.*

sad-guru ("true teacher" or "teacher of the true") is an authentic spiritual *teacher who is *enlightened, or has realized the *Self. The *Kula-Arnava-Tantra* (XIII.104ff.) has these pertinent stanzas:

> There are many teachers (*guru), like lamps in house after house; but hard to find, o *Devī, is the teacher who lights up all like the sun.

> There are many teachers who are proficient in the *Vedas and the textbooks (*shāstra); but hard to find, o Devī, is the teacher who has attained to the supreme *Truth.

> There are many teachers on earth who give what is other than the *Self; but hard to find in all the worlds, o Devī, is the teacher who reveals the *Self.

> Many are the teachers who rob the disciple of his wealth; but rare is the teacher who removes the *disciple's afflictions.

> He is a [true] teacher by whose very contact there flows the supreme bliss (*ānanda). The intelligent man should choose such a one as his teacher and none other.

sādhu ("virtuous") is a saintly person who may or may not be a practitioner of *Yoga. Association (*sanga or sangama) with saintly folk has traditionally been considered to be one of the most rewarding practices. *Sādhu-sanga,* as the *Yoga-Vāsishtha* (II.16.9) notes, "removes the darkness in one's *heart and is the lamp for the right *path in the world." See also *sat-sanga.*

Sage. See *muni;* cf. *keshin, rishi.*

saguna-brahman ("qualified Absolute") is the phenomenal dimension of *Reality composed of the three "primary constituents" (*guna*) of *nature. See also *brahman*; cf. *nirguna*.

sahaja ("innate," "spontaneous"). The word *sahaja* means literally "together born" or "coemergent." It signifies the idea that *freedom is not external to us but our very condition; that the phenomenal reality (*samsāra*) arises simultaneously with, and within, the transcendental *Reality (*nirvāna*); and that the conditional *mind and *enlightenment are not mutually exclusive principles. According to this teaching, true spontaneity of naturalness is an expression of *Reality, and enlightenment is always close at hand. The great Buddhist adept Sahajapāda calls this the "straight path" (*uju-patha*) or "royal path" (*rāja-patha*). This is a key notion of Mahāyāna *Buddhism and the *Sahajiyā movement.

sahaja-karman ("innate action") is a phrase found in the *Bhagavad-Gītā* (SVIII.48). It refers to *action that is in keeping with one's essential nature (*sva-bhāva*). The *Gītā* is adamant that it is preferable to perform, even if only imperfectly, actions that are true to oneself rather than to perform perfectly actions that are true to another person's inner law (*sva-dharma*). See also *karma-yoga*.

sahaja-samādhi ("spontaneous enstasy") is explained in the *Tri-Pura-Rahasya* (XVII.107), an exceptional *Vedānta work, as the realization of unbroken transconceptual enstasy (*nirvikalpa-samādhi*) while being engaged in external activities. Supraconscious enstasy (*asamprajnāta-samādhi*) implies an extreme focusing of *attention with a concomitant withdrawal of one's awareness from the physical *body. As a result, this condition has often been confused with trance. However, the external "stonelike" existence fails to convey the *yogin's inner realization of the transcendental *Consciousness. By contrast, the *sahaja-samādhi* brings that realization down into the *body. The *yogin lives as it were in both worlds—the dimension of unqualified (*nirguna*) existence and the dimension of relativity. *Sahaja-samādhi* is equivalent to full and permanent *enlightenment, or "liberation while being alive" (*jīvan-mukti*). Within that condition, the liberated *yogin* may experience a variety of states of consciousness, including *savikalpa- or *samprajnāta-samādhi* and *nirvikalpa- or *asamprajnāta-samādhi*. See also *sahaja*, *samādhi*.

Sahajiyā movement is a development within the medieval *Vaishnava tradition, which originated in Bengal and was associated with Sahajayāna *Buddhism on the one hand and Hindu *Tantrism on the other. As the name suggests, this movement was dedicated to the cultivation of the *sahaja state, primarily through the transmutation of sexual pleasure (*rati) into transcendental bliss (*ānanda, *mahā-sukha). *Yoga, in the form of *bhakti-yoga as spiritual eroticism, played a significant role in this movement. The ideal of sexual pleasure with a *woman other than one's wife—parakīya-rati—best expresses the spirit of the Sahajiyā teachings. The greatest figure of this movement is the fourteenth-century adept-poet *Candīdāsa. The *Bauls also belong to this remarkable manifestation of *Hindu spirituality, though they conceive of the sexo-spiritual union as occurring within one's own *heart rather than externally through intercourse (*maithunā). See also rasa, sama-rasa.

sahajolī-mudrā ("sahajolī seal") is described in the *Hatha-Yoga-Pradīpikā (III.92ff.). This technique, which is a variation of the *vajrolī-mudrā, consists in besmearing the *body, after intercourse (*maithunā), with a mixture of water and ashes obtained from the burning of cow dung. This process is said to succeed only in the case of a virtuous practitioner who is brave and free from *jealousy. See also mudrā; cf. amarolī-mudrā.

sāhasa ("boldness") is, according to the *Hatha-Yoga-Pradīpikā (I.16), one of the six factors that promote *Yoga. Timidity clearly has no place in Yoga, which is experiential and even experimental—one's own body-mind being the laboratory. Boldness is not, however, recklessness.

sahasrāra-cakra ("thousand-spoked wheel") is the topmost center (*cakra) of psychospiritual energy (*prāna). It is situated at the crown of the *head, and is also called the "thousand-petaled lotus" (sahasra-dala-padma), the "great seat" (mahā-pītha), or "ether wheel" (*ākāsha-cakra). The *Kaula-Jnāna-Nirnaya (V.8) describes it as a white lotus floating in the middle of the "milk ocean" in whose center resides the *Self. The *Shiva-Samhitā (V.102, 122f.) gives three different locations for it: the root of the palate (*tālu), the "brahmic fissure" (*brahma-randhra), and outside the *body (above the head). Only the last two locations are generally accepted.

The *Shaiva adherents visualize the sahasrāra-cakra as Mount Kailāsa, the abode of God *Shiva and his spouse *Pārvatī (or simply *Devī). For the *Vaishnavas, it is the locus of the "supreme person" (parama-

purusha). This is the upper terminal point of the central channel (**sushumnā-nādī*) and the final destination of the awakened "serpent power" (**kundalinī-shakti*). When the *kundalinī*, the force of Devī, reaches this center, this signals the merging of **Shiva and **Shakti.

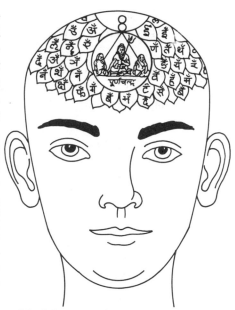

The thousand spoke or petals of this bell-shaped psychospiritual center are arranged in twenty layers, with fifty petals each. Each petal has one letter (**mātrikā*) of the Sanskrit alphabet inscribed in it forming a ring, which is known as "five-crested garland" (*panca-shikhā-mālā*). In the pericarp of the lotus is the "lunar region" (*candra-mandala*), which emits nectarine **light. It contains a luminous triangle within which is the void

56. Sahasrāra-cakra, the psychoenergetic center at the crown of the head.

(**shūnya*), also called "supreme seed point" (*parama-bindu*), the abode of transcendental **Consciousness-Bliss. See also *dvādasha-anta*.

sahita-kumbhaka ("combined retention") is one of the eight types of **breath control mentioned in the **Gheranda-Samhitā* (V.47f.). It is of two kinds—*sagarbha* ("with womb") and *nigarbha* ("without womb"), the "womb" being the sacred syllable **om*. The former is practiced together with the **recitation of the syllable *om* (as *aum*), whereby one inhales—reciting *a*—for sixteen measures, retains the breath—reciting *u*—for sixty-four measures, and exhales—reciting *m*—for thirty-two measures. One should alternate between nostrils. *Nigarbha-kumbhaka* consists simply in controlling the **breath without repetition of the **bīja-mantra*, and inhalation, retention, and exhalation can be regulated from one to one hundred measures (**mātrā*), which are to be counted by circling the left knee with the palm of the left hand. See also *kumbhaka, prānāyāma*.

sākshāt-kārana or **sākshāt-kāra** ("sensing with the eyes"), which is also known as "yogin's perception" (**yogi-pratyaksha*), is the unmediated **perception of things in the state of enstasy (**samādhi*). No sensory input is involved but the **yogin*, through the enstatic process, becomes identical with the *object, thereby experiencing it from "within." This term is often applied to *Self-realization. Cf. *grahana*.

sākshin ("witness") is a common designation for the transcendental *Self. The *witness consciousness has been hailed as the great discovery of Indian spirituality. See also *drashtri*.

sama ("same," "equal") is a favorite term in the *Bhagavad-Gītā*, where it is used on its own and in conjunction with nouns, especially as *sama-darshana*. The underlying idea is conveyed in stanza IX.29 thus: "I [*Krishna] am the same in all beings. To Me none is hateful or dear . . ." The *Absolute, or *Divine, is omnipresent. All things are arising in and as it. Hence nothing in the world is alien to it, and notions like hateful rejection or passionate favoritism do not apply. The *yogin is asked to emulate this spirit of perfect equality (*samatva*). Thus, the *Bhagavad-Gītā* (XII.18f.) states:

> He who is the same toward friend and foe and also toward fame and ill fame, the same in cold and heat, *pleasure and *suffering, without *attachment;

> who is the same toward blame and praise, is silent and content with everything, "homeless" and of steady *mind, and who loves [Me]— that man is dear to Me.

On the surface, this statement seems to contradict *Krishna's claim to flawless impartiality. However, what is spoken of here is an esoteric fact rather than a theological doctrine: Through love devotion (*bhakti*), the *yogin can directly participate in the blissful being of the *Divine. He opens himself to the ever-present grace (*prasāda*), experiencing the love of *Krishna.

sama-buddhi ("same-mindedness") is the attitude of inner aloofness by which the *yogin comes to regard a clod of earth or a piece of gold with equal *tranquility. This yogic ideal is balanced by the positive orientation toward the common weal (*sarva-bhūta-hita*), which is likewise recommended in the *Bhagavad-Gītā* (XII.4).

sama-cittatva ("equal-mindedness") is a synonym for *sama-buddhi*. The *Bhagavad-Gītā* (XIII.8–9) regards this as a manifestation of wisdom (*jnāna*).

sama-darshana ("even vision" or "vision of the same") refers to the state or the person who beholds the *Self in everything. The *Bhagavad-Gītā* (VI.32) celebrates such a person as the foremost of *yogins*.

samādhāna ("collectedness") is a synonym for *samādhi*.

samādhi ("enstasy") is the final "limb" (*anga*) of the yogic *path. The *Gheranda-Samhitā* (VII.1) speaks of *samādhi* as a "great Yoga," which is acquired through good fortune and through the *grace and kindness of one's *teacher and by virtue of one's *devotion to him. The *Tri-Shikhi-Brāhmana-Upanishad* ((II.31), describes enstasy as the "perfect forgetting" of the state of *meditation, which precedes it. The *Yoga-Sūtra* (III.3) speaks of it as that condition in which consciousness (*citta*) shines forth *as* the intended object. That is to say, in *samādhi* there is a merging of subject and object. The *Kūrma-Purāna* (II.11.41) explains this state as being one of "uni-formity" (*eka-ākāra*). The *Paingalā-Upanishad* (III.4) offers this explanation: "Enstasy is [that condition where] *consciousness ranges only with the object of meditation (*dhyeya*) and, like a lamp laced in a windless [spot], is oblivious of meditator (*dhyātri*) and meditation (*dhyāna*)."

Ordinarily, enstasy is accompanied by complete sensory inhibition, as effected through the techniques of sense withdrawal (*pratyāhāra*) and meditation (*dhyāna*). Some works, like the *Mani-Prabhā* (III.12) and various *Purānas, explain that *samādhi* has the duration and intensity of twelve *meditations, which implies abstraction from the external environment. Enstasy is thought to have magical properties as well. This is made clear in the *Hatha-Yoga-Pradīpikā* (IV.108ff.):

> The *yogin* yoked by enstasy is not devoured by time (*kāla*), is not bound by [his] actions (*karman*), and cannot be overpowered by others.

> The *yogin* yoked by enstasy knows neither himself nor others, and does not [experience] smell, taste, sight (*rūpa*), touch, or *sound.

> The *yogin* yoked by enstasy does not experience cold or heat, *sorrow or *joy, honor or contempt.

> The *yogin* yoked by enstasy is immune to [magical influences from] *mantras and *yantras, and is invulnerable to any weapon and unassailable by any person.

All traditions distinguish at least between two major types of enstasy. First, there is the *samādhi* involving identification with an *object and accompanied by higher thought forms (called *prajñā*), and, second, there is the *samādhi* that consists in one's identification with the transcendental *Self and that is devoid of any content of *consciousness. The former type is known as *savikalpa- or *samprajñāta-samādhi*, and the latter as *nirvikalpa- or *asamprajñāta-samādhi*. Only the second variety of enstasy can lead to *Self-realization, or *liberation, by way of the complete transmutation of consciousness. Some schools also know of a third type of enstatic condition, namely "spontaneous enstasy" or *sahaja-samādhi*, which is equivalent to liberation while still in the embodied state, or *jīvan-mukti*.

According to the *Yoga-Cūḍāmany-Upanishad (110), *samādhi* leads first to "wondrous consciousness" (*caitanya-adbhuta*), and subsequently to liberation (*moksha*). The wonders of *consciousness are indeed accessed through the various states of *samprajñāta-samādhi*. In fact, these states are the *yogin's way of doing research, as is evident from the third chapter of the *Yoga-Sūtra*, which introduces examples of the method of enstatic "constraint" (*samyama*). But, ultimately, all forms of gnosis (*prajñā*) must be transcended as well, so that only the vision of the *Self remains. As the *Garuda-Purāna* (49.36) puts it, *samādhi* is the condition where the *yogin realizes "I am the *Absolute." Hence *samādhi* is often defined in the *Vedānta and Vedānta-dependent schools as the "union of the psyche (*jīva*) with the Self (*ātman*)." For "union" (*samyoga*), some authorities substitute "sameness" (*samatva*) or "identity" (*aikya*). The *Hatha-Yoga-Pradīpikā (IV.5ff.) has the following famous simile:

> As salt mingles with and dissolves in water, similarly the merging of the *mind and the *Self is enstasy.

> When the life force (*prāna*) is compressed [in the central channel, or *sushumnā-nādī] and the mind is dissolved, then there is "coessentiality" (*sama-rasatva*), which is designated as enstasy.

> That equilibrium (*sama*) or identity of the individual self and the supreme Self [in which] all volition is absent is designated as enstasy.

This event of *Self-realization alone destroys, in the words of the *Yoga-Yājnavalkya* (X.1), the "noose of existence" (*bhava-pāsha*). Therefore, *samādhi* is occasionally equated with *liberation, or *enlightenment.

The most complete model of enstatic states is that of *Classical Yoga. The following forms of *samādhi* are given in descending order. (1) Supraconscious enstasy (*asamprajnāta-samādhi*); (2) Conscious enstasy (*samprajnāta-samādhi*) with its subforms suprareflexive clarity (*nirvicāra-vaishāradya*), suprareflexive enstasy (*nirvicāra-samāpatti*), reflexive enstasy (*savicāra-samāpatti*), supracogitative enstasy (*nirvitarka-samāpatti*), cogitative enstasy (*savitarka-samāpatti*).

The different forms of conscious enstasy bear the technical designation of "coincidence" (*samāpatti*). Some authorities, like *Vācaspati Mishra, insert the following additional states before the above subcategories of conscious enstasy: Enstasy beyond I-am-ness (*nirasmitā-sampatti*), enstasy with I-am-ness (*sa-asmitā-samāpatti*), enstasy beyond bliss (*nirānanda-samāpatti*), and enstasy with bliss (*sa-ānanda-samāpatti*).

The term *samādhi* is also used to denote the circular grave of the *yogin. In India, ascetics are buried in the cross-legged position, whereas the ordinary person is cremated. Cremation is seen as a rite of passage for those who have not been purified by the fire of Yoga.

sama-drishti ("even vision") is a synonym for *sama-darshana.

samāna is one of the principal currents of the life force (*prāna*), which pervades all limbs and is reponsible for nourishing the *body by distributing food as *rasa. According to the *Linga-Purāna (I.8.65), it normalizes the bodily functions. Many *hatha-yoga texts place it in the region of the *navel, but the *Mahābhārata epic (XII.177.24) assigns it to the *heart. According to the *Yoga-Sūtra (III.40), mastery of the *samāna* leads to "effulgence" (*jvalana*).

samāpatti ("coincidence") is a technical term of *Classical Yoga signifying the enstatic identification with the object of *contemplation. See also *ananta-samāpatti, nirānanda-samāpatti, nirasmitā-samāpatti, sa-ānanda-samāpatti, sa-asmitā-samāpatti, samādhi.*

samarasa ("even essence" or "equilibration") is an important concept of the *Siddha movement, especially *hatha-yoga. It stands for the process and state of resonating bodily in harmony with the *Divine. According to the *Siddhi-Siddhānta-Paddhati (V.4), this condition presupposes yogic *knowledge of the *body's structure and the *grace of one's *teacher.

sama-samsthāna ("even position") is a posture (*āsana) mentioned in the *Yoga-Bhāshya (II.46). It is described by *Vācaspati Mishra in his commentary thereon as follows: One should pull in the feet and press them against each other at the heels and the toes.

samatva or **samatā** ("evenness," "equanimity"). The notion of sameness is an important concept in the *Bhagavad-Gītā, which (II.47) defines *Yoga as "equability" (*samatva*). Because the same transcendental *Absolute underlies all phenomenal forms, to realize that fundamental sameness through the attitude of equanimity and even-mindedness is deemed the greatest spiritual virtue. The *Shiva-Samhitā (III.18), a late work on *hatha-yoga, regards this orientation as a precondition for success in Yoga. According to the *Laghu-Yoga-Vāsishtha (IV.5.12), *samatā* is what remains when all volitional activity (*samkalpa) has ceased. The *Yoga-Tattva-Upanishad (107) understands the term as the "sameness," or union, of the individual psyche with the transcendental *Self.

Sāma-Veda. See *Veda*.

Samhitā *("collection") is the title given to a genre of sacred works in the tradition of *Vaishnavism. Also, the four *Vedic hymnodies carry this designation, as do a number of *Yoga works.

samkalpa ("volition," "intention," or "fancy") is sometimes listed as one of the functions of the "inner instrument" (*antahkarana), or *mind. According to the *Shvetāshvatara-Upanishad (V.8), volition and "I-maker" (*ahamkāra) characterize the finite personality. The *Yoga-Vāsishtha (VIb.1.27) defines it as "mental bondage" (*mano-bandha*), while the absence of volition is said to be *liberation (*vimuktatā*). The *Bhagavad-Gītā (VI.2) notes that one becomes a *yogin by renouncing all volitonal activity, which breeds desire (*kāma). The *Varāha-Upanishad (II.45), again, speaks of *samkalpa* as the real origin of the universe and states that it should be abandoned in favor of *nirvikalpa (*samādhi*).

samkata-āsana ("critical posture") is described in the *Gheranda-Samhitā (II.28) thus: One should place the left foot on the ground and encircle the left leg with the right leg, placing the hand on one's knees.

samketa ("convention") is a technical term employed in the *Yoga-Shāstra* (41ff.) of *Dattātreya to denote specific foci of *concentration, such as the *contemplation of the void (*shūnya) or the space in front of one's *nose. See also *desha*.

Sāmkhya refers to both the tradition by that name and an adherent of Sāmkhya. The word *sāmkhya* is commonly derived from *samkhyā* meaning "number," which is explained by the fact that the Sāmkhya authorities enumerate the categories (*tattva) of existence. Sāmkhya is an archaic form of ontology, distinguishing between twenty-four or twenty-five major ontic categories. The two principal categories are that of the transcendental *Self (called *purusha), and that of *Nature (called *prakriti). The remaining categories pertain to the different levels of manifestation in Nature. The spiritual *path of Sāmkhya consists in the careful differentiation between *purusha* and *prakriti* and the complete *renunciation of everything that is other than the Self, which is the only principle endowed with *consciousness. This practice of discernment (*viveka) hints at the other meaning of the term *sāmkhya*, which is "insight" or "investigative understanding."

Like *Yoga, the Sāmkhya tradition has a protracted history whose beginnings cannot be precisely determined. Proto-Sāmkhya elements can be found already in the hymns of the *Rig-Veda and *Atharva-Veda. The *Mahābhārata (notably the *Bhagavad-Gītā and *Moksha-Dharma sections) and such esoteric texts as the *Katha-, *Shvetāshvatara-, and *Maitrāyanīya-Upanishad represent Pre-Classical schools of Sāmkhya, which developed in the period between 500 and 200 B.C. These schools show a close connection with the tradition of Yoga, to the degree that both are often mentioned together—as Sāmkhya-Yoga. However, there are also passages in the *Moksha-Dharma that make a clear distinction between Sāmkhya and Yoga, though emphasizing that both lead to the same goal. Thus, one passage of the *Mahābhārata epic (XII.289.7) delineates the two traditions by stating that whereas Yoga relies on perception (*pratyaksha), Sāmkhya is based on tradition. In the *Bhagavad-Gītā (V.4), Yoga is equated with *karma-yoga and Sāmkhya with the path of renunciation (*samnyāsa), though in the next stanza their essential unity is stressed.

The sage *Kapila is celebrated as the founder of Sāmkhya, though nothing definite is known about him. This ramified and once obviously influential tradition reached its zenith in the classical formulations of *Īshvara Krishna, author of the *Sāmkhya-Kārikā. There is also an aphoristic (*sūtra), compilation, the *Sāmkhya-Sūtra* ascribed to Kapila, but this is of a later date (probably the fourteenth century A.D.), and it differs philosophically in many respects from Īshvara Krishna's teachings. From about A.D. 1000 on, the Sāmkhya tradition declined, until *Vijnāna Bhikshu's valiant attempts at reviving Sāmkhya metaphysics in the light of *Vedānta nondualism. Often, *Patanjali's *yoga-darshana is wrongly held to have been crafted onto Sāmkhya metaphysics, whereas in fact his teachings represent an original yogic point of view.

sāmkhya-yoga describes a spiritual approach based on insight into the nature of worldly existence and the transcendental *Self, as characteristic of Pre-Classical *Sāmkhya. In the *Matsya-Purāna* (LII.2), it is equated with *jnāna-yoga and contrasted with *karma-yoga, or "ritual *Yoga." In the *Laghu-Yoga-Vāsishtha* (VI.7.13), the *samkhya-yogin* is juxtaposed to the *yoga-yogin*. The same distinction is made in the *Anna-Pūrna-Upanishad* (V.49), where the former is said to awakend by means of enstasy (*samādhi) and the complete restriction of *knowledge, whereas the latter reaches *liberation through the tranquilization of the life force (*prāna).

sammoha ("confusion") arises, according to the *Bhagavad-Gītā* (II.63), from contact with the sense objects (*vishaya). The *Maitrāyanīya-Upanishad* (III.2), which employs the synonym *sammūdhatva*, declares that as a result of this fundamental confusion, one cannot behold the *Lord. See also *moha*.

samnidhi ("proximity") is a technical term used in the *Yoga-Bhāshya* (I.4) to describe the transcendental closeness between the *Self and consciousness (*citta) by virtue of which it is possible for the Self to apperceive the cognitions (*buddhi) of the finite *mind. See also *samyoga*.

samnyāsa ("renunciation") is a fundamental orientation within *Hinduism, which, like *Yoga, has produced its own values, practices, and literature (e.g., the *Samnyāsa-Upanishads). It is as old as the oldest *Upanishads. The *Bhagavad-Gītā* (XVIII.2) explains *samnyāsa* as the *renunciation, or inner *sacrifice, of *actions dictated by *desire, or (in VI.2) as the renunciation of volition (*samkalpa). This is contrasted with *tyāga, or the relinquishing of the fruit (*phala) of all one's actions, which is essential to *karma-yoga. Mere renunciation is held (V.2) to be inferior to *karma-yoga. See also Abandonment.

samnyāsa-yoga ("Yoga of renunciation") is a compound found in several works of *Pre-Classical Yoga, including the *Bhagavad-Gītā (IX.28) and the *Mundaka-Upanishad (III.2.6). It simply means the "practice of *renunciation."

Samnyāsa-Upanishads are *Upanishads that specifically expound renunciation (*samnyāsa). Generally, nineteen such works are mentioned, several of which belong to the late pre-Christian era.

samnyāsin ("renouncer") is typified in the *Bhagavad-Gītā (V.3) as the person who neither hates nor desires anything and who is above the "pairs of opposites" (*dvandva). See also samnyāsa.

samprajnāta-samādhi ("conscious enstasy") designates, in *Classical Yoga, a range of enstatic experiences that have an objective prop (ālambana) with which consciousness (*citta) becomes identified and which is associated with superknowledge (*prajnā). According to the *Yoga-Sūtra (I.17), the principal forms of conscious enstasy are *vitarka-, *vicāra-, *ānanda-, and *asmitā-samāpatti (or -samādhi). The *Yoga-Bhāshya (I.17) proposes the following schema to understand the composition of each of these four forms:

vitarka ("cogitation") = vitarka + vicāra + ānanda + asmitā
vicāra ("reflexion")   =   vicāra + ānanda + asmitā
ānanda ("bliss")   =   ānanda + asmitā
asmitā ("I-am-ness")   =   asmitā

Vācaspati Mishra suggests in his *Tattva-Vaishāradī (I.47) that the focus of the first two types are the "coarse" (*sthūla) and the "subtle" (*sūkshma) objects of existence, whereas the focus of the third type are the *senses and of the fourth type the ego principle (*asmitā). Vācaspati further argues that each of these four forms has a higher form in which all conscious contents is stilled: nirvitarka-, nirvicāra-, nirānanda- and nirasmitā-samāpatti. However, this typology of eight forms of conscious *enstasy is explicitly denied by *Vijnāna Bhikshu, who admits of only six types. He states that the object of "coinciding with bliss" (*ānanda-samāpatti) is *bliss itself, and of "coinciding with 'I-am-ness' " (*asmitā-samāpatti) is the intuition (samvid) of the absolute *Self (kevala-purusha). Thus, there are no nirānanda and nirasmitā forms.

These six or eight types of samprajnāta-samādhi correspond to the *savikalpa-samādhi in *Vedānta. Superior to them is supraconscious enstasy (*asamprajnāta-samādhi), which reveals the transcendental *Self. See also *samādhi*.

samrambha-yoga ("Yoga of hatred"). In the *Vaishnava tradition, the strong emotion of hatred—like *love—is sometimes regarded as a means of *Self-realization. A classic example is Hiranyakashipu, the father of *Prahlāda, whose abiding hatred of the *Divine finally led to his spiritual *liberation. Hatred can thus be a form of involuntary spiritual practice, based on the esoteric principle that one becomes what one deeply meditates on. See also *dvesha*.

samsāra ("flow") is the phenomenal world, as opposed to the transcendental or noumenal *Reality, whether it be called *nirvāna, *brahman, or *ātman. The word *samsāra* conveys well the idea that finite existence is a constant flux of events in which no permanence and security can be found. The eternal, transcendental *Self alone serves as a refgue to those wishing to escape the changeability of nature (*prakriti). *Samsāra* is, above all, the domain of *karma and *rebirth and thus of unmitigated suffering (*duhkha). The *Varāha-Upanishad (II.64) describes it as a long dream (*svapna), a protracted delusion of the *mind, and a sea of *sorrow. As the *Maitrāyanīya-Upanishad (VI.28) puts it, those who are *liberated look down upon the *samsāra* as upon a dizzily revolving wheel (*cakra*). The *Yoga-Bhāshya (IV.11) explains that this world wheel, which turns due to the power of spiritual ignorance (*avidyā), has six spokes, namely virtue (*dharma) and vice (*adharma), pleasure (*sukha) and pain (*duhkha), as well as attachment (*rāga) and aversion (*dvesha).

samsārin ("worldling") is the being, or psyche (*jīva), who is entrapped in the ever-changing world (*samsāra) of natural and moral *causation. Cf. Self.

samshaya ("doubt") is a major obstacle (*antarāya) on the yogic *path. It is named in the *Yoga-Kundaly-Upanishad (I.59) as one of the ten obstructions (*vighna) foiling spiritual growth. The *Yoga-Bhāshya (I.30) defines it as a kind of thought (*vijnāna*) that touches both alternatives of a dilemma. This work (I.35) also claims that doubt can be effectively dispelled by suprasensory awareness (*divya-sampad*), which creates *faith in the practitioner. According to the *Bhagavad-Gītā (IV.40), doubt afflicts the person who lacks faith (*shraddhā) and ultimately can destroy him or her. As the *Matsya-Purāna* (CX.10) notes laconically, a person who is inclined toward doubt merely reaps *pain, not *Yoga. Availing itself of a popular image, the *Bhagavad-Gītā* (IV.42) states that only the sword of wisdom (*jñāna*) can cut through the doubts harbored in one's *heart.

samskāra ("activator"). The general meaning of the term *samskāra* is "ritual," and in this sense it is widely applied to such rites of passage as the birth ceremony, tonsure, and marriage. In *Yoga, however, the word has a psychological significance. It stands for the indelible imprints in the subconscious left behind by our daily experiences, whether conscious or unconscious, internal or external, desirable or undesirable. The term *samskāra* suggests that these imprints are not merely passive vestiges of a person's *actions and *volitions but highly dynamic forces in his or her psychic life. They constantly propel *consciousness into action. The *Yoga-Sūtra* (III.9) distinguishes two varieties of subliminal activators: those that lead to the externalization (*vyutthāna*) of consciousness and those that cause the inhibition (*nirodha*) of the processes of consciousness. The *yogin* must cultivate the latter type of *samskāras* in order to achieve the condition of enstasy (*samādhi*), which prevents the renewed generation of subliminal activators. According to the *Yoga-Sūtra* (I.50), at the highest level of conscious enstasy (*samprajnāta-samādhi*) a subliminal activator is generated that obstructs all others and thus leads over into the condition of supraconscious enstasy (*asamprajnāta-samādhi*). See also *āshaya, karma, vāsanā*.

samtosha ("contentment") ranks among the constituent practices of self-discipline (*niyama*) in *Classical Yoga and, according to the *Yoga-Sūtra* (II.42), leads to unexcelled joy (*sukha*). The *Darshana-Upanishad* (II.4–5) explains it as delight with whatever *fate may bring. This medieval work also speaks of supreme contentment (*para-samtosha*), which is that agreeable condition that results from perfect indifference (*virakti*) and which terminates in the realization of the *Absolute. The *Mahābhārata* epic (XII.21.2) praises contentment as follows: "Contentment is indeed the highest *heaven. Contentment is supreme joy. There is nothing higher than satisfaction (*tushti*). It is complete in itself." The *Laghu-Yoga-Vāsishtha* (II.1.73) explains it as the "evenness" (*samatā*) toward hardship and ease, as well as toward things one has obtained and those that are far from one's reach.

samyag-darshana ("perfect vision"), is, according to the *Yoga-Bhāshya* (II.15), the means to *liberation from pain (*duhkha*), following upon the obliteration of the five "causes of suffering" (*klesha*). The *Manu-

Smriti (VI.74), a prominent late pre-Christian on ethics, declares that he who is endowed with perfect vision is never bound by his *actions. See also *jnāna*, *vidyā*, *viveka*.

samyama ("constraint") is explained in the *Yoga-Sūtra* (III.4) of *Patanjali as the continuous practice of concentration (*dhāranā*), meditation (*dhyāna*), and enstasy (*samādhi*) upon the same *object. This technique is the *yogin's way of doing research, since it yields all kinds of suprasensuous knowledge (*prajnā*). The term *samyama* is also sometimes used in the sense of "control," particularly in connection with the mastery of the *senses.

samyoga ("connection" or "correlation"). In *Classic Yoga, *samyama* denotes the correlation that exists between the transcendental Self (*purusha*) and Nature (*prakriti*), or consciousness (*citta*). This correlation, or connection, is at the root of all suffering (*duhkha*). It is caused by spiritual nescience (*avidyā*), and it is removed through wisdom (*prajnā*). *Patanjali maintains that the contact between the *Self and the experienced object (*drishya*) is merely an apparent junction, since both the Self and experiencable *Nature are by definition utterly distinct. He does not analyze this epistemological problem further. This has led to a great deal of speculation in the commentarial literature on the *Yoga-Sūtra. Thus, *Vācaspati Mishra speaks of that enigmatic relationship in terms of a special fitness (*yogyatā*) between the Self and *consciousness. As he elucidates in his *Tattva-Vaishāradī (II.17), the *sattva aspect of the *mind contains the reflection (*bimba*) of the transcendental Awareness (*caitanya*), which yields the illusions of the empirical consciousness. *Vijnāna Bhikshu even speaks of a "counter-reflection" (*pratibimba*) of the mental states in the Self.

The historical germ for these philosophical speculations can be found in the literature of *Pre-Classical Yoga. Thus, the *Bhagavad-Gītā (XIII.26) mentions the connection between the "field" (*kshetra*) and the "field knower" (*kshetra-jna*), which underlies the coming into being of all creatures. This scripture (V.14) also employs the word *samyoga* in regard to the causal "nexus" between action (*karman*) and its fruit (*phala*). See also *samnidhi*.

sanātana-dharma ("eternal teaching" is the traditional name given to *Hinduism by its adherents.

Sanatkumāra is mentioned in the *Mahābhārata* (XII.327.64), together with Sana, Sanaka, Sānandana, Sanātana, and Sanatsujāta, as a knower of *Yoga and *Sāmkhya. He also figures as a renowned teacher in some of the *Purānas and later *Upanishads.

sancita-karman ("accumulated karma"). See *karma*.

sanga means first of all "attachment," which is considered a great stumbling block on the spiritual *path. In the *Bhagavad-Gītā* (II.47), *sanga* denotes specifically the "clinging" to the fruit (*phala*) of one's *actions, which produces adverse *karmic effects and is therefore to be renounced. In some contexts, *sanga* stands for "socializing," which, according to the *Shiva-Samhitā* (V.185), must simply be abandoned. Cf. *nihsangatā, sat-sanga*.

sankata-āsana ("dangerous posture") is described in the *Gheranda-Samhitā* (I.26) thus: Placing the left foot on the ground, one should twine the right leg around the left leg and place one's hands on the knees. Modern manuals on *hatha-yoga observe that this practice should be repeated while standing on the right foot.

sapta-anga-yoga ("seven-limbed Yoga"). See *sapta-sādhana*.

saptadha-prajnā ("sevenfold wisdom") is a phrase occurring in the *Yoga-Sūtra* (II.27), which is left unexplained by *Patanjali. However, the *Yoga-Bhāshya* (II.27), the oldest extant commentary, supplies a probable elucidation, stating that at the culmination of conscious enstasy (*samprajnāta-samādhi*), the *yogin has the following immediate insights: (1) That which was to be prevented, namely future suffering (*duhkha*) has been prevented. (2) The causes of *suffering have been eliminated. (3) Complete "cessation" (*hāna*) has been accomplished. (4) The means for effecting cessation, namely the "vision of discernment" (*viveka-khyāti*) has been applied successfully. (5) Sovereignty of the highest mental faculty, namely the *buddhi, has been achieved. (6) The primary constituents (*guna*) of *Nature have lost their foothold and, "like rocks rolling down the mountain slope," incline toward dissolution (*pralaya*). (7) The *Self abides in its essential nature as primordial light (*jyotis*), undefiled and "alone" (*kevalin*).

Vyāsa further explains that the first four insights, or spontaneous realizations, are called "release of the tasks" (*kārya-vimukti*), while the last three insights are known as "release of consciousness" (*citta-vimukti*).

sapta-jnāna-bhūmi ("seven stages of wisdom") is a model associated with some schools of *Post-Classical Yoga, notably the *Yoga-Vāsishtha in its shorter and longer versions. Thus, according to the *Laghu-Yoga-Vāsishtha (VI.13.56ff.), the seven levels are as follows: (1) *Shubha-icchā* ("desire for the auspicious") is the impulse on the part of the *Yoga novice (*nava-yogin*) to cultivate a positive spiritual attitude and outlook through the *study of the sacred teachings and the application of understanding. (2) *Vicārana* ("discrimination") is the practice of discernment in daily life, leading to the gradual abandonment of self-will (*abhimāna*), *pride, *jealousy, *delusion, and so on, and yielding the ability to comprehend the hidden (*rahasya*) meaning of the sacred teachings. (3) *Asanga-bhāvanā* ("cultivation of nonattachment"): At this level, the practitioner lives in a hermitage (*āshrama*) and seriously engages the practice of "listening" (*shravana*) to the sacred lore about self-knowledge and *self-transcendence. This naturally leads to the pacification of the *mind and the inclination to perform only virtuous *actions. (4) *Vilāpinī* ("lamenting"): Here the practitioner looks with *tranquility upon everything, and his *mind will "perish like a bank of clouds in autumn." (5) *Shuddha-samvin-maya-ānanda-rūpa* is, as the name indicates, the level "formed of *bliss and composed of pure awareness." On this stage, the *yogin lives in the perpetual certainty of the truth of nonduality (*advaita*). This level coincides with the condition known as "living liberation" (*jīvan-mukti*). (6) *Asamvedana-rūpa* is the level that goes beyond sensation (*samvedana*) and yields the constant experience of massive bliss (*ānanda*). This stage is said to resemble deep sleep (*sushupti*). (7) *Turya-avasthā-upashānta* is the stage of the "tranquil fourth state," coinciding with "disembodied liberation" (*videha-mukti*) or supreme extinction (*para-nirvāna*).

Following one of three versions found in the *Yoga-Vāsishta, the *Varāha-Upanishad (IV.1.1ff.) gives the seven stages as follows: (1) *Shubha-icchā* (see above); (2) *vicārana* (see above); (3) *tanu-mānasī* ("fine-minded [stage]"); (4) *sattva-āpatti* ("acquisition of *sattva"); (5) *asamsakti* ("[perfect] detachment"); (6) *padārtha-bhāvanā* ("realization of the essence [of existence]"); (7) *turīya-ga* ("entering the *Fourth").

The last four stages are said to pertain to the *adept who is liberated while yet alive (*jīvan-mukta*).

sapta-sādhana ("sevenfold discipline") consists, according to the *Gheranda-Samhitā (I.9), of cleanliness (*shodhana*), firmness (*dridhatā*), stability (*sthairya*), constancy (*dhairya*), lightness (*lāghava*), perception (*pratyaksha*), and nondefilement (*nirlipta*). Vedānta, *sapta-sādhana* refers to a different set of disciplines.

sarasvatī-cālana ("stirring the *sarasvatī*") is the practice in **kundalinī-yoga* of forcing the life energy (**prāna*) into the central channel (**sushumnā-nādī*). The **Yoga-Kundaly-Upanishad* (I.10ff.) describes this esoteric process as follows: Seated in the lotus posture (**padma-āsana*), one should, while the life force is circulating through the **idā-nādī*, lengthen the life force (i.e., the **breath*) from the normal four digits to twelve digits and "surround" the *sarasvatī-nādī* with that elongated breath. Then one should hold the life force (through breath retention) in that *nādī*, closing all apertures of the **head* with one's fingers and forcing the **prāna* repeatedly from the right *nādī* into the left *nādī* for forty-five minutes. Next, one should "draw up" the **sushumnā-nādī*, which forces the **kundalinī-shakti* toward the mouth of the *sushumnā*. Then one should practice the throat "lock" (**jālandhara-bandha*) and the abdominal "lock" (**uddīyāna-bandha*), referred to in the text as *tāna*. This will force the **prāna* upward. Finally, one should expel the life force through the "solar" channel, that is, the **pingalā-nādī*. See also *shakti-cālana*.

sarasvatī-nādī ("*sarasvatī* channel") is a channel (**nādī*) of the life force (**prāna*) that is generally said to be situated in front of the central channel (**sushumnā-nādī*) and to extend to the tongue. This channel, or flow of life energy, must be activated before the "serpent power" (**kundalinī-shakti*) can ascend along the central channel. Sarasvatī, the Goddess of speech and learning in **Hinduism*, is also associated with the esoteric center at the base of the spine called **mūlādhāra-cakra*.

sarga ("creation"). The **Hindu* philosophers have always been acutely interested in the origins of the **cosmos*, because they have rightly intuited that **knowledge* of this kind will provides important clues about our personal origins and functions, since **microcosm* and **macrocosm* are mirrored in each other. See also world ages.

sarva-anga-āsana ("all limbs posture") is what modern manuals of **hatha-yoga* call the shoulder stand. It has a number of variations, depending on the position of the legs and arms. Cf. *shīrsha-āsana*.

sarva-arthatā ("all-objectness") is a technical expression found in the **Yoga-Sūtra* (III.11), which describes the status of the ordinary **consciousness*. Cf. *eka-agratā*.

sarva-bhāva-adhisthātritva ("supremacy over all states [of existence]") is, according to the *Yoga-Sūtra* (III.49), acquired by that *adept who is constantly aware of the distinction between the transcendental *Self and the *sattva aspect of *Nature.

sarva-bhūta-hita ("the good of all beings") is according to the *Mahābhārata* epic (XII.187.3), one of the outcomes of realizing the *Self. As the *Bhagavad-Gītā* (XII.4) insists, the sage should actually take delight (*rati) in promoting the weal of everyone. This does not conflict with the call for even-mindedness (*sama-buddhi). See also *loka-samgraha*.

sarva-jnātva or **sarva-jnātritva** ("omniscience"). According to the *Yoga-Sūtra* (III.49) of *Patanjali, omniscience is the product of the perfected "vision of discernment" (*viveka-khyāti). The *Shiva-Samhitā* (V.65), however, claims that it results from contemplating the

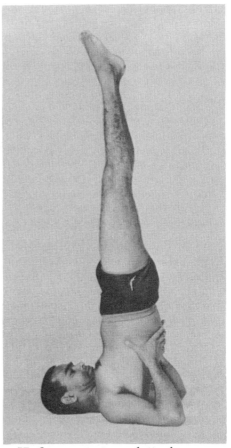

57. Sarva-anga-āsana, better known as the shoulderstand.

psychoenergetic center (*mūlādhāra-cakra) at the base of the spine. The *Yoga-Shikhā-Upanishad* (III.25) regards omniscience as the fruit of one's remembrance of the *Absolute. This work makes the same claim for omnipotence (*sarva-sampūrna-shakti*).

sat. See Being, *sac-acid-ānanda*.

Sat-Karma-Samgraha ("Compendium of Right Action") is a work authored by Cidghanānanda, a disciple of Gaganānanda of the *Nātha sect. It is concerned with the therapeutic aspects of *hatha-yoga and describes a whole range of purificatory techniques, especially for *illnesses resulting from carelessness in the execution of yogic practices or laxity in observing the dietary and other rules. Cidghanānanda advises the *yogin to first try postures (*āsana) and occult remedies to cure himself before resorting to the practices disclosed in his work.

sat-kārya-vāda means "doctrine of the (pre-)existent effect" and refers to the *Sāmkhya and *Yoga teaching according to which all effects are potentially contained in their causes (*kārana). The sat-kārya doctrine explicitly rejects the notion of creation ex nihilo. Creation is always only the manifestation (āvirbhāva) of latent possibilities. The ultimate cause is thought to be *prakriti ("creatrix"), or *Nature. All unmanifest (invisible) and manifest (visible) forms are simply transformations (vikriti, vikāra, *parināma) of that primal supersubstance. See also Evolution.

sat-sanga ("contact with the Real") is the practice of associating with *adepts and saintly folk (*sādhu). Contact with them is thought to be purifying and uplifting and to stimulate the spiritual process. See also shakti-pāta.

satta-mātra ("mere being"). In the *Yoga-Bhāshya (II.19), this is a synonym for *linga-mātra or what the *Tattva-Vaishāradī (II.19) calls the "great mind" (mahad-buddhi). It is the first evolute of Nature (*prakriti). However, the Yoga-Vāsistha (V.10,86) employs this term to designate the transcendental *Reality itself. Sattā-mātra is said to have two aspects, namely homogeneity (eka-rūpa) and heterogeneity (vibhāga). The latter is created by temporality (kāla-sattā), fragmentation (kalā-sattā), and objective existence (vastu-sattā).

sattva ("beingness") can mean "being" in general or "a being" in particular. In the *Yoga and *Sāmkhya traditions, the term also stands for one of the three primary constituents (*guna) of Nature (*prakriti). The *Bhagavad-Gītā (XIV.6) characterizes it as "immaculate, illuminating, without ill." However, sattva—by virtue of being one of the *gunas—also has a binding effect and, as the Gītā notes, can cause attachment to *joy and *knowledge. Nevertheless, it is only by overcoming rajas and tamas through the magnification of sattva that *liberation, or *enlightenment, is possible.

Sattva is the psychocosmic principle of lucidity or sheer existence devoid of conceptual filters and emotional overlays. *Classical Yoga seeks to purify the sattva aspect of the psyche to the point where its lucidity matches the inherent clarity of the transcendental Self (*purusha), which is pure *Consciousness. See also sapta-jnāna-bhūmi.

sāttvika is the adjectival form of *sattva* and is generally rendered as "sattvic."

satya ("truth" or "truthfulness"). *Satya* in the sense of truthfulness is one of the constituent practices of moral observance (*yama*). The *Mandala-Brāhmana-Upanishad* (I.4) lists it among the practices of self-restraint (*niyama*). This shows the high regard in which truthfulness is held in the spiritual traditions. The *Mahānirvāna-Tantra* (IV.75ff.) extols truthfulness thus:

> No virtue (*dharma*) is more excellent than truthfulness, no *sin greater than [telling] the untruth. Therefore, the [virtuous] man should see refuge in truthfulness with all his *heart.

> Without truthfulness, worship (*pūjā*) is futile. Without truthfulness, the recitation (*japa*) [of sacred *mantras*] is useless. Without truthfulness, [the practice of] asceticism (*tapas*) is as unfruitful as seed [that has fallen] on barren soil.

> Truthfulness is the form of the supreme Absolute (*brahman*). Truly, truthfulness is the best *asceticism. All *actions [should be] rooted in truthfulness. Nothing is more excellent than truthfulness.

According to the *Yoga-Sūtra* (II.36), the *yogin* who is grounded in this virtue acquires the paranormal power (*siddhi*) by which the fruit of his actions depends entirely on his will. The *Yoga-Bhāshya* (II.36) takes this to mean that whatever the *adept says comes true. Elsewhere in this work (II.3), *Vyāsa states that if one speaks at all it should be in order to communicate one's *knowledge and as a *service to others, and hence the communication should not be deceitful, erroneous, or barren. This definition combines personal integrity with fidelity to facts. Expressing a common sentiment, the *Garuda-Purāna* (XLIX.30) similarly understands truthfulness as "speech that is beneficial to beings (*bhūta-hita*)." The *Darshana-Upanishad* (I.9f.) notes that true is what is based on the evidence of the *senses but that the highest truth is the conviction that everything is the Absolute (*brahman*).

saumanasya ("gladness") is, according to the *Yoga-Sūtra* (II.41), one of the fruits of purity (*shauca*). Cf. *daurmanasya*.

Saunaka is mentioned in the *Mahābhārata* epic (III.2.14) as a sage learned in both *Sāmkhya and *Yoga.

savicāra-samāpatti ("reflexive coinciding") is a subtype of conscious enstasy (*samprajnāta-samādhi*), in which *attention is focused on a "subtle" (*sūkshma*) object. See also *samādhi*; cf. *nirvicāra-samāpatti*.

savikalpa-samādhi ("enstasy with form") is the *Vedānta equivalent of *samprajnāta-samādhi*. The word *vikalpa* can mean both "form" and "concept." This type of *enstasy involves higher mental process that can be called thinking, though the thoughts that spontaneously arise have a clarity and an immediacy that distinguishes them markedly from the thoughts of our ordinary, discursive *mind. See also *samādhi*; cf. *nirvikalpa-samādhi*.

savitarka-samāpatti ("cogitative coinciding") is the lowest form of conscious enstasy (*samprajnāta-samādhi*). Here, *attention is concentrated on the coarse or "gross" (*sthūla*) aspect of a thing, such as the visible shape of a *deity as represented iconographically. See also *samādhi*; cf. *nirvitarka-samāpatti*.

Scripture. See *shruti*, *smriti*.

Secrecy is enjoined by many texts. Those who do not heed this injunction are often threatened with dire consequences, not least ultimate spiritual misfortune. For instance, the *Brahma-Vidyā-Upanishad* (47) demands that its teachings should only be imparted to a devoted *disciple, lest the *teacher should be cast into hell (*nāraka*). Similarly, the *Mahā-Vākya-Upanishad* (2) asks that its most esoteric knowledge should be divulged only to a sattvic (*sāttvika*) student who is introspective (*antar-mukha*). Secrecy is frequently enjoined regarding specific practices, notably the *khecarī-mudrā*. The *Yoga-Shikhā-Upanishad* (I.156) demands it with respect to the paranormal powers (*siddhi*), which should not be displayed. The *Hatha-Yoga-Pradīpikā* (I.11) declares that the *yogin who wishes for perfection (*siddhi*) should keep the science of *hatha-yoga carefully concealed, for it is potent only so long as it is kept secret but becomes quite inefficacious when disclosed to unworthy people. This demand for secrecy is characteristic of initiatory traditions in general.

Seed. See *bija*, *bindu*.

Seer. See *rishi*.

Self, transcendental. The Self (*ātman*, *purusha*) is the essential core of one's being or what in the Christian tradition is known as the soul. It is one's authentic identity apart from all one's roles. The Self is deemed immortal and immutable. Moreover, in most spiritual traditions of *Hinduism, it is considered to be suprasensuous (*atīndriya*) and pure Consciousness (*cit*, *citi*, *cetana*, or *caitanya*—words that all have the same root).

The transcendental Self is distinct from but lies hidden within or behind the empirical self, or ego (*ahamkāra*, *asmitā*). It is also different from C. G. Jung's notion of the Self, which is a psychic archetype that is responsible for the psychospiritual maturation of the personality to the degree that the *ego is sensitive and willing to respond to the messages of the Self. Jung's notion corresponds more to the idea of the "inner controller" (*antaryāmin*), one of the aspects of the transcendental Self according to *Vedānta.

All Hindu traditions are agreed that the realization of the transcendental Self is the noblest and worthiest object of human aspiration. See also *purusha-artha*.

Self-realization, which is called *ātma-jnāna* ("Self-knowledge) or *ātma-darshana* ("Self-vision") in Sanskrit, is the recovery of one's authentic identity as the transcendental *Reality, rather than the ego personality. This is not a cognitive process, or mere experience, but a radical shift at the root of *consciousness, which involves the transcendence of the human *mind as well as the *body. It is synonymous with *enlightenment, *liberation.

self-transcendence is the practice of going beyond the limitations of the *ego habit in all matters. It is the ideal and foundation process of spiritual life. A self-transcending attitude is to be applied not only to ordinary situations but also in regard to visions, paranormal abilities (*siddhi*), and the different forms of enstasy (*samādhi*). This orientation of self-sacrifice fulfills itself in the great event of *Self-realization, or *liberation.

Semen. See *bindu, retas, shukra*; cf. *rajas*.

Sense control. See *indriya-jaya, indriya-nigraha*.

Senses. See *indriya*.

Sense withdrawal. See *pratyāhāra*.

Serpent power. See *kundalinī-shakti*.

Service. See *sevā*.

sevā, sevana ("service") is an important aspect of discipleship. Since ancient times, the pupil (*shishya*) hoping for higher initiation (*dīkshā*) had to prove himself or herself through steadfast service to his or her teacher (*guru*). See also *ācārya-sevana, guru-sevā, pada-sevana, panca-anga-sevana*.

Sexuality. The spiritual traditions of India fall into two categories: those that espouse a body- and sex-positive orientation, like most schools of *Tantrism, and those that look upon sexuality as an inevitable stumbling block on the spiritual *path. The latter, which are in the majority, demand that the aspirant should abstain from all sexual activity and cultivate chastity (*brahmacarya*) in the strict sense. Concessions are usually made for the householder (*grihastha*) who endeavors to engage spiritual life. However, even he or she should strive toward perfect sexual abstinence in thought, word, and deed. The reason for this counsel is that the discharge of one's sexual energies in orgasm involves a loss of life energy (*prāna*), or vitality, which is needed for the arduous and lifelong task of transforming the personality through the yogic disciplines. Sublimation is understood as a psychosomatic process that leads to the actual refinement of the seminal substance into what is known as *ojas*.

The sex-positive schools are not merely hedonistic, licentious adventures. They also do not favor orgasm and the concomitant loss of vitality. Yet they permit and even recommend sexual activity as a valid means of spiritual transmutation. Sexual desire (*kāma*) is seen as a normal, if particularly potent, function of the finite personality, which should not be repressed but properly harnessed. In fact, the left-hand branch of *Tantrism offers a battery of methods that specifically seek to stimulate the sexual urge. The core ritual of this Tantric orientation is known as the "five m's" (*panca-ma-kara*), of which sexual intercourse (*maithunā*) is the fifth and final ceremonial practice. Its purpose is to achieve the enstatic state (*samādhi*) through physical union. This approach is based on the notion that sexual pleasure (*sukha, *rati*) is a manifestation of transcendental bliss (*ānanda*) and hence can be experienced as such. This orientation is epitomized in the religious motif of the love play between *Krishna and the shepherdesses (*gopī*).

India's predominant mood has always been puritanical, and the sex-positive schools for the most part have had to exist underground.

Today, a decidedly anti-Tantric attitude prevails. On the other side, Tantrism has come West, and a number of neo-Tantric schools have sprung up. In most cases, however, these have little more in common with traditional Tantrism than the name. See also *bindu, rasa*, Sahajiyā.

Shābara is mentioned in the *Hatha-Yoga-Pradīpikā* (I.5) as a master of *hatha-yoga*. Nothing is known about him.

shabda ("sound") is one of the principal and oldest means by which *yogins* have sought to focus their *attention. Their hard-won experimental findings and theories about the transformative nature of sound are embodied in what is known as *mantra-vidyā*, or the "science of sacred utterances."

Shabda can be lettered (*varna-ātmaka*) and endowed with meaning or it can be meaningless sound (*dhvani*), such as the roar of a waterfall. In addition, there is suprasensuous or inner sound (*nāda*). The ultimate ground in and from which all types of sound arise is called the *shabda-brahman*. Audible sound is the end product of a whole process of *evolution by which the transcendental vibration (*spanda*) of shabda-brahman is gradually made manifest. Generally, four stages are distinguished: (1) *Para-shabda* ("supreme sound"), which is the most subtle form of sound and which is associated with the psychoenergetic center at the base of the spine (i.e., the *mūlādhāra-cakra*). (2) *Pashyantī-shabda* ("visible sound"), which is associated with the *heart, can be heard as the sacred syllable *om (or *pranava). (3) *Madhyama-shabda* ("middle sound") refers to a variety of basic sounds, such as the fifty sound values (*varna*) of the Sanskrit alphabet known as "matrices" (*mātrikā*). This is also the level on which *mantras are revealed to the *adept. Each of these sound units has three aspects: *bīja, *nāda, and *bindu. (4) *Vaikhāra-shabda* ("manifest sound"), which is the coarsest aspect of sound, is expressed in speech. See also *mantra-yoga*; cf. *mauna*.

shabda-brahman ("Absolute as sound") is the ground of all sound (*shabda*), whether audible or unmanifest. In *Hinduism, it is indicated by the sacred sound *om. See also *akshara*; cf. *para-brahman*.

shad-anga-yoga ("six-limbed Yoga") is first taught in the *Maitrāyanīya-Upanishad* (VI.18), a work of *Pre-Classical Yoga. It consists of breath control (*prānāyāma*), sense withdrawal (*pratyāhāra*), meditation (*dhyāna*), concentration (*dhāranā*), examination (*tarka*), and enstasy (*samādhi*). Noteworthy are the switching of *concentration and *meditation in this sequence and the mention of *tarka*. Similar sixfold arrangements are presented in a variety of scriptures of *Post-Classical Yoga. An interesting variant is found in the *Garuda-Purāna* (CCXXVII.18), which includes recitation (*japa*) as the second component, following *breath control. All these schemas have in common the absence of any mention of moral observance (*yama*) and self-discipline (*niyama*), which are the foundation of the "eight-limbed Yoga" (*ashta-anga-yoga*) of *Patanjali. However, this does not mean that the moral rules of *yama* are disregarded; they are merely not formalized.

shad-vimsha or **shad-vimshaka** ("twenty-sixth [principle]"). This is a term of *Pre-Classical Yoga, which is used in several places in the *Mahābhārata* epic. It denotes the transcendental *Reality, the "Lord" (*īshvara*). It is the assumption of a twenty-sixth ontic principle (*tattva*) that distinguishes the *Epic Yoga schools from the rival *Sāmkhya schools of that era. The adherents of Sāmkhya know of only twenty-five principles; twenty-four pertain to insentient Nature (*prakriti*), and the twenty-fifth is the supraconscious transcendental Self (*purusha*). See also *budhyamāna*.

shaiva ("pertaining to *Shiva") is an adherent of *Shaivism.

Shaiva-Siddhānta is the southern branch of the ramifying tradition of *Shaivism. Partly based on the (twenty-eight) Sanskrit *Āgamas* composed in the north, it has spawned a huge literature of its own in the Tamil language, beginning with the poetry of such Shaiva saints as *Tirumūlar, *Sundarar, and *Manikkavācaka. The first systematic Tamil exposition of the doctrines of Shaivism is the thirteenth-century *Shiva-Jnāna-Bodha* ("Awakening to the Knowledge of Shiva") of *Meykandar, which is a commentary on the *Shaiva-Siddhānta*, a work consisting of twelve *sūtras* apparently excerpted from the Sanskrit *Raurava-Āgama*.

The Shaiva-Siddhānta, which espouses a nondualist (*advaita*) metaphysics, distinguishes between the *Divine called *pashupati* (i.e., *Shiva), the individual psyche called *pashu*, and insentient *Nature, which is referred to as the "fetter" (*pāsha*). This religiophilosophical system also recognizes thirty-six principles (*tattva*) of existence, which include the twenty-four principles of the *Sāmkhya tradition. The other twelve principles are said to be "pure," or transcendental, categories.

Although this school, which is still active today, emphasizes devotional *worship and *ritual, *Yoga also plays a significant role, as can be seen from such works as the *Shiva-Jnāna-Siddhi* and the *Shiva-

Yoga-Ratna ("Jewel of Shiva-Yoga") of *Jnānaprakāsha. See also Pā-shupata, Pratyābhijna school, Vīra-Shaivism.

Shaivism is the name given to a number of schools—notably *Kāpālika, *Kālāmukha, *Pāshupata, *Pratyābhijna, *Shaiva-Siddhānta, and *Vīra-Shaivism (or Lingāyata)—which cover a wide range of doctrinal outlooks and practical approaches. The common denominator is the *worship of the transcendental *Reality as *Shiva. The origins of Shaivism lie in the obscure past. The earliest evidence of the sectarian worship of God Shiva is found in the pre-Christian *Shvetāshvatara-Upanishad. The *Mahābhārata epic reflects the emergent importance of Shiva, who begins to seriously rival *Vishnu. The post-Christian era witnessed the gradual flowering of both Shaivism and its rival *Vaishnavism, reaching its culmination around the turn of the first millennium A.D. The adherents of Shaivism—called Shaivas—produced a vast literature, only a fraction of which is extant today and which is still only poorly researched. They were instrumental in the development of *Yoga, especially along more ascetical lines. Not surprisingly, the Jaina writer Rājasekhara styles Shaivism a "Yoga tradition" (*yoga-mata*) in his *Shad-Darshana-Samuccaya* ("Compendium of Six Systems"). See also Vaishnavism, Shaktism.

shakti ("power") is the dynamic or creative principle of existence, envisioned as being feminine. This concept is intended to explain how the undifferentiated singular *Reality can produce the multidimensional *cosmos with its infinite forms. The transcendental static principle, personified as *Shiva, is in itself incapable of creation. As a popular doctrinal maxim has it: "Shiva without *Shakti is unable to effect anything." Shiva apart from Shakti is likened to a corpse. The *Shiva-Purāna* (VII.2.4.10) resorts to this poetic metaphor: "Just as the moon does not shine without moonlight, so also Shiva does not shine without [the principle of] *shakti*."

*Shiva is called *shaktimān*, or the "possessor of power," whereas *shakti* is like the bride whose life is made complete by the bridegroom. Shiva and *shakti* are inseparable principles, and the *Kaula-Jnāna-Nirnaya* (XVII.8) compares their relationship to that between fire and smoke. Some authorities explain that the *Absolute includes an infinite number of *shaktis*. However, frequently three or more principal types of *shakti* are differentiated. Thus, the (*Kaula-Jnāna-Nirnaya* (II.6) reiterates a popular *Shaiva teaching when it speaks of three fundamental aspects of *shakti*: the *kriyā-shakti* ("power of action"); the *icchā-shakti* ("power of intention"), whose essence is sometimes said to be astonishment (*camatkāra*); and the *jnāna-shakti* ("power of knowledge"). These respectively represent the conative, volitional, and cognitive side of the incomprehensible being of *Shiva. At the time of the dissolution of the universe, the former two aspects resolve into the third aspect. Occasionally, two more aspects are listed—the *cit-shakti* ("power of awareness") and the *ānanda-shakti* ("power of *bliss"). In another passage, the *Kaula-Jnāna-Nirnaya* (XX.10) mentions nine kinds of *shakti*, and other works offer yet different and still more complicated models.

The *Siddha-Siddhānta-Paddhati* (I.5ff.) mentions the following five aspects of the *shakti*: the *nija-shakti* ("innate power"); the *para-shakti* ("higher power"); the *apara-shakti* ("lower power"); the *sūkshma-shakti* ("subtle power"); and the *kundalinī-shakti* ("serpent power"). Elsewhere this scripture (IV.2) furnishes a different list: the *para-shakti* ("higher power"); the *sattā-shakti* ("power of being"); the *ahantā-shakti* ("power of 'I-ness' "); the *sphurattā-shakti* ("power of manifestation"); the *kalā-shakti* ("power of partial existence"). All these refer to the *shakti* as it relates to specific levels of the process of psychocosmic *evolution.

The *Laghu-Yoga-Vāsishtha* (VI.2.28) makes the important point that all these *shaktis* reside within the human *body. That is to say, they are both cosmological and psychological realities. However, the *shakti* is not only responsible for *creation; it is also the agent of change and destruction. It is the power behind cosmic existence as well as *liberation. Practically speaking, the most significant form of the *shakti* is the *kundalinī-shakti*.

The term *shakti* is also used in *Tantrism to refer to the female initiate into the sexual practices. See also *cit-shakti citi-shakti*.

Shakti is the personification of the feminine form of the *Divine. Cf. Shiva.

shakti-cala- or **shakti-cālana-mudrā** ("seal of stirring the power") is described in the *Gheranda-Samhitā* (III.49ff.) thus: One should smear the *body with ashes and then wrap a piece of soft cloth four digits (about three inches) wide and one span (about nine inches) long around one's waist and hold it firmly in place with a piece of string. Sitting in the "adept's posture" (*siddha-āsana*), one should inhale and energetically mingle the in-breath (*prāna*) with the out-breath (*apāna*). Then one should contract the anus slowly by means of the *ashvinī-mudrā* until the breath (*vāyu*) reaches the central channel (*sushumnā-nādī*). The *Hatha-Yoga-Pradīpikā* (III.104.ff.) offers a different description: Seated in the "adamantine posture" (*vajra-āsana*), one should hold one's ankles and press them against the "bulb" (*kanda*). Next,

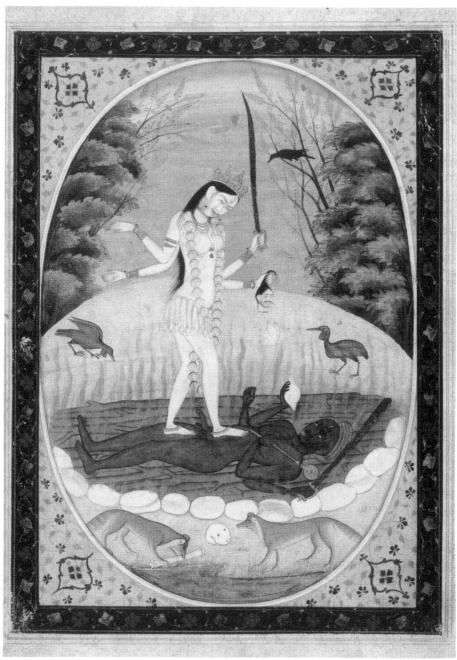

58. *Shakti, the Goddess of Power, who is associated with the cremation ground symbolizing the finitude of all creation.*

one should perform the "bellows breathing" (*bhastrikā-prānāyāma*) and contact the "sun" (i.e., the *navel region). In this manner, one should fearlessly stir the "serpent power" (*kundalinī-shakti*) for an hour and a half until the *kundalinī* enters the central channel. Celibate practitioners are said to gain perfection (*siddhi*) within forty days. According to the *Yoga-Kundaly-Upanishad* (I.8), this "seal" (*mudrā*) involves the rousing of the *sarasvatī-nādī* followed by *breath retention. This is said to make the *kundalinī* "erect" (*rijvi*).

Essentially, the *shakti-cālana-mudrā* utilizes the *apāna* form of the life force to awaken the *kundalinī*. The *Goraksha-Paddhati* (I.74) notes that this brings about the union of "semen" (*shukla*) and "blood" (*rajas*). See also *sarasvatī-cālana*.

shakti-pāta ("descent of power") is the *transmission of psychospiritual energy (*shakti*) from the *adept to the disciple (or even any person). This is generally effected by touch, as in the case of *Ramakrishna, who placed his foot on his favorite disciple Naren (the later Swami *Vivekanada) and plunged him into deep enstasy (*samādhi*). But transmission can also take place through a mere glance. See also *dīkshā*, *satsanga*.

Shaktism refers to a large number of schools and traditions within *Hinduism that revolve around the cultic *worship of the *Divine in its feminine form as *shakti. Going back into the dim prehistorical past, Goddess worship has always flourished among the lower classes of Indian society but, from about the fifth century A.D. on, also won the hearts of a large section of the literate population. The Goddesses are understood as the active spouses of the transcendental *Reality that is essentially quiescent and unapproachable. Some of the most popular Goddesses (*devī*) of the Hindu pantheon are *Kālī, *Durgā, Sarasvatī, Annapūrnā, Candī, Lakshmī, Pārvatī, Umā, Satī, and *Rādhā. The sacred scriptures of the *shaktas*, or followers of Shaktism, are generally known as the *Tantras, but *Tantrism should be distinguished from Shaktism.

shalabha-āsana ("locust posture") is described in the *Gheranda-Samhitā* (II.39) thus: Lying belly down on the ground, with one's hands placed near the chest, one should raise one's legs in the air by a span (about nine inches).

shama ("quiescence") is regarded as one of the gatekeepers to *liberation in the *Laghu-Yoga-Yāsistha* (II.1.64), where it is described as follows: "He who upon hearing, touching, seeing, tasting, and smelling pleasant or unpleasant [things] neither delights in nor regrets them, is said to be tranquil (*shānta*)."

According to the *Bhagavad-Gītā* (VI.3), *shama* is the very essence of the spiritual practice of the accomplished *yogin*, whereas *karma-yoga* is said to be the way for the aspirant. The *Uddhāva-Gītā* (XIV.36) explains it as the mind's (*buddhi*) "intentness on Me" (*man-nishthatā*), the "Me" being god *Krishna, the transcendental *Reality.

shāmbhavī-mudrā ("seal pertaining to Shambhu"). Shambhu is another name for God *Shiva. This is one of the most important "seals" (*mudrā*) of *Tantrism and *hatha-yoga, and the texts typically enjoin complete *secrecy about it. For instance, the *Gheranda-Samhitā* (III.65) says of this *mudrā* that it should be "guarded like a bride of noble lineage" and that, by comparison with it, the *Vedas, textbooks (*shāstra*), and *Purānas are "like courtesans." The same work (III.64ff.) offers the following description: One should fix one's *gaze between the eyes and behold the *Self "grove" (*ārāma*). The *Gheranda-Samhitā* (I.54) also notes that this *mudrā* can be induced by means of steady gazing (*trātaka*). The *Hatha-Yoga-Pradīpikā* (IV.36) adds that *mind and *breath should be absorbed in the "inner sign" (*antar-lakshya*), with one's open pupils fixed and unseeing. In another verse, this scripture (IV.39) refers to a variant practice, which involves gazing at the *light (at the tip of the nose). This is otherwise known as the "external sign" (*bahir-lakshya*). This technique is claimed to quickly yield the realization of the state of exaltation (*unmanī*). See also *vaishnavī-mudrā*.

Shame. See *lajjā*.

Shāndilya is the name of several teachers, including a famous authority of the *Pāncarātra tradition. He lived prior to *Rāmānuja, who defended the *Vedic legitimacy of the teachings of that stage. He is mentioned already by *Shankara in his commentary on the *Brahma-Sūtra* (II.2.45), where a stanza is cited that states that Shādilya turned to the Pāncarātra tradition because he did not find the highest *bliss through the *Vedas. Probably a different Shāndilya authored the *Bhakti-Sūtra*, and the teachings of yet another well-known *adept by that name are recorded in the ancient *Chāndogya-Upanishad* (III.14).

Shāndilya-Upanishad is one of the
*Yoga-Upanishads. It consists of
three chapters and comprises well
over thirty printed pages. This
scripture is named after *Shāndilya, who figures in it as the disciple of Atharvan (who is
associated with the *Atharva-
Veda). The first chapter defines the
"limbs" (*anga) of the eightfold
*path (*ashta-anga-yoga), mentioning ten components each for
moral observance (*yama) and self-
discipline (*niyama) and describing
five phases of sense withdrawal
(*pratyāhāra) and five types of concentration (*dhāranā), as well as
two forms of meditation (*dhyāna).
It also discusses esoteric *anatomy
and the appropriate environment

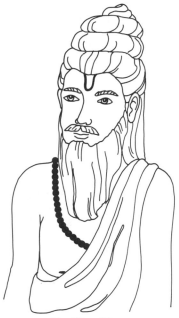

59. Shandilya.

(*desha) for yogic practice at some length. The short second chapter
and the third chapter contain an exposition of *Vedānta metaphysics,
which forms the philosophical basis of its teachings. Many of the
stanzas are also to be found in the *Yoga-Yājnavalkya, and the text
generally has the appearance of being a composite with probably numerous interpolations.

Shankara, the celebrated teacher (*ācārya*) of *Advaita-Vedānta, was
born probably in the village of Kaladi in Kerala, South India. He is
traditionally said to have lived from A.D. 788 to 822, though some
modern scholars take the first date to be his year of initiation as a
renunciate. Legend describes him as a precocious child who could read
at the age of two and had mastered the *Vedas at the age of eight.
Shankara's *Advaita-Vedānta teacher was Govinda, the disciple of
*Gaudapāda. Shankara, who traveled widely in India, founded four
monastic orders: at Dvarāka in the west, at Pūri in the east, at Badrī
in the north and at Shringeri in the South. His expositions of Advaita-
Vedānta, as preserved in many extant works of great erudition, were
mainly responsible for the renaissance of that ancient tradition and
the decline of *Buddhism in India. In addition to his scholarly commentaries on the *Brahma-Sūtra*, the principal *Upanishads, and the

Bhagavad-Gītā, he also apparently wrote a number of popular didactic works, notably the *Upadesha-Sahasrī* ("Thousand Instructions"). There is also a large number of devotional hymns that are attributed to him. Shankara's (legendary) life-story is related in the famous biography by Mādhava, which is entitled *Shankara-Dig-Vijaya*.

The German indologist Paul Hacker (1968) put forward good reasons for assuming that prior to his conversion to *Advaita-Vedānta, Shankara had been a follower of *Yoga, more specifically of *Patanjali's school. This would support the indigenous claim that Shankara Bhagavatpāda authored the important but little known (and probably suppressed) sub-commentary on the *Yoga-Sūtra, entitled *Vivarana.

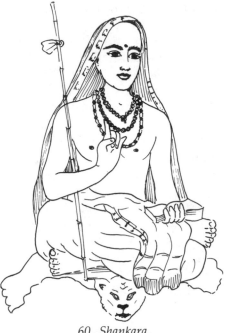

60. Shankara.

Shankara is also one of the many names of God *Shiva of whom Shankara the sage is widely regarded as a partial incarnation (*avatāra). The name is also occasionally spelled Shamkara, which is explained in the *Spanda-Kārikā* (I.1) as "he who makes *sham*," with the word *sham* being a synonym for *anugraha, or "grace."

shankhinī-nādī ("mother-of-pearl channel") is one of the principal channels of the life force (*prāna), which is situated between the *gāndhārā- and the *sarasvatī-nādī and extends to the right (or to the left) ear. See also *nādī*.

shan-mukhī-mudrā ("six-openings seal") is referred to, for instance, in the *Goraksha-Paddhati* (II.16), where it is said to consist in the blocking of one's ears, eyes, and nostrils with one's fingers. This "seal" (*mudrā) is correctly executed by covering the ears with one's thumbs, the eyes with one's index fingers, and the nostril with the remaining fingers. This practice is recommended for the manifestation of the inner sound (*nāda).

shānti ("peace") is sometimes cited as one of the components of moral observance (*yama*) and in this context denotes mental equilibrium. However, as is clear from the *Bhagavad-Gītā* (V.29), the word can also stand for the highest condition of "extinction in the *Absolute" (*brahma-nirvāna*).

sharīra ("body") is derived from the verbal root *shrī*, meaning "to fall apart", and denotes the "wretched *body." The *Maitrāy-anīya-Upanishad* (II.3ff.) compares

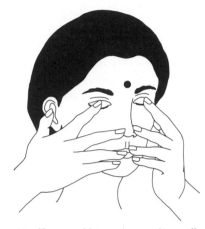

61. Shan-mukhī-mudrā: sealing off the six openings of the head.

the body to an insensate cart and to a potter's wheel that is whirled about by the *Self. This *Upanishad (III.4) also offers the following classic denunciation of *embodiment:

> This body, arising from sexual congress (*maithunā*), grows in the [uterine] *hell and emerges from the urinary opening. It is made up of bones, smeared over with flesh, covered the skin, filled with feces, urine, *bile, *phlegm, marrow, fat, grease, and [endowed] with numerous *diseases, like a treasury with wealth.

As the *Shiva-Purāna* (V.23.9) puts it succinctly: There is not a single clean spot on the body. See also *deha*, *kosha*, *pinda*.

sharīrin ("embodied one") is a synonym for *dehin*.

shashi-mandala ("lunar circle") or shashi-sthāna ("lunar place"). See *candra*; cf. *sūrya*.

shāstra ("teaching," "textbook"). While most Hindu authorities consider the *study of the textbooks essential to successful spiritual practice, some question or even outright deny the value of written teachings. Thus, the *Laghu-Yoga-Vāsishtha* (VI.2.130) observes that the *Self cannot be realized without a qualified teacher (*guru*) and knowing the content of the textbooks. The *Bhagavad-Gītā* (XVI.24) states that the *shāstras* should guide a person in determining appropriate (*kārya*) and inappropriate behavior, because those who live as they please can never find perfection (*siddhi*) or joy (*sukha*). The *Mahābhārata* epic

(XII.245.12) even has the phrase *shāstra-yoga* ("Yoga of the textbooks"). By contrast, the *Yoga-Shikhā-Upanishad* (I.4) warns of the "snare of textbooks" (*shāstra-jāla*, that is, mere book learning). See also *grantha*.

shat-cakra-bheda ("piercing the six centers"). The most common model of psychoenergetic centers (*cakra*) distinguishes six such centers, with a seventh center serving as the terminal for the ascending "serpent power" (*kundalinī-shakti*). On its upward path, the *kundalinī* is pictured as "piercing" (*bheda*) the six lower centers or "lotuses" (*padma*), rather like a string pierces the flowers of a garland.

Shat-Cakra-Nirūpana ("Investigation of the Six Centers") is the sixth chapter of Pūrnānanda Svāmin's *Shrī-Tattva-Cintāmani*, a late voluminous treatise on *Tantrism consisting of twenty-five chapters. The Nirūpana, which comprises fifty-five (or fifty-six) stanzas, is the best-known work dealing with the process of *shat-cakra-bheda*.

shat-karma ("six acts"). According to the *Gheranda-Samhitā* (I. 12), this is the first step of *ghatastha-yoga*. It consists of the following practices: (1) *dhauti* ("cleansing"), which has four constituent techniques; (2) *vasti* ("bladder"), which is the yogic equivalent to an enema; (3) *neti* (untranslatable), which is nasal cleansing; (4) *naulī* or *laulī* or *laulikī* ("to and fro movement"), consisting in rolling the addominal muscles; (5) *trātaka* (untranslatable), which is steady conscious gazing; (6) *kapāla-bhāti* ("skull luster"), which has three constituent techniques. The *Hatha-Yoga-Pradīpikā* (II.21) recommends these six practices specifically for initiates who suffer from an excess of fat or phlegm (*kapha*).

   The term *shat-karma* can also refer to the following six *Tantric magical practices: (1) *marana* ("killing"); (2) *uccātana* ("repelling"); (3) *vashī-karana* ("bringing under one's control"); (4) *stambhana* ("arresting"), such as arresting a storm, for instance; (5) *vidveshana* ("creating enmity") (6) *svastyayana* ("causing warfare"). Most of these practices belong to black *magic. See also *ashta-siddhi, siddhi*.

shat-sthāla ("six stages") is a central doctrine of *Vīra-Shaivism (or *Lingāyata). It refers to the six levels of spiritual maturation: (1) *bhakti* ("devotion"), as expressed in ritual *worship at the temple or in the home; (2) *mahā-īsha* ("great Lord"), which is the phase of disciplining one's *mind; (3) *prasāda* ("grace"), which is the peaceful stage in which the *devotee recognizes the *Divine working in and through everything; (4) *prāna-linga* ("phallus of the life force"), or the stage at which the devotee begins to experience the Divine within the *body (as a consecrated temple); (5) *sharana* ("[taking] refuge"), which is the phase in which the devotee becomes a "fool of God," longing for God *Shiva as a woman yearns for her lover; (6) *aikya* ("union"), or the consummate state at which ritual worship is at an end because the devotee has *become* the Lord.

In some contexts, *shat-sthāla* refers to the six psychoenergetic centers (*cakra*).

shauca ("purity" or "cleansing") is, according to *Classical Yoga, one of the techniques of self-discipline (*niyama*). It is also listed in some scriptures of *Post-Classical Yoga as one of the ten practices of moral observance (*yama*). The *Yoga-Sūtra* (II.40) states that when *purity is perfectly cultivated, it leads to "aversion" (*jugupsā*) toward one's own *body and a desire to avoid "contamination" through contact with others. The *Yoga-Bhāshya* (II.32) notes that cleansing is twofold: external (*bāhya*) and internal (*abhyantara*). The former is effected by the use of water, earth, and other similar substances, as well as the consumption of pure *food. Inner cleansing is the washing away of the "blemishes" (*mala*) of the mind. According to the *Bhagavad-Gītā (XIII.7), *shauca* is a manifestation of knowledge (*jnāna*) and (XVII.14) forms part of bodily asceticism (*tapas*). See also *dhauti*, *shodhana*, *shuddhi*.

shava-āsana ("dead posture") is a synonym for *mrita-āsana*.

Shesha. See Ananta.

shikhin ("tuft wearer") is an epithet of fire (*agni*). According to the *Tri-Shikhi-Brāhmana-Upanishad* (II.56), the *shikhin* situated in the center of the human *body is "lustrous like molten gold." The location of the *shikhin* is generally envisioned as being of triangular (*trikona*) shape. This scripture further mentions that it is quadrangular in the case of quadrupeds, hexagonal in the case of snakes, octagonal in the case of insects, and circular in the case of birds. These ideas belong to the realm esoteric *anatomy.

shīla ("disposition," "behavior"). The *Yoga-Bhāshya* (I.2) speaks of three fundamental dispositions of consciousness (*citta*), resulting from the predominance of one or the other of the three primary constituents (*guna*) of *Nature: luminosity (*prākhya*), activity (*pravritti*), and inertia (*sthiti*).

shīrsha-āsana ("head posture") is the headstand described in modern manuals of *hatha-yoga*. In the earlier literature of this school of *Yoga, it goes by the name of *viparīta-kāranī* Cf. *sarva-anga-āsana*.

shishya ("pupil," "disciple"). *Yoga is an initiatory tradition that, as a rule, calls for a period of apprenticeship during which a spiritual aspirant submits himself (or, more rarely, herself) not only to rigorous self-discipline but also to a teacher (*guru*). After a potential disciple has presented himself or herself to a master (*svāmin*), that *teacher applies certain personal and traditional criteria to the applicant to see whether he or she has the necessary qualifications or competence (*adhikāra*) for a life of spiritual practice. A teacher might, of course, accept an un-

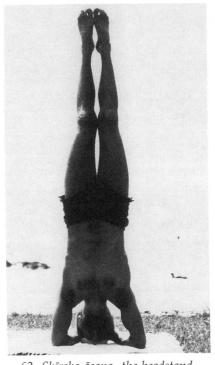

62. *Shīrsha-āsana, the headstand.*

prepared student because he senses that the applicant has promising potential.

The *Shiva-Samhitā* (V.10ff.) distinguishes four types of students, depending on the practitioner's commitment to spiritual life: (1) The weak (*mridu*) practitioner is unenthusiastic, foolish, fickle, timid, ill, dependent, rude, ill-mannered,and unenergetic. He is only fit for *mantra-yoga. (2) The mediocre (*madhya*) practitioner is endowed with even-mindedness, *patience, a desire for virtue, kind speech, and the tendency to practice moderation in all undertakings. He is fit for *laya-yoga. (3) The exceptional (*adhimātra*) practitioner demonstrates firm understanding, an aptitude for meditative absorption (*laya*), self-reliance, liberal-mindedness, bravery, vigor, faithfulness, the willingness to *worship the teacher's lotus feet (both literally and figuratively), and delight in the practice of *Yoga. He is capable of practicing *hatha-yoga. (4) The extraordinary (*adhimātratama*) practitioner displays energy, enthusiasm, charm, heroism, scriptural knowledge, the inclination to practice, freedom from delusion, orderliness, youthfulness, moderate eating habits, control over the *senses, *fearlessness, *purity, skillfulness, liberality, the ability to be a refuge for all people, general capability, stability, thoughtfulness, the willingness to do whatever is desired by the teacher, *patience, good manners, observance of the moral and spiritual law (*dharma), the ability to keep his struggle to himself, kind speech, *faith in the scriptures, the willingness to worship *God and the teacher (as the embodiment of the *Divine), knowledge of the vows (*vrāta) pertaining to his level of practice, and, lastly, the practice of all types of Yoga.

Traditionally, the student was expected to live with, and serve, the *teacher during the period of pupilage. Such a student is known as an antevāsin ("one who dwells near"). The reason for this is undoubtedly to give the teacher the frequent opportunity to break down the student's self-will. Additionally, discipleship gives the student the opportunity not only to see the teacher's good example but also to benefit from the *adept's psychophysical "radiation," which is a primary form of spiritual *transmission. This is why the scriptures recommend the great principle of "communion with the Real" (*sat-sanga). The disciple assimilates the teacher's state of being, both by intention and by physical contagion, until—ideally—the disciple reaches *liberation, or at least the same level of spiritual accomplishment as the teacher, if the teacher happens to be not yet liberated. It is widely held that only a teacher who is himself (or herself) fully *Self-realized, or *enlightened, can guide the student to Self-realization. See also dīkshā, guru-yoga.

shītali ("cooling") is one of the eight types of breath control (*prānāyāma) taught in *hatha-yoga. It is described in the *Gheranda-Samhitā (V.73f.) thus: One should draw in the air by means of the (extended and curled) tongue and gradually fill one's abdomen. Retaining it there for an instant, one should exhale again through both nostrils. This is said to cure indigestion and disorders arising from an imbalance of bile (*pitta) and phlegm (*kapha).

shīt-krama ("process [causing the sound] shīt") is one of the three processes of *kapāla-bhāti, as described in the *Gheranda-Samhitā (I.59f.). It gets its name from the sound shīt produced when water is sucked up through the mouth and expelled through the *nose. This practice is said to make one as beautiful as the God Kāma, the *Hindu equivalent of Cupid. According to the *Shāndilya-Upanishad (I.7.13.3), which calls this practice *sīt-karī, the practitioner should, after inhalation, retain the air for as long as possible. Here it is also stated that shīt-krama defeats *hunger and *thirst as well as *sleep and *languor.

Shiva is the personification of the static, masculine form of the *Divine. The word means "benevolent." Paradoxically, however, Shiva is generally conceived as the destroyer of the universe. But, from a spiritual perspective, his destructive power is the essential process of breaking down (deconditioning) the ego-personality so that it becomes pervious to the divine *light. In countless myths, told in the *Mahābhārata epic and the *Purānas, Shiva emerges as the God of *yogins par excellence. He combines within himself the possibilities of both fierce asceticism (*tapas) and orgiastic excess. See also *deva, shakti*.

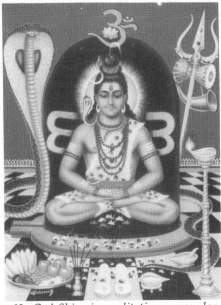

63. God Shiva in meditation; a popular Hindu representation.

Shiva-Jnāna-Siddhi ("Perfection of Shiva Wisdom") is a classic exposition of southern *Shaivism (*Shaiva-Siddhānta) by Arulnanda, the foremost of *Meykandar's forty-nine disciples. It has a brilliant commentary by *Jnānaprakāsha.

shiva-mantra is the most revered sacred *mantra of *Shaivism, which reads: *om namah shivāya* or "*Om. Obeisance to *Shiva!" The *Shiva-Purāna (III.5.6.25f.) gives the text of the full *mantra*: *om namah shivāya shubham shubham kuru kuru shivāya namah om* or "Om. Obeisance to Shiva! Do [us] good! Do [us] good! To Shiva [be] obeisance! Om."

Shivananda, Swami (A.D. 1887–1963) was one of the great modern masters of *Yoga. After a successful practice as a physician, he renounced the world in 1923, founded his own hermitage in 1932, and four years later established the Divine Life Society, which has meantime won an international reputation. He has over three hundred publications attributed to him. Among his best-known disciples are Swami Cidananda, who is the head of the Divine Life Society, Swami Satyananda (whose Tantra-Oriented *āshrama is in Bihar), and Swami Shivananda Radha (a German-born woman whose Yoga school is in Canada).

Shiva-Purāna is one of the major works of the *Purāna genre, comprising seven chapters with over 24,000 stanzas. As the title suggests, this scripture belongs to *Shaivism and so *Yoga is defined as restraint in all one's activities and concentration upon God *Shiva. In section 17 of the first chapter, *mantra-yoga* is introduced, involving the recitation (*japa*) of the *shiva-mantra. Adherents of this type of Yoga are said to be of three kinds: the *kriyā-yogin*, who engages in sacred rites (*kriyā*); the *tapo-yogin*, who pursues asceticism (*tapas*); and the *japa-yogin*, who, in addition to observing the practices of the other two kinds of *yogin*, also constantly recites the *shiva-mantra*. Yoga is again dealt with at length in sections 37–39 of the seventh chapter. Five types of Yoga are differentiated: (1) *mantra-yoga*; (2) *sparsha-yoga* ("tangible Yoga"), which is a form of *mantra-yoga* coupled with breath control (*prānāyāma*); (3) *bhāva-yoga* ("Yoga of being"), which is a higher form of *mantra-yoga* where contact with the *mantra is lost and *consciousness enters a subtle dimension of existence; (4) *abhāva-yoga* ("Yoga of non-being"), which is the *contemplation of the universe in its entirety, associated with the transcendence of object-related awareness; (5) *mahā-yoga* ("great Yoga"), which is the contemplation of *Shiva without any limiting conditions.

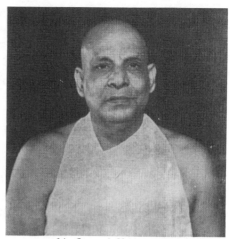

64. Swami Shivananda.

Shiva-Samhitā ("Collection on [the Wisdom of] *Shiva") is one of the principal manuals in *hatha-yoga. It was probably written in the late seventeenth or early eighteenth century A.D. and consists of 645 stanzas distributed over five chapters. This work begins with a review of various schools of thought, which are judged to be inferior to nondualist *Yoga. It is clear from this opening section that the author was thoroughly familiar with the metaphysics of *Advaita-Vedānta. The second chapter deals with esoteric *anatomy. This subject matter is taken up again in the concluding chapter in regard to actual yogic practice. The third chapter describes the five types of life force (*prāna) and the means of its regulation, including breath control (*prānāyāma) and several postures (*āsana). The fourth chapter treats the "seals" (*mudrā). The fifth chapter appears to be a later appendage. It is presented as a discourse between *Īshvara (the Lord) and *Devī (the Goddess). Its content is mixed, ranging from definitions of different types of Yoga to descriptions of various esoteric practices. In several places, this work emphasizes that also householders (*grihastha) can obtain success in Yoga through diligent practice.

Shiva-Sūtra ("Aphorisms of *Shiva") is a source text of Kashmiri (or northern) *Shaivism. It was composed ("discovered") by *Vasugupta in the early ninth century A.D. and has given rise to an extensive commentarial literature, the most important commentary being Kshemarāja's *Vimarshinī*. Vasugupta's work consists of three sections with a total of 77 *sūtras. Similar to *Patanjali's *Yoga-Sūtra*, the *Shiva-Sūtra* can be regarded as an extremely terse exposition of *Yoga, with a fully developed technical vocabulary. See also Pratyābhijna.

Shiva-Svarodaya ("Production of *Shiva's Sound"). The Sanskrit word *svarodaya* is composed of *svara meaning "sound" and *udaya* meaning "rising," "production," and "success." The "production of sound" refers specifically to the sound made by the *breath so that *svara* is almost synonymous with *prāna. The *Shiva-Svarodaya* is a late work of 395 stanzas. It deals with the flow of the life force/breath through the three principal pathways: the *idā-nādī on the left, the *pingalā-nādī on the right, and the *sushumnā-nādī in the middle. The *yogins have noted that the life force alternates between the left and the right channel (*nādī) and that, when switching from the one to the other, it flows for a short period of time through the central pathway. This can be determined by checking which nostril is blocked. When both are open, the *prāna is thought to flow through the *sushumnā-nādī. The cycle is said to last for approximately one hour per nostril. The flow can be changed in a few minutes by lying on the opposite side of the nostril that is blocked. Each flow is associated with certain auspicious and inauspicious moments. The *Shiva-Svarodaya* is largely concerned with divination on the basis of the breath.

shiva-yoga is equated in the *Shiva-Purāna* (VII.1.33.25) with *pāshupata-yoga. According to this work (I.3.27), *shiva-yoga* is painful at first but subsequently auspicious. It consists of *shravana ("listening"), *kīrtana ("chanting"), and *manana ("pondering").

Shiva-Yoga-Ratna ("Jewel of Shiva-Yoga") is an important treatise on southern *Shaivism consisting of 192 stanzas and a short prose appendix. It is one of the nine works ascribed to *Jnānaprakāsha. The

*Yoga taught in this work closely resembles *asparsha-yoga, but unlike *Gaudapāda, Jnānaprakāsha also outlines the practical techniques of *breath control and *meditation.

Shiva-Yoga-Sāra ("Essence of Shiva-Yoga") is one of the works of *Jnānaprakāsha, which is a digest of the yogic teachings of southern *Shaivism.

shodasha-cakra ("sixteen[-petaled] center"), mentioned in the *Yoga-Kundaly-Upanishad* (I.69), is better known as the *indu-cakra.

shodhana ("cleansing, cleanliness") is the first member of the "sevenfold discipline" (*sapta-sādhana). According to the *Gheranda-Samhitā* (I.10) it is accomplished by means of the "six acts" (*shat-karma). See also Purity, *shuddhi*.

shoka ("grief") is considered as one of the "defects" (*dosha). The teaching about the futility of grief figures prominent in the *Bhagavad-Gītā*, where *Arjuna is depicted as grieving at the thought of having to slay his kinsmen. The God-man *Krishna instructs him in the secret of the indestructibility of the *Self and encourages him to practice *karma-yoga.

shonita ("reddish") is a synonym for *rajas, the female sexual secretion.

shoshana ("desiccation") is generally regarded as the essence of asceticism (*taps). In *hatha-yoga, it sometimes signifies the "drying up" of the life liquid (*rasa), as effected through the practice of the "great seal" (*mahā-mudrā). See also *upavāsa*.

Shoulder stand. See *sarva-anga-āsana*; cf. *viparīta-karanī-mudrā*.

shraddhā ("faith"), which is sometimes deemed one of the practices of self-discipline (*niyama), is crucial to spiritual life. *Faith is often explained as a "positive frame of mind" (*āstikya-buddhi). The *Yoga-Bhāshya* (I.20) defines the word as "mental repose" (*cetasah samprasādah*) and likens faith to a caring mother, since it protects the *yogin. As such, faith is the exact opposite of the mood of doubt (*samshaya), which saps a person's energies and disrupts the spiritual process. "Faith," states *Vācaspati Mishra in his *Tattva-Vaishāradī* (I.20), "is the root of *Yoga." The *Yoga-Sūtra* (I.20) treats faith as a prerequisite for the induction of the supraconscious enstasy (*asamprajnāta-samādhi).

The *Bhagavad-Gītā* (IV.39) speaks of the "man of faith" (*shraddhāvāms*), who wins first wisdom (*jnāna*) and then peace (*shānti*). The same scripture (XVII.2f.) declares that faith can be of three kinds, depending on the prevalence of one or the other *guna*.

> The faith of embodied beings (*dehin*) is threefold, springing from [their] very being (*sva-bhāva*): *sattva*-natured, *rajas*-natured, or *tamas*-natured. Hear [more about] them.

> The faith of everyone is in accordance with his essence (*sattva*), o son of Bharata. This person (*purusha*) is of the form of faith. Whatever his faith is, that verily is he.

Cf. Reason.

shravana ("listening") is an aspect of *bhakti-yoga*. It also stands for attentive listening to the sacred teachings, which is followed by pondering (*manana*). In some contexts, *shravana* denotes auditory phenomena associated with *meditation practice, and as such is sometimes considered to be one of the "obstacles" (*upasarga*, *vighna*). See also *siddhānta-shravana*.

shrī-yantra ("blessed device"), also called *shrī-cakra* ("blessed wheel"), is the best known *yantra employed in Hindu *Shaktism and in Tantric *Buddhism. It is composed of nine interlocking triangles, commonly depicted with five triangles pointing downward and four pointing upward. These represent the feminine principle (*shakti*) and the male principle (*shiva*) respectively. The arrangement of these interpenetrating triangles is such that they yield a total of forty-three small triangles

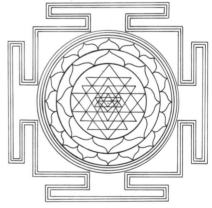

65. Shrī-yantra.

that house the deities (*devatā*) associated with particular aspects of existence. This is sometimes indicated by inscribing in Sanskrit letters the names of the deities or their appropriate "seed sounds" (*bīja-mantras*). This complex geometrical structure is usually enclosed by two circular lotus patterns of eight and sixteen petals respectively, as well as four concentric circles. The whole design is placed in a square surround of three parallel lines, forming what is known as the protective "world-house" (bhū-griha). Cf. mandala.

shruta ("that which has been heard"). In *Classical Yoga, this is a synonym for "tradition" (*āgama).

shruti ("revelation"), which is the feminine form of shruta, refers to the sacred literature of *Hinduism, comprising the four ancient *Vedic collections and the *Upanishads. As opposed to the *smriti literature, the revealed scriptures are thought to be of nonhuman, or divine, origin. They have been "seen" by the sages (*rishi, *muni) during extraordinary states of *consciousness. See also āgama.

shubhā-nādī ("auspicious channel"), which is mentioned in the *Tri-Shikhi-Brāhmana-Upanishad (II.73), extends from the "bulb" (*kanda) to the glans penis (medhra-anta).

shuddhi ("purity, purification"). See bhūta-shuddhi, Purity.

Shuka is an *adept who is said in the *Mahābhārata epic (XII.319.9) to have flown through the air. According to the *Varāha-Upanishad (IV.2.34), Shuka is a representative of instantaneous *liberation (sadyo-mukti) as opposed to gradual liberation (krama-mukti). See also Levitation.

shukla ("white") is a synonym for shukra (semen). See also bindu, retas; cf. rajas.

shukla-dhyāna ("white meditation") is explained in *Upanishad Brahmayogin's commentary on the Jābāla-Upanishad as *meditation on the white brilliance of the *Absolute.

shukra ("semen"), which is sometimes called *shukla, is a synonym for *bindu. As the *Shiva-Purāna (V.22.49) notes, the strength of living beings depends on the semen.

shūnya ("void"). The idea of the ultimate *Reality as the Void originated in Mahāyāna *Buddhism. It is also expressed in some *hatha-yoga scriptures, though is given a different meaning. In the *Hatha-Yoga-Pradīpikā (IV.56), the highest state of enstasy (*samādhi) is described as being void and full (pūrna) at the same time. The term is also occasionally employed to denote the suspension of the *breath after exhalation. The term *shūnyatā* ("voidness") is used in the sense of "absentmindedness" in the *Tejo-Bindu-Upanishad* (I.41), and is considered to be one of the "obstacles" (*vighna*). See also *sahasrāra-cakra*.

shūrā-nādī ("valiant channel") extends, according to the *Yoga-Shikhā-Upanishad* (V.22), to the place at the middle between the brows (*bhrū-madhya*).

shushka-vasti ("dry enema"), also called *sthala-vasti*, is one of the two forms of *vasti*. It is described in the *Gheranda-Samhitā* (I.48f.) thus: One should assume the *pashcima-uttāna-āsana* and gently push the intestines downward and then contract and dilate the sphincter muscle by means of the *ashvinī-mudrā*. This is said to cure constipation and flatulence, and to stimulate the gastric fire (*jāthara-agni*). Cf. *jala-vasti*.

shushrūshā ("obedience"). See *guru-shushrūshā*.

shvāsa ("inhalation") is used in *Classical Yoga both in the sense of inhalation and faulty breathing, being one of the obstacles (*antarāya*). The latter connotation is found already in the *Mahābhārata* (XII.290.54), which lists *shvāsa* as one of the five "defects" (*dosha*) and states (vs. 55) that it can be conquered by a scant diet (*laghv-āhāra*). In another passage (XII.266.6), *shvāsa* is said to be overcome by cultivating the "field knower" (*kshetra-jna*), that is, by magnifying the principle of pure *Consciousness in one's life. Cf. *nishvāsa*.

Shvetāshvatara-Upanishad ("Whitest Horse Upanishad"), which belongs to the third or fourth century B.C., has been hailed as one of the more beautiful creations of the *Upanishadic genre. Consisting of six chapters with a total of 113 stanzas, this work is the earliest document of *Shaivism. Its curious title is left unexplained. According to *Shankara's learned commentary on this scripture, *shveta-ashva-tara* ("most white horse") is the title of a sage whose *senses (also esoterically referred to as "horses") are purified and under control.

In its theistic metaphysics, this work is rather similar to the *Bhagavad-Gītā*. However, it knows nothing about *karma-yoga*, and its yogic teachings center on meditation (*dhyāna*). It introduces a sixfold *path (*shad-anga-yoga*) that has God *Rudra-*Shiva-Hara as the priceless goal of the spiritual aspirant. The following stanzas capture the orientation and tone of this early *Yoga scripture:

Following the Yoga of meditation, they perceived the self-power (*ātma-shakti*) of the *God hidden by His own qualities (*guna*). He is the One who presides over all the causes connected with time and self (*ātman*). (I.3)

The Lord (*īsha*) supports this universe, composed of the perishable and the imperishable, the manifest and the unmanifest. The [individuated] self, [which is] not the Lord, is bound by [its notion of] being the enjoyer. But on knowing God, it is released from all fetters. (I.8)

The "foundation" (*pradhāna*) [i.e., Nature] is perishable. Hara [*Shiva] is immortal and imperishable. The one God rules over the perishable and the selves. By meditating on Him, by uniting with and becoming the Real (*tattva*), there is finally the cessation of all illusion (*māyā*). (I.10)

By knowing God, the falling away of all fetters [is swiftly accomplished]. Upon the waning of the afflictions (*klesha*) [i.e., spiritual *ignorance and its results], the falling away of birth and *death [is accomplished]. By meditating on Him, there is a third [state], universal lordship, upon separating from the *body. [Thus, the *yogin becomes] the solitary (*kevala*) [Self], whose *desires are satisfied. (I.11)

The meditative process, which involves *recitation of the sacred syllable *om, is described as a kind of churning by which the inner *fire is kindled, which then leads to the revelation of the *Self's intrinsic splendor. Successful meditation (*dhyāna*) inevitably gives rise to a variety of inner visions that, warns the text, must not be confused with *enlightenment. This is how the anonymous author of the *Shvetāshvatara-Upanishad* (III.8) describes the ultimate realization: "I know that great Self (*purusha*) who is effulgent like the sun beyond darkness. Realizing Him alone, one passes beyond *death. There is no other way for passing [beyond the cycle of repeated births and deaths]."

This work has in rough outline all the basic elements of the yogic *path, and even includes the devotional (*bhakti*) aspect.

siddha ("accomplished" or "adept") is a spiritual master who is generally held to be *enlightened, or to have reached perfection (*siddhi*). According to the *Yoga-Shikhā-Upanishad* (I.159), an *adept can be recognized by his possession of paranormal powers (*siddhi*). In the same work (I.50), it is also stated that the grace (*prasāda*) of an adept is essential for a practitioner of *jñāna-yoga (or *jñānin) of inferior standing in order to become a full-fledged *yogin. See also *mahā-siddha, *shakti-pāta.

siddha-anganā ("adept's companion") is a female *siddha.

siddha-āsana ("accomplished posture") is a *meditation posture that is described in the *Gheranda-Samhitā (II.7) as follows: One should place the (left) heel at the anus and the other heel above the genitals, while resting the chin on the chest and gazing at the spot between the eyebrows. This posture (*āsana) is said to lead to *liberation. The *Hatha-Yoga-Pradīpikā (I.40) promises perfection in twelve years through the proper practice of this technique. It also mentions (I.36) an alternative version in which the left ankle is placed above the penis. This practice is also sometimes referred to as *vajra-āsana, *mukta-āsana, and *gupta-āsana. In the *Yoga-Mārtanda (5), it is also called svastha-āsana.

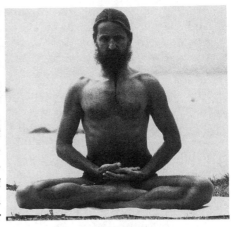

66. Siddha-āsana.

Siddha cult. This cult, which flourished between A.D. 800 and 1200, sprung up around the recognition and *worship of a group of perfected beings known as the *siddhas. The northern Indian tradition recognizes eighty-four great adepts (*mahā-siddha) who not only enjoy the superlative condition of liberation (*moksha) but are also in possession of great paranormal powers (*siddhi). They are venerated as deified humans. Best known among these extraordinary beings are *Matsyendra (known as Luipā in Tibet) and *Goraksha. As is clear from this roster of eighty-four spiritual notables, the Siddha cult or movement straddled both *Hinduism and *Buddhism. The southern Indian tradition knows of a pantheon of eighteen such adepts, notably *Agastya, *Tirumūlar, and *Civavākkiyar. This second list also includes several non-Indian individuals, of Chinese, Singhalese, and even Egyptian origin. Countless legends have been woven around the lives and miraculous deeds of these figures. However, their teachings have been only imperfectly preserved. In addition to some writings—mostly of dubious authenticity—there are also numerous didactic songs (dohā).

The *veneration of spiritual personages, as focal points of sacred presence or power, is of course a time-honored practice, dating back to pre-Christian times, as is evident from the *Mahābhārata* and other early works. Teacher worship (*guru-pūjana*) is an aspect of this practice.

Integral to the Siddha cult or movement was a concern for bodily perfection, even physical *immortality. This orientation of "cultivating (the potential of) the body" (*kāya-sādhana*) led to the creation of *hatha-yoga. However, the historical connections between the Siddha cult and *hatha-yoga, *Nāthism, and *Kaulism are still rather obscure.

siddha-darshana ("vision of the adepts"). According to the *Yoga-Sūtra (III.32), one can induce a visionary experience of the *adepts by practicing "constraint" (*samyama) upon the "light in the head." The *Shiva-Samhitā (V.87) states that this vision can be obtained through *contemplation of the heart center (*anāhata-cakra).

siddhānta ("doctrine") is derived from the words *siddha* ("accomplished," "established") and *anta* ("end," "conclusion"). The teachings, or doctrines, are a "settled matter," because they are based on the experiences and realizations of *adepts. See also Shaiva-Siddhānta.

siddhānta-shravana ("listening to the doctrines") is, according to the *Darshana-Upanishad (II.9), one of the ten components of self-discipline (*niyama). It is defined as "(the study of) the true, infinite knowledge (*jñāna), the supreme bliss (*ānanda), the supreme certainty, the 'innermost' (*pratyak)." The *Yoga-Tattva-Upanishad introduces it as one of the constituent practices of *hatha-yoga. Listening to the esoteric teachings creates right understanding and instills faith (*shraddhā) and thus motivates the student to devote himself or herself to the ordeal of self-discipline and *self-transcendence. See also *shravana*.

Siddhapāda is mentioned in the *Hatha-Yoga-Pradīpikā (I.6) as a master of *hatha-yoga. Nothing is known about him.

Siddha-Siddhānta-Paddhati ("Tracks of the Doctrines of the Adepts") is an important work of early *hatha-yoga. It is ascribed to *Goraksha and consists of six chapters with a total of 353 stanzas. This text develops the philosophy of *Nāthism, especially the teachings about the body (*pinda). In the first chapter, six types or levels of *embodiment are distinguished, beginning with the transcendental (*para*) *body and ending with the "embryonic" (*garbha*), or physical, body. Subsequent chapters deal extensively with esoteric *anatomy. In one verse

(II.32), the genuine *yogin* is defined as someone who knows firsthand the nine centers (*cakra*), the sixteen "props" (*ādhāra*), the three "signs" (*lakshya*), and the five "ether-spaces" (*vyoman*). The nine psychoenergetic centers include the well-known series of seven, except that the *sahasrāra* is here called *nirvāna-cakra*. The eighth center is the *tālu-cakra*, which is situated at the *palate and is the location of the mysterious "bell" (*ghantikā*), or uvula, or "royal tooth" (*rāja-danta*), the point from which the divine nectar (*amrita*) drips. The ninth center is the *ākāsha-cakra*, which is described as having sixteen spokes and is situated at the "brahmic fissure" (*brahma-randhra*) at the crown of the head.

The fourth chapter introduces the "serpent power" (*kundalinī-shakti*), which is stated to exist in two forms—unmanifest (cosmic) and manifest (individuated). In the former state it is known as *akula*, in the latter as *kula*. This scripture further distinguishes between the lower, middle, and upper forces (*shakti*), respectively located at the base of the spine, the *navel, and the crown of the *head. In the fifth chapter, the important point is made that success in *Yoga depends on the teacher's grace (*prasāda*). It empowers the practitioner to renounce all the paranormal powers (*siddhi*) that he or she has obtained and to proceed to the "nonemergent" (*nirutthāna*) state where the *body unites with the "supreme estate" (*param-pada*), or *Shiva.

There is another work by this name, which consists of one hundred stanzas and is attributed to a certain Parameshvara Yogin.

Siddha-Siddhānta-Samgraha ("Compendium of the Doctrines of the Adepts"), ascribed to Balabhadra, is a work of 306 stanzas purporting to be a summary of the *Siddha-Siddhānta-Paddhati* of Nityanātha.

siddhi ("accomplishment") is used in the yogic scriptures in a number of ways. In the most general sense, it means "attainment" or "success." More specifically, the term is equivalent to *samsiddhi*, signifying "*perfection," that is, *liberation. This is also occasionally referred to as the "great accomplishment" (*mahā-siddhi*). The *Shiva-Samhitā (III.18) speaks of six specific preconditions for success in Yoga: (1) *vishvāsa, or confidence that the spiritual *path and one's efforts are fruitful; (2) *shraddhā, or faith; (3) *guru-pūjana, or *worship of the *teacher; (4) *samatā-bhāva, or the sense of *equanimity, the condition of psychic balance; (5) *indriya-nigraha, or control of the *senses; and (6) *pramita-āhāra*, or moderate *diet.

A third, important connotation of the term *siddhi* is "paranormal attainment" or "magical ability." As we read in the *Yoga-Bīja (54): "The *yogin is possessed of unthinkable powers. He who has conquered the *senses can, by his own will, assume various shapes and make them vanish again." Since ancient times, yogins have been not only been venerated as saintly folk but also feared as thaumaturgists, whose powers were many and whose curses were potent. The word siddhi stems from the same root as the word for "adept" (*siddha). An *adept is someone who is master of his own *body and *mind as well as master of the forces of *Nature.

The *yogin's powers are considered a by-product of the spiritual process, especially of enstatic "constraint" (*samyama). The *Yoga-Shikhā-Upanishad (I.151ff.) speaks of two fundamental types of paranormal powers, namely those that are artificial (kalpita) and those that are nonartificial (akalpita). The former are produced by herbs (*aushadhi), ritual (kriyā), magic (jāla), *mantra practice, and alchemical elixirs (*rasa). In an aphorism that is probably an interpolation, the *Yoga-Sūtra (IV.1) similarly explains that the powers can spring from five possible causes, namely birth (janman), herbs (aushadhi), *mantra recitation, asceticism (*tapas), and enstasy (*samādhi). They are transient and have little efficacy. The second kind of siddhis, however, spring from self-reliance (svatantrya) and are permanent, greatly efficacious, and pleasing to the Lord (*īshvara). They manifest naturally in those who are free from desire (*vāsanā). They are the mark of a true adept (*siddha). These powers are encountered in the course of one's spiritual practice, just as a pilgrim on the way to the sacred city of Kāshī (modern Benares) passes by a number of sacred spots (*tīrtha). This *Upanishad (I.160) observes that the person lacking these powers is bound.

The literatures of *Hinduism, *Buddhism, and *Jainism are filled with references to, and examples of, paranormal abilities. Best known is the set of eight "great powers" (mahā-siddhi), which are thought to accompany *liberation. According to the *Yoga-Bhāshya (III.45) these are: *animan ("miniaturization"), *mahiman ("magnification"), *laghiman ("levitation"), *prāpti ("extension"), *prākāmya ("[irresistible] will"), *vāshitva ("mastery"), *īshitritva ("lordship [over the universe]"), and *kāma-avasāyitva ("fulfillment of [all] desires"). Some scriptures provide a slightly different list of mahā-siddhis. The *Purānas often group them according to the five material elements (*bhūta) that serve as props for *concentration and enstatic "constraint" (*samyama). Thus, the *Linga-Purāna (I.9.30ff.) furnishes a detailed catalogue of paranormal powers. These range from the ability to make oneself bulky or lean, prophesize or see the future to the power of producing *fire from the body, to the magical ability of assuming any form at will, or even of dissolving the entire *cosmos.

So long as one has a fickle *mind, advises the *Yoga-Shikhā-Upanishad (V.54), one should not dwell on the attainment of paranormal powers. The *Yoga-Tattva-Upanishad (75) regards them as one of the obstacles (*vighna) on the spiritual *path. The *Varāha-Upanishad (III.29) notes that they are not important to the aspirant who seeks to realize the *Self. The "seers of the Self" (ātma-darshin), announces the *Laghu-Yoga-Vāsishtha (VI.14.4), do not long for them. The *Linga-Purāna (I.9.14) states that the initial obstacles (*antaraya) disappear through devoted spiritual practice, but then new obstacles (*upasarga) arise, namely the magical powers. According to the *Yoga-Sūtra (III.37), certain paranormal powers—called *pratibhā—are to be looked upon as obstacles in attaining enstasy (*samādhi). However, *Patanjali was obviously favorably inclined to the use of the siddhis in order to gain a higher understanding of oneself and the cosmos, or else he would not have dedicated the entire third chapter of his work to what he calls the *vibhūtis, or "manifestations (of power)." The *Tattva-Vaishāradī (III.55) declares that the siddhis are not necessary for attaining liberation (*kaivalya) but neither are they completely useless, because they can strengthen the practitioner's faith (*shraddhā).

Many texts, as for instance the *Yoga-Tattva-Upanishad (76f.), state that these powers should not be demonstrated but be kept secret. The reason for this is that any public display would interfere with the *yogin's life of quietude and, if he is not fully *enlightened, possibly ensnare him in *pride, causing all kinds of *karmic entanglements. Indian folklore and mythology know of numerous stories in which ascetics or yogins have come to fall through their misuse of magical powers. Rarely do they end as happily as the story of Tibet's favorite adept Milarepa, who, in his youth, used his magical abilities with devastating results, which is why his discipleship under Marpa was particularly difficult. *Secrecy is, therefore, enjoined more for the protection of the practitioner than for the innocent bystander. The widespread and consistent claims for the existence of paranormal powers in *Yoga deserve careful study through the empirical means available to *Parapsychology. Given the extraordinary understanding and also control of the workings of the nervous system and the *mind demonstrated by *yogins, we should not be surprised if at least some of the paranormal phenomena claimed in the spiritual literature of Yoga and indeed of other traditions are based in reality. Yet, how much of the traditional claims are pious fiction and how much solid fact remains to be discovered. See also cihna, pratibhā, pravritti.

Siddhi is mentioned in the *Hatha-Yoga-Pradīpikā* (I.6) as an *adept of *hatha-yoga. No biographical information about him is available.

Sight. See *darshana, drishti*.

Sign. See *cihna*, Omens.

Silence. See *mauna*.

simha-āsana ("lion posture") is described in the *Gheranda-Samhitā* (II.14f.) as follows: One should place the crossed and upturned heels under the scrotum, with one's knees on the ground and hands placed on the knees. Keeping the mouth open and applying the throat "lock" (*jālandhara-bandha*), one should gaze steadily at the tip of the nose (*nāsa-agra*).

Sin. See *pāpa*; cf. *punya*.

sīt-karī ("making the [sound] *sīt*") is one of the basic forms of breath control (*prānāyāma*). It is taught in the *Hatha-Yoga-Pradīpikā* (II.54) as follows: One should make a

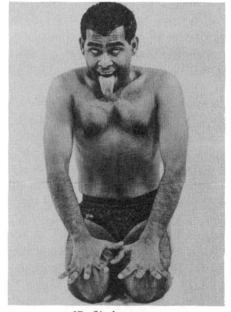

67. Simha-āsana.

hissing sound (i.e., *sīt*) during inhalation through the mouth, whereas the exhalation should be done quietly through the nose. See also *shīt-krama*.

Sleep. See *nidrā, sushupti, svapna*.

smarana ("recollection"), or remembrance of the *Divine, is one of the aspects of *bhakti-yoga. It is the loving regard for one's "chosen deity" (*ishta-devatā*).

smaya ("pride") may, according to the *Yoga-Sūtra (III.51), arise as a result of the flattering attention paid to the *adept by higher beings. It must be overcome in order to prevent renewed entanglement with worldly existence. See also Pride.

smriti is derived from *smri* ("to remember"). In the sense of "mindfulness," *smriti* is mentioned in the *Yoga-Sūtra (I.20) as one of the factors that precede the supraconscious enstasy (*asamprajnāta-samādhi). In his commentary on this aphorism, *Vācaspati Mishra equates the word with *dhyāna ("meditation"). A less specialized meaning of *smriti* in *Classical Yoga is that of "memory." As such, it figures as one of the five types of mental fluctuation (*vritti). In some of *Patanjali's aphorisms the term is used in the sense of "depth memory," that is, the deep structure of consciousness (*citta), which is composed of the "subliminal activators" (*samskāra) responsible for the *karmic continuity in one's life and also between the present existence and future *embodiments.

A further connotation of *smriti* is "remembered (knowledge)," or authoritative traditional literature as opposed to revealed literature (*shruti). See also *āgama*.

Snake charming can be understood as a symbolic representation of *kundalinī arousal, whereby the snake is looked upon as a device (*yantra) for focusing *attention.

snāna ("bathing, ablution") is sometimes, as in the *Hatha-Ratna-Āvali (III.3), considered to be a component of self-discipline (*niyama). The ritual of bathing is described in detail in the *Brihad-Yogi-Yājnavalkya (VII.1ff.). The *Garuda-Purāna* (L.8) distinguishes six types of ablutions: (1) *brāhma-* ("brahmic"), by means of sprinkling water on oneself; (2) *āgneya-* ("fiery"), by means of smearing ashes on the body; (3) *vāyavya-* ("airy"), by means of use of cow dung; (4) *divya-* ("divine, resplendant"), by means of bathing in sunshine; (5) *vāruna-* ("watery"), by means of bathing in water; and (6) *yaugika-snāna* ("yogic bathing"), by means of *meditation on the *Divine.

The *Shiva-Samhitā (V.4) considers bathing as one of the obstacles (*vighna) but mentions (V.134) "mental bathing" (*mānasa-snāna*) at the sacred junction of the "inner rivers"—Ganges, Yamunā, and Sarasvatī—which represent the three principal channels (*nādī) through which the life force circulates and which come together at the *ājnā-cakra. This mental bathing is to be resorted to particularly at the time of *death.

sneha ("attachment") is a synonym for **rāga*.

soma ("extract") is the draft of *immortality, used as a libation in the daily sacrificial ritual of *Vedic times. Some scholars have identified it as an extract from the fly agaric mushroom. During the era of *Tantrism, a new conception of the *soma* juice emerged according to which it is an inner secretion produced by the *body as a result of spiritual practice. It is also known as **amrita* and *sudhā*. The **Hatha-Yoga-Pradīpikā* (III.44) claims that he who drinks the inner *soma* continually by means of the practice of **khecarī-mudrā* conquers *death in fifteen days.

Sorrow. See *duhkha, shoka*.

Sound. See *nāda, shabda*.

Space. See *ākāsha*.

spanda ("quiver," "vibration") is a prominent technical concept in Kashmiri (or northern) *Shaivism. It is the "throb" of utter *bliss of the ultimate *Reality. It is not movement as ordinarily understood but the transcendental cause of all motion. This philosophical notion is elaborated at length in *Vasugupta's ninth-century *Spanda-Kārikā*, which is also often ascribed to his disciple Kallata.

sparsha ("touch") is one of the cognitive senses (**jnāna-indriya*) related to the *water element. In the **Mahābhārata* epic (XII.232.21), the term denotes a superperception in the tactile field, which is a by-product of *meditation.

sparsha-yoga ("Yoga of contact"). In the **Shiva-Purāna* (VII.2.37.9), this phase refers to **mantra-yoga* coupled with *breath control. Cf. *asparsha-yoga*.

sphota ("bursting forth") is an esoteric linguistic notion according to which the concept underlying a configuration of *sounds is eternal. This idea was taught by the grammarian *Patanjali and has traditionally been ascribed to the author of the **Yoga-Sūtra* on the strength of aphorism III.17. However, a closer examination of this **sūtra* does not lend support to such an interpretation. All discussion about the *sphota* is actually confined to *Vācaspati Mishra's commentary entitled **Tattva-*

Vaishāradī (III.17). The word *sphota* is not even mentioned in the *Yoga-Bhāshya*.

sphurana ("throbbing") is the pulsing of the life force (*prāna*) as experienced by the *yogin*. Sometimes this term is used synonymously with *spanda*.

Spine. See *meru-danda*.

Spirit. See *ātman, purusha*, Self.

Spontaneity. See *sahaja*.

Stability. See *sthairya*.

stambha ("stoppage") refers in the *Yoga-Sūtra* (III.21) to the suspension of the *breath. This word also denotes the paranormal ability (*siddhi*) to paralyze another being, as mentioned in the *Kaula-Jnāna-Nirnaya* (IV.14). See also *kumbhaka*.

Steadfastness. See *dhairya, dhriti*.

Steadiness. See *sthairya*.

sthairya ("stability") is sometimes counted among the practices of moral observance (*yama*), and it is the third member of the "sevenfold discipline" (*sapta-sādhana*) of *hatha-yoga*. According to the *Gheranda-Samhitā* (I.10), it is also called *sthiratā* ("firmness"). The *Bhagavad-Gītā* (XIII.7) treats it as a manifestation of wisdom (*jnāna*), while the *Yoga-Sūtra* (III.31) sees it as the fruit of "constraint" (*samyama*) upon the "tortoise channel" (*kūrma-nādī*).

sthāla. See *shat-sthāla*.

sthala-vasti is a synonym for *shushka-vasti*.

sthāna ("place," "abode") is sometimes employed for *desha* ("location"). Thus, the *Gheranda-Samhitā* (V.3–7) observes that one should not take up the practice of *Yoga in a far-off country, a forest, a metropolis, or in the midst of a crowd, since this would only frustrate one's endeavors. In a distant country, one loses faith (*shraddhā*); in the forest, one has no protection; and in the "wilderness" of the public, one is exposed.

The term *sthāna* can also refer to "places" in the *body that serve as props for *concentration and *meditation. Thus, the *Goraksha-Paddhati* (II.75f.) mentions nine such loci. Other scriptures mention five bodily regions governed by the five elements (*bhūta*). According to the *Tri-Shikhi-Brāhmana-Upanishad* (II.135f.), the area from the soles to the knees is the "earth place" (*prithivī-sthāna*); from the knees to the hips, the "water place" (*ap-sthāna*); from the hips to the center of the *body, the "fire place" (*agni-sthāna*); from the *naval to the *nose, the "air place" (*vāyu-sthāna*); and from the nose to the "brahmic cave" (*brahma-bila*), that is, the crown of the *head, the "ether place" (*vyoma-sthāna*). See also *marman*.

sthita-prajnā ("he who is steadied in wisdom") is, according to the *Bhagavad-Gītā* (II.54), the sage who is content abiding in the *Self alone, who has repelled all desire (*kāma*), and who is neither dismayed by sorrowful events nor elated by joyous experiences. Such an *adept is constantly immersed in the "vision of sameness" (*sama-darshana*). He is also known as a *sthita-dhī* ("he who is steadied in visionary thought").

sthiti ("state," "condition"). In some contexts, the word *sthiti* stands for the mental disposition (*shīla*) of inertia, as a manifestation of *tamas*. The *Tattva-Vaishāradī* (I.2) states that this term covers undesirable states like heaviness, concealment, and dejection.

sthūla ("gross," "coarse") denotes the outermost, or visible material, aspect of a thing. Thus, the "coarse body" (*sthūla-deha*) is the mortal physical frame, the "sheath composed of food" (*anna-maya-kosha*). The opposite is *sūkshma*. See also Cosmos.

sthūla-dhyāna ("coarse meditation") is *meditation on the "coarse" aspect of a thing, such as the iconographic form of one's "chosen deity" (*ishta-devatā*). Cf. *jyotir-dhyāna*, *sūkshma-dhyāna*.

strī. See Woman.

Study. See *svādhyāya*.

styāna ("languor") is recognized in *Classical Yoga as one of the obstacles (*antarāya) on the spiritual *path. The *Yoga-Bhāshya (I.30) defines it as "inactivity of the mind" (akarmanyatā cittasya). It is a
manifestation of *tamas. See also ālasya, tandrā.

Subconscious. See samskāra, vāsanā.

sudhā ("beverage") is a synonym for *amrita and *soma.

Suffering. see duhkha.

sukha ("joy," "pleasure," "ease"). In combination with the word
*duhkha, the word sukha stands for "pleasure." Pleasure, as the *Yoga-
Bhāshya (IV.11) notes, gives rise to attachment (*rāga). The *Bhagavad-
Gītā (XVIII.36ff.) distinguishes three kinds of pleasure, depending on
the prevalence of one or the other *guna: (1) Sāttvika-sukha is that which
seems like *pain at first but then turns out to be nectar and generates
serenity (*prasāda). (2) Rājasa-sukha is that which seems like nectar at
first but then turns into poison; it springs from the contact of the
senses (*indriya) with the sense objects (*vishaya). (3) Tāmasa-sukha is
that which arises from *sleep, *sloth, and *inattention and simply leads
one astray. According to the ascetical tradition of India, all forms of
sukha—like all forms of duhkha—must be overcome. In *Tantrism, pleasure need not be anxiously shunned, because it conceals or contains
the ultimate *bliss. Rather, the spiritual practitioner is advised to find
the "great joy" (*mahā-sukha) in all ordinary moments of pleasure. See
also ānanda, kāma, rati

sukha-āsana ("pleasant posture"). According to the *Shiva-Samhitā
(III.97), this posture (*āsana), which is also often rendered as the "easy
posture," is synonymous with the *svāstika-āsana. The *Tri-Shikhi-
Brāhmana-Upanishad (II.52) describes it as that posture through which
*steadiness can be gained. It is said to be suitable for those who cannot
perform the other *āsanas. Generally, the sukha-āsana corresponds to
the tailor seat.

sūkshma ("subtle") denotes the inner or psychic dimension of existence, which is not visible to the physical eyes but which can be
experienced in *meditation. The subtle dimension extends all the way
to the transcendental foundation (*pradhāna) of *Nature. Cf. sthūla.

sūkshma-dhyāna ("subtle meditation") is equated in the *Gheranda-Samhitā* (VI.9f.) with the *shāmbhavī-mudrā*, which is the experience of the union of *Shiva and *Shakti. Cf. *jyotir-dhyāna, sthūla-dhyāna*.

sūkshma-sharīra ("subtle body") is the entire psychomental complex that, according to *Yoga metaphysics, can exist independent of the physical or coarse *body. This is the bodily "field" that remains after *death and that serves as the precondition for a furture *embodiment. The existence of such a body is rejected by *Vācaspati Mishra in his *Tattva-Vaishāradī* (IV.10), on the grounds that there is no proper scriptural support for it and also because it is not necessary to postulate a subtle body in order to explain the process of rebirth (*punar-janman*). See also *ātivāhika-deha, deha, sharīra*.

Sulabhā is a *yoginī mentioned in the *Mahābhārata (XII.308.3ff.), who entered the *consciousness of King Videha in order to ascertain whether he was truly *enlightened.

Sun. See *sūrya*.

Surānanda is mentioned in the *Hatha-Yoga-Pradīpikā* (I.6) as a master of *hatha-yoga*. Nothing else in known about him.

sūrya ("sun") refers to an esoteric phenomenon or subtle anatomical structure that is thought to be situated in the region of the *navel. The scriptures of *hatha-yoga* describe it as devouring the "nectar of immortality" (*amrita*) that drips from the "moon" (*candra*) located in the *head. It turns the ambrosia that is naturally produced by the *body into poison, which then flows through the *pingalā-nādī*. Various techniques are proposed for stopping this solar generator and for enhancing and exploiting the lunar flow. See also Anatomy.

sūrya-bheda or -bhedana ("sun piercing") is one of the eight types of breath control (*prānāyāma*), which is described in the *Gheranda-Samhitā* (V.58f.) as follows: One should energetically inhale through the "solar channel" (i.e., the right nostril), carefully retain the *breath while performing *jālandhara-bandha* (the throat "lock") until one perspires heavily. In another passage (V.66f), the following technique is recommended: One should raise from the navel (*nābhi*) the various forms of the life force (*prāna*) that are cut off from the solar channel, and then slowly exhale through the *idā-nādī* (i.e., the left nostril). This should be done repeated for the awakening of the "serpent power" (*kundalinī-shakti*). See also *kumbhaka*.

sūrya-grahana ("solar eclipse") occurs, according to the *Darshana-Upanishad* (IV.47), when the life force (*prāna*) reaches, via the right channel (or *pingalā-nādī*), the place of the "serpent power" (*kundalinī-shakti*), namely the *mūlādhāra-cakra*. Cf. *candra-grahana*.

sūrya-namaskara ("obeisance to the sun") is a series of twelve dynamic postures (*āsana*) described in contemporary manuals of *hatha-yoga*. This series is so called becuase it should be practiced in the morning while facing the benign rays of the sun.

Sundarar (Sanskrit: Sundara) is one of the great Tamil saints of *Shaivism, who came to be known as the "insolent devotee" because of his familiar (and to some offensive) behavior toward the *Divine. He lived in the first half of the eighth century A.D., and we know of his life and teachings primarily from his own passionate poetry. See also Crazy adept.

sushumnā-nādi ("most gracious channel") is the central conduit through which the life force (*prāna*) flows from the psychoenergetic center (*cakra*) at the base of the spine to the crown of the *head. Already mentioned in the *Maitrāyanīya-Upanishad* (VI.21), this is the most important of all the *nādīs* of the *body. The *Yoga-Vishaya* (11) declares that it is of the form of delight (*sukha*). The reason for this is that the *sushumnā-nādī*, in the words of the *Hatha-Yoga-Pradīpikā* (IV.17), "devours *time, which is created by the sun and the moon." That is to say, it is the secret pathway through which the *yogin transcends the polar dynamic between the left and the right psychoenergetic currents—the *idā-nādī* and the *pingalā-nādī*—and wins the immortal condition of *Self-realization. Hence it is called the "way to liberation" (*moksha-mārga*) in the *Yoga-Yājnavalkya* (IV.30). The *sushumnā-nādī* originates, like all *nādīs*, in the "bulb" (*kanda*), but it alone proceeds to the "brahmic fissure" (*brahma-randhra*) at the crown of the head. It runs along the spine, which is variously called *meru and *vīnā-danda* ("fiddlestick"). According to the *Shat-Cakra-Nirūpana* (2), this axial channel is composed of several layers—the *vajrā-nādī* within which is the *citrinī-nādī* within which is the *brahma-nādī*.

The *sushumnā* must be purified of all defilements (*mala*) so that the "serpent power" (*kundalinī-shakti*) can ascend in it. This process is sometimes referred to as *sushumnā-yoga* or *mahā-yoga* ("great Yoga").

Staff posture. See *danda-āsana*.

sushupti ("sleep"). See *nidrā, svapna*.

sūtra ("thread") is literally the thread worn by male members of the upper three social estates of *Hinduism. It is also a terse aphorism serving as a device for memorizing the sacred teachings. According to Kumārila Bhatta's *Shloka-Vārttika* (I.1.22f.), there are six kinds of such aphorisms, depending on their purpose: definition (*samjnā*), interpretation (*paribhāshā*), general rule (*vidhi*), restrictive rule (*niyama*), original statement (*adhikāra*), and analogy (*atidesha*). This style of writing is employed in the source books of the six systems (*darshana*) of Hindu philosophy, such as the *Yoga-Sūtra* of *Patanjali. In *Buddhism, the term *sūtra* (Pali: *sutta*) refers to the memorable and memorized utterances of the *Buddha and other *adepts.

Sūtra-Artha-Bodhinī ("Illumination of the Content of the [Yoga] aphorisms") of *Nārāyana Tīrtha is an original commentary on the *Yoga-Sūtra*, consisting of about twenty-four folios. The same author also wrote the longer *Yoga-Siddhānta-Candrikā*.

sva-dharma ("own norm") is the moral law or order (*dharma*) as it applies to oneself. This concept plays an all-important role in the teachings of the *Bhagavad-Gītā* (XVIII.47), which has this memorable saying:

> Better is [one's] own norm imperfectly [carried out] than another's norm well performed. By performing the action prescribed by [one's] own being (*sva-bhāva*), one does not accumulate guilt (*kilbisha*).

> One should not relinquish "congenital" (*sahaja*) action, defective though it be, o son of Kuntī [*Arjuna], because all undertakings are veiled by fault (*dosha*), as fire by smoke.

Here the God-man *Krishna instructs his disciple *Arjuna that a warrior (*kshatriya*) should defend the moral order by military force, if necessary. It would be inappropriate for a warrior to live the life of a merchant or a brahmin, and vice versa. One must be true to one's innate (*sahaja*) obligations. According to the ethics of *Hinduism, these largely derive from one's place in society, which is determined by one's *karma. *Sva-dharma* has a double aspect. It is both the moral "categorical imperative" of one's essential being (*sva-bhāva*), and also the formalization of this inherent moral standard in terms of the caste laws. It is through the fulfillment of his or her *sva-dharma* that a person can actualize himself or herself. See also *karma-yoga*.

svādhishthāna-cakra ("own-base center," from *sva* and *adhishthāna*) is, in ascending order, the second psychoenergetic center of the *body. It is depicted as a crimson six-petaled lotus situated at the genitals. Its "seed syllable" (*bīja-mantra*) is *vam*, pertaining to the water (*ap*) element. The center's presiding deities are *Vishnu and the Goddess Rākinī. The center is associated with the sense of taste (*rasa*), the hands, and fertility symbolized by the image of an aquatic monster resembling a crocodile. This center contains an "inward-facing" phallus (*linga*) shining like coral. Through *con-templation of this center, the *yogin* becomes attractive to the world, especially to the other sex. See also *linga-cakra*.

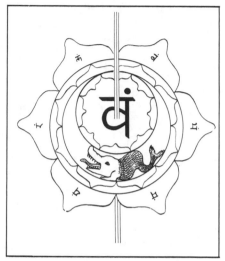

68. *Svādhishthāna-cakra, the psycho-energetic center located near the genitals.*

svādhyāya ("study") means literally "one's own (*sva*) going into (*adhyāya*)." In the *Yoga-Sūtra* (II.1), *svādhyāya* is mentioned as one of the constituent practices of *kriyā-yoga* and (in II.32) as one of the components of self-discipline (*niyama*). The *Yoga-Bhāshya* (II.1) explains it as the recitation (*japa*) of the sacred syllable *om* and other similar *mantras* and as the *study of the sacred love on *liberation (*moksha-shāstra*). This dual meaning has a historical explanation: In *Vedic times, study meant the memorization of the sacred tradition through repeated *recitation. Study was recognized early on as a viable means of self-understanding and *self-transcendence. This is borne out in the *Shata-Patha* ("Hundred Paths")-*Brāhmana* (XI.5.7.1):

> The study and the interpretation [of the sacred lore] are [a source] of *joy. [The serious student] becomes yoked-minded and independent of others, and day by day he gains [spiritual] power. He sleeps peacefully and is his own best physician. He controls the *senses and delights

in the One. [His] insight (*prajñā) and [inner] glory (yashas) grow, [and he acquires the ability] to promote the world (loka-pakti) [literally, "world cooking"].

Svādhyāya is more than mere intellectual learning. It approaches the quality of *meditation. It complements the practice of spiritual exercises, as is clear from the following passage from the *Vishnu-Purāna* (VI.6.2f.): "From study one should proceed to *Yoga and from Yoga to study. Through perfection in study and Yoga, the supreme *Self becomes manifest. Study is one eye with which to behold that [Self], and Yoga is the other." See also *grantha*, *shāstra*.

svāmin ("owner" or "lord") is a common title of respect for a spiritual personage, and is often written "Swami" in English. The *svāmin* is understood to be a master of himself rather than over other people, though he is popularly thought to possess all kinds of paranormal powers (*siddhi) as well. In *Classical Yoga, the word also stands for the *Self, whereas *sva* signifies *Nature.

svapna ("dream") has been recognized since ancient times as a distinct state of *consciousness. Often the word means "sleep" in general and as such is a synonym for *nidrā or *sushupti. But in numerous contexts it stands for "dream" in particular. The *Varāha-Upanishad (II.61) explains this condition as being the result of the mind's (*buddhi), traveling in the "subtle channels" (sūkshma-nādī). That is to say, the dream state is based on the focusing of *attention on the inner environment of the *body. The *Hamsa-Upanishad (8) states that dream results when the psyche (*jīva) enters the pericardium of the *heart, while deep sleep (sushupti) comes about when it is focused on the "phallus" (*linga) in the heart.

In the *Mahābhārata epic (XII.232.4), svapna is regarded as one of the "defects" (*dosha). But according to the *Yoga-Sūtra (I.38), dream sleep can yield useful insights that may be suitable for *meditation. Also, the *yogin's dreams may contain important omens (*arishta).

svara ("sound") is sound in general but specifically the sound made by the *breath. The *Amrita-Bindu-Upanishad (7) contrasts the svara with the asvara, the "soundless" *Absolute. This is a key concept of *mantra-yoga. See also *shabda*.

Svara-Cintāmani ("Thought Gem on the Sound [of the Breath]") is a late work of twenty-four short chapters dealing with divination through the flow of the breath. It is more detailed than the *Shiva-Svarodaya*.

svara-saushthava ("pleasantness of voice") is, according to the *Shvetāshvatara-Upanishad* (II.12), one of the signs (*cihna*) of initial progress (*pravritti*) in *Yoga. This is also referred to as "softness of the voice" (*svara-somyatā*).

svarga ("heaven"), or *svarga-loka* ("heavenly realm"), is the domain of the *deities and, as the *Bhagavad-Gītā* (IX.20f.) reminds us, of virtuous folk who worship the *Divine by means of sacrifices (*yajna*) but who will nonetheless be reborn as soon as their merit (*punya*) is exhausted. *Heaven thus offers no permanent security from the pain of change. It is not equivalent to *liberation.

svarodaya-vijnāna ("knowledge of the rising of the sound [of the breath]") is the art of diagnosing and predicting a person's *health and future well-being and destiny by means of the *breath. This is thought to be possible simply because the breath is intimately connected with the *mind, and the mind is equally closely associated with the *body.

Svarodaya-Vivarana of Bhāva Shāstrin of Baroda (Gujarat) is a late work of 125 verses on the subtle channels (*nādī*) of the life force (*prāna*).

sva-rūpa ("own form") is, in *Classical Yoga, the essential nature of a thing, such as solidity is the characteristic property of the *earth element. The *Yoga-Bhāshya* (III.47) defines it as the conglomerate of the generic (*samānya*) and the particular (*vishesha*). An example of the generic would be audibility; of the particular, sound.

svāstika. The word *svāstika*, which has entered the European languages as a symbol of destruction, is composed of *su* ("well") and *asti* ("it is") and means "fortunate" or "auspicious" in Sanskrit. An ancient symbol of the sun, it came to be associated in *Yoga with the

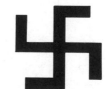

69. *Svastika, symbol of good fortune.*

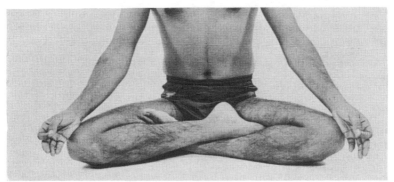

70. Svastika-āsana.

psychoenergetic center at the *navel, which is the place of the microcosmic "sun" (*sūrya).

svāstika-āsana ("fortunate posture"), which is mentioned already in
the *Yoga-Bhāshya (II.46), is described in the *Gheranda-Samhitā (II.13)
thus: One should place one's feet between knee and thigh (of either
leg) while sitting straight (*riju-kāya). The Shiva-Samhitā (III.96) notes
that this posture wards off disease and brings paranormal control over
the wind (*vāyu), presumably externally and internally (as the *breath).
The svāstika-āsana is specifically recommended in the *Shiva-Purāna
(VII.2.16.55) for the samaya ritual during which the teacher (*guru)
enters the *body of the *disciple. This posture is also called *sukha-
āsana.

svātantrya ("self-reliance") is an important quality in a spiritual practitioner. As the *Yoga-Shikha-Upanishad (I.154) asserts, self-reliance is
essential in order to procure permanent perfection (*siddhi). At the
same time, however, a student must not be so self-willed that he or
she is incapable of *obedience to the teacher (*guru).

Svātmārāma Yogīndra is the author of the *Hatha-Yoga-Pradīpikā. Although he venerates *Matsyendra and *Goraksha as his *gurus, he did
not study with them personally. Little is known about his life, though
it is likely that he lived in the fourteenth century A.D.

svayambhū-linga ("self-existent phallus") is the phallic symbol associated with the *mūlādhāra-cakra. It faces downward and is encircled
by the "serpent power" (*kundalinī-shakti). See also linga.

sveda ("sweat"), or *prasveda*, is a phenomenon particularly associated with the initial stages of breath control (**prānāyāma*). The **Hatha-Yoga-Pradīpikā* (II.3) recommends that one should rub one's perspiration (*jala*) into the *body to give it "firmness" and "lightness." The **Tejo-Bindu-Upanishad* (I.41) sees sweating as one of nine obstacles (**vighna*).

Swami. See *svāmin*.

Sympathy. See *dayā*.

T

tādāgī-mudrā ("tank seal") is described in the *Gheranda-Samhitā* (III.61) thus: Assuming the back stretch (*pashcima-uttāna*) position, one should make the belly like a water tank. In the opinion of the traditional commentators, this exercise is to be done while lying on one's back with the stomach made hollow. However, according to some contemporary authorities, this practice is to be performed by bending forward in the sitting position and inhaling so as to expand the stomach. This "seal" (*mudrā*) is said to prevent aging and *death.

Tailor seat. See *sukha-āsana*.

Taittirīya-Upanishad, which counts among the earliest *Upanishads, belongs to the school of the ancient *Vedic teacher Tittiri, whose name means "partridge." This work contains many archaic notions, notably a primitive "ecological" interpretation of life. According to this teaching, which is associated with the name of the sage *Bhrigu, everything is "food" (*anna*) for everything else: life feeding upon life in order to perpetuate itself. As one passage (II.21) has it: "From food, verily, creatures are produced—whatsoever [creatures] dwell on earth. Moreover, by food, in truth, they live, and into it they finally pass."

  This potentially dreadful vision of life is balanced by another doctrine, according to which existence is essentially blissful (*ānanda*). The *Taittirīya-Upanishad* speaks of levels of bliss that can be experienced— from simple *pleasure to unexcellable *bliss. Spiritual life consists in discovering the culmination of bliss, which is inherent in the Absolute (*brahman*). This scripture also contains the first reference to the doc-

361

trine of the five "sheaths" (*kosha*), of which the fifth and final sheath is composed of pure bliss. Here (II.4.1), we also find the first recorded mention of the word *yoga* in the technical sense, as the control of the fickle senses (*indriya*).

Talkativeness. See *prajalpa*.

tālu ("palate") is an important locus of the life force (*prāna*). Its yogic significance was recognized already in the *Taittirīya-Upanishad* (I.6.1), which mentions the "nipple"—that is, the uvula—that hangs down from the palate and is "Indra's exit." Here the word *indra* stands for the individual psyche (*jīva*). Later works even speak of a *tālu-cakra*, as the place of the "royal tooth" (*rāja-danta*) or the "bell" (*ghantikā*). Thus, the *Saubhāga-Lakshmy-Upanishad* (III.6) states that from this psychoenergetic center (*cakra*) flows the "nectar of immortality" (*amrita*).

tālu-mūla ("root of the palate") is mentioned in the *Tri-Shikhi-Brāhmana-Upanishad* (II.132) as one of the eighteen sensitive zones (*marman*) of the *body. It also notes that this locus is associated with *consciousness in the state of deep sleep (*sushupti*).

tamas ("darkness"). In the *Yoga and *Sāmkhya traditions, this term refers to one of the three primary constituents (*guna*) of Nature (*prakriti*). It is the psychocosmic principle of inertia. As the *Bhagavad-Gītā* (XIV.8) declares, it springs from spiritual nescience (*ajnāna*) and deludes all beings, binding them by heedlessness (*pramāda*), sloth (*ālasya*), and sleep (*nidrā*). The *Tejo-Bindu-Upanishad* (I.41) counts it among the nine obstacles (*vighna*). The *Maitrāyanīya-Upanishad* (III.5) supplies a long list of characteristics of *tamas*, or *tamo-guna*. These include, among others, *fear, *confusion, *despondency, *grief, as well as *hunger and *thirst. Cf. *rajas, sattva*.

tandrā or **tandra** ("sloth") is listed in the *Yoga-Tattva-Upanishad* (12) as one of the "defects" (*dosha*). See also *ālasya, styāna*.

tanmātra ("that only"). It is possible that this word is a distortion of *tanu-mātra* ("fine matter"). According to the cosmology of the *Yoga and *Sāmkhya traditions, the term denotes the subtle (*sūkshma*) aspect of the material elements (*bhūta*). They are the *potentials* of sound (*shabda*), sight (*rūpa*, literally, "form"), touch (*sparsha*), taste (*rasa*), and smell (*gandha*). The *Sāmkhya-Kārikā* (38) describes them as being "nonspecific" (*avishesha*). In *Classical Yoga, these five potentials pertain, together with *asmitā-mātra, to the level of "unparticularized" (*avishesha) existence. They arise from the *linga-mātra and, in turn, give rise to the sixteen categories (*tattva) of "particularized" (*vishesha) existence, namely the mind (*manas), the ten senses (*indriya), and the five material elements (*bhūta).

tantra ("loom"), derived from the root *tan* ("to extend, expand"), is most generally used as a synonym for *shāstra ("textbook"). Specifically, however, the term refers to a work belonging to a genre of sacred writing in *Shaktism and *Shaivism but also in the tradition of *Buddhism. There are scores of *Hindu Tantras, which often take the form of a dialogue between God *Shiva and his divine spouse *Devī (or Parvatī, etc.). The two best-known *Hindu Tantras are the *Kula-Arnava-Tantra and the *Mahānirvāna-Tantra. Like the *Āgamas (of *Shaivism), the *Samhitās (of *Vaishnavism) and the *Purānas, the Tantras cover a wide range of subjects. They contain accounts of psychocosmology and the history of the world (divided into ages, or *yugas), descriptions of the *deities and their appropriate *rituals of worship, and of rites for the acquisition of a battery of *magical powers. There are also instructions about the esoteric process of activating the psychospiritual power called *kundalinī-shakti, which is crucial to the spiritual *path of *Tantrism.

tāntrika ("tantric") is an adjective that is also used as a noun referring to the practitioner of *Tantrism.

Tantrism is the religious philosophy and culture expounded in the scriptures known as *tantras. The origins of Tantrism are still obscure. Some scholars trace the beginnings of Tantrism back to ancient cults current in the *Vedic period, while others detect Tantric elements in the pre-Vedic *Indus civilization. Tantrism emerged as a distinct tradition within *Hinduism, *Buddhism, and *Jainism in the early post-Christian era. Tantrism purports to be a new teaching, or revelation (*shruti), that is particularly suited for the "dark age" (*kāli-yuga). Because of its long history and great diversity in the doctrinal and practical dimensions, it is very difficult to define or even generalize about Tantrism. What can usefully be said is that the pivot of most Tantric schools is the idea of *shakti, the feminine principle of cosmic existence, the *Goddess. The *tāntrika seeks to enlist the help of this principle in his quest for *liberation. This is expressed in ceremonies of external worship (*pūjā) of the feminine *Divine but also in inner or symbolic rituals, notably the whole orientation of *kundalinī-yoga.

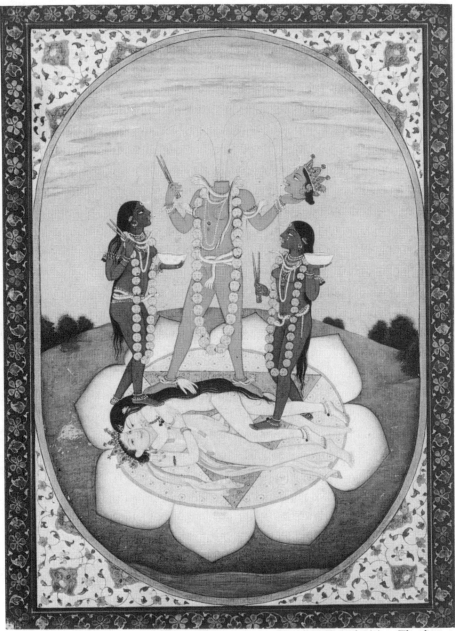

71. *Tantrism makes use of sexual symbolism to express ultimate polarities. The decap-itated Goddess Chinnamastā represents the spiritual law of self-sacrifice.*

This rediscovery of the feminine cosmic principle was accompanied by a reappraisal of the human *body and bodily existence in general, which have a largely negative significance in the non-Tantric traditions. In contrast to the ascetical, world-denying schools of *Hinduism, the Tantric *adepts affirmed the body as the temple of the Divine and as an immensely valuable instrument for reaching *liberation. But this reevaluation of the body and *shakti-focused rituals also opened the gates to *occultism and *magic, which surprisingly parallels the contemporary renaissance of Goddess worship and the arcane arts.

Generally, three great approaches are distinguished within Tantrism: (1) the *dakshina-mārga, or right-hand *path; (2) the *vāma-mārga, or left-hand path; and (3) the kula-mārga, or path of the prominent *Kaula sect. The first approach is the conservative mainline of Tantrism. The second approach, which has brought Tantrism into disrepute, involves the infamous *panca-tattva rite that makes use of traditionally forbidden elements, especially sexual intercourse (*maithunā). The third approach can roughly be equated with *kundalinī-yoga, the exploitation of the *body's inherent psychospiritual potential. See also vīra.

tapas ("heat" or "glow") signifies asceticism, which the *Yoga-Bhāshya (II.32) explains as the endurance of extremes (*dvandva). *Patanjali, the founder of *Classical Yoga, regards tapas as one of the three constituents of *kriyā-yoga, and he also counts it among the components of self-discipline (*niyama). He further states in his *Yoga-Sūtra (III.43) that tapas leads to perfection (*siddhi) of the *body and the *senses. This contradicts the characterization of tapas given in many scriptures, including the *Yoga-Yājnavalkya (II.3), which understand it as the "desiccation" (*shoshana), or emaciation, of the *body. Endorsing Patanjali's positive interpretation of asceticism, the *Tattva-Vaishāradī (II.1) notes that tapas should only be practiced so long as it does not imbalance the bodily humors (*dhātu).

Similarly, the *Bhagavad-Gītā (VII.5f.) speaks against exaggerated asceticism, which springs from ostentation (*dambha) and selfishness (*ahamkāra) and which ignores the fact that the Lord (*īshvara) resides within the body. According to this scripture (XVII.14ff.), tapas is threefold: (1) sharīra-tapas, or "bodily austerity," consisting of reverence (*pūjana) for the *deities, the "twice-born" (dvija), the *teachers and the sages, and comprising purity (*shauca), rectitude (*ārjava), chastity (*brahmacarya), and nonharming (*ahimsā); (2) van-maya-tapas, or "vocal austerity," consisting of speech that does not cause disquiet and that is truthful, kind, and pleasing, as well as study (*svādhyāya); (3) mānasa-

tapas, or "mental austerity," consisting of serenity (*prasāda*), friendliness (*saumyatva*), silence (*mauna*), self-restraint (*ātma-vinigraha*), and purity of feeling (*bhāva-samshuddhi*). These three kinds of *tapas* are *sāttvika.* However, when asceticism becomes tinged with ostentation or the desire to win honor or fame, it is *rājasa.* Finally, when *tapas* turns into self-torture or is performed in order to harm another being, it is *tāmasa.* The *Uddhāva-Gītā* (XIV.37), again, defines *tapas* as the abandoning of *desires (*kāma-tyāga*).

tapasvin is a practitioner of *tapas.*

tapo-yogin is a synonym for *tapasvin.*

tāraka ("deliverer") generally refers to the transcendental *Reality in its salvific aspect. In *Classical Yoga, however, the word designates not the *Absolute but the "wisdom born of discernment" (*viveka-ja-jnāna*), which appears at the culmination of the enstatic (*samādhi*) condition. The *Pāshupata-Brāhmana-Upanishad* (I.32) uses the term to denote the sacred syllable *om. In *tāraka-yoga,* again, it signifies the manifestation of the *Self in the form of *light.

tāraka-yoga ("Yoga of the delivering [sign]") is a *Vedānta-based Yoga taught in the *Advaya-Tāraka-Upanishad* and the *Mandala-Brāhmana-Upanishad,* which appears to have been widespread in medieval India. Central to this approach are photistic phenomena that occur during *meditation and that are considered to be a manifestation of the *Absolute as "deliverer" (*tāraka*). Three kinds of phenomena are distinguished: The *antar-lakshya* ("inner sign"), the *bahir-lakshya* ("external sign"), and the *madhya-lakshya* ("intermediate sign"). The three "signs" (*lakshya*) are known as "corporeal deliverers" (*mūrti-tāraka*), while the higher realization of the *Self is styled "incorporeal" (*amūrti*) and "transmental" (*amanaska*). The intermediate sign leads to the experience of the five types of luminous consciousness-space (*ākāsha*).

tarka ("reflection," "pondering") is defined in the *Amrita-Nāda-Upanishad* (16) as inference (*ūhana*) in keeping with tradition (*āgama*). In the context of the sixfold *path (*shad-anga-yoga*), however, this term has a different meaning, and may correspond to the experience of *savitarka-samāpatti* in *Classical Yoga. See also Reason.

tarpana ("satisfaction") is one of the "limbs" (*anga*) of *mantra-yoga.* See also *tushti.*

tat ("that") is a cryptic reference to the *Absolute, or *Self in such doctrinal sayings (*vākya*) as "That art thou" (*tat tvam asi*) or "I am the Absolute" (*aham brahma asmi*).

tattva ("thatness") can denote either *Reality or a category of cosmic existence. The relationship between these two connotations is well expressed in the *Shiva-Samhitā* (II.54), which states that "when all the *tattvas* have disappeared, then the *tattva* itself becomes manifest." Classical *Sāmkhya distinguishes twenty-four such categories, which are the principal levels or principles of Nature (*prakriti*): (1) *prakriti*, which is the transcendental ground of (insentient) existence; (2) *mahat* ("great one"), which is also known as *buddhi; (3) *ahamkāra* ("I-maker"), the principle of individuation, (4–14) the mind (*manas*) and the ten senses (*indriya*), (15–19) the five subtle elements (*tanmātra*), (20–24) the five material elements (*bhūta*). Separate and above these categories is the principle of pure *Consciousness, the *purusha. In some schools of *Shaivism, thirty-six categories are recognized; the *Brahma-Vidyā-Upanishad* (62) hints at fifty-one, while the *Varāha-Upanishad* (I.7ff.) mentions as many as ninety-six. See also Cosmos, *shad-vimsha*.

Tattva-Vaishāradī ("Autumnal Clarity on the Categories [of Existence]") is a major subcommentary on the *Yoga-Bhāshya. Authored by the renowned scholar *Vācaspati Mishra, this gloss is a work of considerable scholastic achievement, which contains many illuminating philological observations. However, it does not match the appeal and authority of *Shankara's *Vivarana*.

tattva-vid ("knower of Reality") is an *enlightened being who, in the words of the *Bhagavad-Gītā* (V.8f.), knows that the *Self transcends all *action and yet engages in activities. Sometimes the appellation refers to the knower of the categories of existence (*tattva*).

Teacher. See *ācārya, guru, upādhyāya*.

tejas ("brilliance") is often cited as one of the effects of intense asceticism (*tapas*), expressed in the shining face of the saint. In the sense of overzealousness, *tejas* is listed in the *Tejo-Bindu-Upanishad* (I.41) as one of the nine obstacles (*vighna*) on the spiritual *path.

Tejo-Bindu-Upanishad ("Brilliance-Point *Upanishad") is one of the *Yoga-Upanishads. It comprises 465 stanzas distributed over six chapters. This is probably a composite work, which is suggested by the clear break after the fourth chapter. The *tejo-bindu* or "radiance point" is said to be found in the *heart of the "All-Self (*vishva-ātman*) during *meditation. This scripture, which is firmly grounded in the nondualist metaphysics of *Vedānta, puts forward a fifteenfold *path (*panca-dasha-anga-yoga*). It mentions nine obstacles (*vighna*) that foil spiritual *progress. The fourth chapter contains a description of the nature of "living liberation" (*jīvan-mukti*) and "disembodied liberation" (*videha-mukti*).

tejo-dhyāna is a synonym for *jyotir-dhyāna*.

Time. See *kāla*.

Tintini is mentioned in the *Hatha-Yoga-Pradīpikā* (I.8) as an *adept of *hatha-yoga*. No biographical information about him is available.

tīrtha is a pilgrimage center. The *Darshana-Upanishad* (IV.48ff.) distinguishes between external (*bahis-*) and internal (*antas-*) pilgrimage centers. The latter, which are deemed superior to the former, are also referred to as *bhāva-tīrthas*, the word *bhāva* meaning "mental condition." These inner *tīrthas* are different auspicious loci for focusing *attention, corresponding to the major psychoenergetic centers (*cakra*) of the *body.

tīrtha-atana ("pilgrimage to a sacred site") is mentioned in the *Uddhāva-Gītā* (XIV.34) as one of the twelve practices of self-restraint (*niyama*). This custom is also called *tīrtha-yātrā*.

Tirumūlar (Tamil), though not widely venerated, is one of the great saints of southern *Shaivism. He is the author of a remarkable work, the *Tiru-Mantiram*, which Kamil V. Zvelebil (1973) has praised as "the greatest treatment of *Yoga in Tamil literature." This work, which forms the tenth book of the *Shaiva canon, consists of over three thousand verses on ethical, philosophical, and religious matters, including the yogic *path. Tirumūlar was a proponent of the devotional (*bhakti*) approach.

titikshā ("forbearance") is defined in the *Uddhāva-Gītā* (XIV.36) as the "patient endurance of suffering" (*duhkha-sammarsha*). See also *kshamā*, *kshānti*.

Tongue lock. See *jihvā-bandha*.

Tradition. See *āgama, smriti;* cf. *shruti.*

Tranquility. See *prasāda, samatva, shānti.*

Transformation, cosmic. See Evolution, *parināma, vikāra.*

Transmission, spiritual. See *shakti-pāta.*

trātaka (untranslatable) is one of the "six acts" (*shat-karma) described in the *Gheranda-Samhitā (I.53f.) thus: One should gaze steadily, without blinking, at a small object until tears begin to flow. This technique is said to cure all eye afflictions and to lead to clairvoyance (*divya-drishti) and the *shāmbhavī-mudrā. See also *dhrishti.*

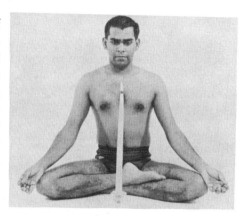

Tree posture. See *vriksha-āsana.*

72. *Trātaka: steady gazing as an aid to concentration.*

tri-granthi ("triple knot"). See *granthi.*

trikona-āsana ("triangle posture") is a posture described in contemporary manuals of *hatha-yoga as follows: Standing upright with legs apart and arms outstretched, one should exhale and bend at the hip to one side. This should be repeated, bending to the other side.

tri-kūta ("triple peak") is an esoteric designation for the spot between the eyebrows where the three principal channels (*nādī) of the life force (*prāna) meet, namely the **sushumnā-*, the **idā-*, and the **pingalā-nādī.*

tri-lakshya ("triple sign"). See *lakshya.*

Tri-Shikhi-Brāhmana-Upanishad ("Triple Tuft Brāhmana-Upanishad") is one of the *Yoga-Upanishads, which gets its title from the recipient of the *Upanishadic wisdom who is a *brāhmana wearing three tufts of hair. This text comprises 165 stanzas in two sections, which are an exposition of the nondualist metaphysics of *Advaita-Vedānta. Its anonymous composer subscribes to an eightfold *path (**ashta-anga-*

yoga) whose goal is union with the *Divine, which is identified with God *Shiva and also with God *Vishnu. The work begins with cosmological speculations, followed by an exposition of the four modes or states (*avasthā*) of consciousness, which are related to the four "sheaths" (*kosha*). Two kinds of Yoga—*jñāna-yoga* and *karma-yoga*— are distinguished. The eightfold path described essentially corresponds to that of *Patanjali. This scripture also lists and describes seventeen postures (*āsana*) and provides details on esoteric *anatomy. Although the "serpent power" (*kundalinī-shakti*) is mentioned, it does not seem to play an important role in the prescribed approach. However, much attention is given to breath control (*prāṇāyāma*) and the purification of the channels (*nāḍī-shodhana*). Enstasy (*samādhi*) is defined, in typical *Vedāntic fashion, as the merging of the psyche (*jīva*) with the *Absolute.

trishā or **trishnā** ("thirst") is often cited as one of the "defects" (*dosha*). Apart from its conventional meaning, the term is also employed metaphorically—as the "thirst" for life. Already the *Mahābhārata* epic (XII.210.34), belonging to the pre-Christian era, presents the "thirst" for conditional experience as the source of unenlightened or *karmic existence and all its attendant suffering (*duhkha*): "As a weaver inserts thread into a cloth by means of a needle, similarly the 'thread of conditioned existence' (*samsāra-sūtra*) is secured to the needle of 'thirst.' "

As another stanza (XII.173.25) of the great epic has it, this thirst cannot be quenched by a sip of water. It can only be eliminated through wisdom (*jñāna*). See also *abhinivesha*; cf. *kshudhā*.

tri-veni ("triple braid") is a synonym for *tri-kūta*.

Truth. See *rita*, *satya*.

turīya ("fourth"). See *caturtha*.

turīya-atīta ("that which transcends the fourth"). According to the *Laghu-Yoga-Vāsishtha* (III.9.124), this term signifies the condition of "living liberation" (*jīvan-mukti*), which is said to go beyond the seven levels of wisdom (*jñāna-bhūmi*).

turya is a synonym for *turīya*.

tushti ("contentment") is sometimes listed as one of the practices of self-discipline (*niyama). See also prīti, samtosha, tarpana.

tyāga ("abandonment") is the third "limb" (*anga) of the fifteenfold *Yoga (*panca-dasha-anga-yoga) taught in the *Tejo-Bindu-Upanishad. In this work (I.19), tyāga is defined as the *abandonment of the "phenomenal world" (prapanca-rūpa) as a result of one's intuition (avalokana) of the *Self. A contrasting explanation is given in the *Bhagavad-Gītā (XVIII.2), which understands tyāga as the relinquishment of the "fruit" (*phala) of one's *actions. This interpretation seeks to combat the popular understanding of tyāga as the total abstention from activities, which, according to the Gītā, is completely impossible. The *Laghu-Yoga-Vāsishtha (V.2.28f.) makes an important distinction between dhyeya-tyāga and jneya-tyāga. The former is characteristic of the liberated being (*jīvan-mukta) who continues to perform actions in the spirit of *play. The latter coincides with the dropping of the *body when all "subliminal traits" (*vāsanā) have been obliterated. See also samnyāsa.

tyāgin ("abandoner") is a practitioner of *tyāga.

U

udāna ("up-breath") is one of the cardinal currents of the life force (*prāna*) in the *body. According to the *Tri-Shikhi-Brāhmana-Upanishad (82), it circulates in all the limbs and joints and is responsible for digestion. But in the much older *Maitrāyanīya-Upanishad (II.6), its functions are stated to be belching and swallowing. The *udāna* is also said to carry the psyche up to the *head in the state of enstasy (*samādhi*) and at *death. Several *hatha-yoga* texts locate it in the throat, while the *Siddha-Siddhānta-Paddhati (I.68) places it in the palate (*tālu*). The *Yoga-Yājnavalkya (IV.55) mentions that the up-breath is responsible for raising the body. According to the *Linga-Purāna (I.8.64) and other *Purānas, the *udāna* stimulates the sensitive zones (*marman*). Mastery of the up-breath (*udāna-jaya*), states the *Yoga-Sūtra (III.39), leads to the paranormal power (*siddhi*) of "nonadhesion" (*asanga*) and levitation (*utkrānti*).

uddāna-kumbhaka ("upward pot") is breath retention (*kumbhaka*) performed after exhalation in conjunction with *uddīyāna-bandha. It is prescribed in the *Gheranda-Samhitā (III.22) as a phase of the "great piercer" (*mahā-vedha*).

Uddhāva-Gītā ("Uddhāva's Song") is an imitation of the *Bhagavad-Gītā, which forms chapters 6–29 of the eleventh book of the *Bhāgavata-Purāna. It is a *Vedāntic tract on Yoga and devotion (*bhakti*), presented as a didactic dialogue between the God-man *Krishna and the sage Uddhāva.

uddīyāna-bandha ("upward lock"), also called *uddāna*, is an important technique of *hatha-yoga*. This "lock" (*bandha*) is described in the *Gheranda-Samitā* (III.10f.) as follows: One should contract the abdomen above and below the navel and toward the back. By this means the "great bird," the life force (*prāna*), is constantly forced to "fly upward" (*uddīna*), that is, ascend along the central channel or *sushumnā-nādī*. The *Gheranda-Samhitā* praises this practice above all the other "locks," calling it "a lion to the elephant of *death*." According to the *Yoga-Shikhā-Upanishad* (I.106ff.), one should perform the upward lock prior to exhalation, and the *Yoga-Kundaly-Upanishad* (I.48f.) specifies that it should be

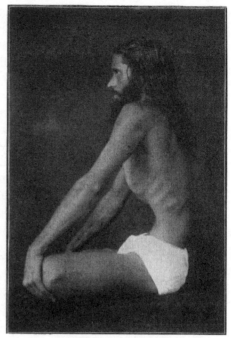

73. *Uddīyāna-bandha.*

done seated in the "adamantine posture" (*vajra-āsana*) and while firmly pressing the "bulb" (*kanda*) near the ankles. The *Varāha-Upanishad* (V.8f.) warns that this practice should not be attempted when one is hungry or is suffering from a weak bladder or bowels.

udgītha ("chant") is a synonym for *pranava*.

urga-āsana ("mighty posture") is described in the *Shiva-Samhitā* (III.92ff.) thus: Stretching out both legs, one should firmly grasp one's head with the hands and push it down into the knees. This posture (*āsana*), the text states, fans the bodily fire and is also called *pashcima-uttāna*.

ujjayī ("victorious") is one of the eight types of breath control (*prānāyāma*) taught in *hatha-yoga*. It is described in the *Gheranda-Samhitā* (V.69ff) as follows: With one's mouth closed, one should inhale through both nostrils, while also drawing up the breath from the *heart* (i.e., the chest) and the throat. One should vigorously retain the breath in the mouth and simultaneously perform the throat "lock" (*jālandhara-bandha*). Drawing the breath from the chest causes a snoring sound, which is characteristic of this technique. According to the *Yoga-Shikhā-Upanishad* (I.94), one should retain the breath in the abdomen and then expel through the left nostril. The texts mention a great number of curative benefits from this exercise, most of them relating to the respiratory system, but this exercise is also said to stimulate the digestive fire (*jāthara-agni*).

Unconsciousness. *Classical Yoga and *Sāmkhya subscribe to the view that Nature (*prakriti*) is inherently unconscious (*acit*) and that *consciousness or awareness (*cit*) pertains only to the transcendental Self (*purusha*). Thus, the entire body-mind complex is thought to be insentient, and the phenomena of consciousness (*citta*) are the product of material Nature reflecting the "light" of the transcendental Self. The *Vedāntic schools of Yoga entertain a similar point of view, according to which all phenomena are (illusory) modifications of the same superconscious *Reality.

The notion of modern psychoanalysis that the psyche includes areas that are not known, or kown only indirectly, to the conscious mind is also not foreign to Yoga. This idea is expressed in the teaching of the "subliminal activators" (*samskāra*), "subliminal traits" (*vāsanā*), and "subliminal deposits" (*āshaya*), which are crucial to understanding the doctrine of *karma and reincarnation (*punar-janman*). However, Yoga approaches these matters from an angle that is strikingly different from that of psychoanalysis. Psychoanalysis employs the concept of the unconscious in order to understand the irrational operations of the conscious mind and to integrate them in a rational manner and thus lead from psychopathology to mental health. By contrast, Yoga has no particular interest in the unconscious aspects of our psyche, except insofar as these interfere with the spiritual process, that is, prevent the stable acquisition of *meditation and *enstasy, and obstruct *liberation. Nor does Yoga seek to rationalize the irrational contents of the human mind but to transcend the entire mechanism by which unconscious Nature—in the form of the body-mind—obscures the fact of our intrinsic *freedom and *bliss.

unmanī ("exaltation"), or **unmany-avasthā** ("exalted state") is also often called *mana-unmanī* or "mental exaltation." The *Gheranda-Samhitā* (VII.17) equates this condition with *sahaja (-samādhi), the state of perfect spontaneity. The *Hatha-Yoga-Pradīpikā* (II.42), however, seems to equate this state with *nirvikalpa-samādhi, because for the duration of this condition the *body becomes rigid like a log of wood and the *yogin cannot hear even the sound of a large drum. It also defines the *unmanī* condition as the steadiness of the *mind, which is effected when the life force (*prāna*) flows through the central channel (*sushumnā-nādī*). In this context, it precedes the supreme enstatic realization called *amanaskatā*.

upādhi ("superimposition") is a *Vedāntic concept that is employed in some of the works on *hatha-yoga*. It denotes a limiting attribution upon the singular *Reality, such as the life force (*prāna*), the mind (*manas*), the senses (*indriya*), the body (*deha*), or the sense objects (*artha*). Upon realization of *nirvikalpa-samādhi*, all these distinctions vanish, and the *Self shines forth in its authentic singularity. The *Goraksha-Paddhati* (II.81f.) notes that the *upādhis* cover up Reality and that they can be removed through constant spiritual practice.

upādhyāya ("instructor") imparts exoteric and esoteric knowledge but, as a rule, does not initiate the disciple (*shishya*) into the mysteries of practical spirituality. This is the function of the *guru*.

Upanishad Brahmayogin, also known as Rāmacandra Indrayogin, was the pupil of Vasudeva Indrayogin and lived in the eighteenth century A.D. He gained fame for his commentaries on 108 Upanishads. His observations on the *Yoga-Upanishads contain many helpful explanations.

Upanishads. The word *upanishad* is composed of the verbal root *sat* ("to sit") prefixed with *upa* and *ni* and means "to sit down close to (one's teacher)." This is a reference to the mode in which esoteric knowledge is transmitted by word of mouth from teacher (*guru*) to disciple (*shishya*). The term designates a particular genre of *Hindu literature. Traditionally, 108 such works are spoken of, though well over 200 Upanishads are extant. The earliest of them were composed in the era prior to *Buddhism, dating as far back perhaps as the ninth century B.C. The youngest Upanishads were composed as recently as our century. They are looked upon as sacred revelation (*shruti*) and are regarded as belonging to the "wisdom part" (*jnāna-kānda*) as opposed to the "ritual part" (*karma-kānda*) of the *Vedic heritage. However, they represent a striking departure from the spirit of the ancient *Vedas, with their pronounced exoteric ritualism. The Upanishads wanted from the beginning to be understood as secret teachings (*rahasya*), and their metaphysical thinking revolves around four closely related themes: (1) the teaching that the transcendental core—the *ātman*—of one's being is declared identical with the transcendental core—the *brahman—of the universe itself; (2) the doctrine of repeated embodiment (*punar-janman) of human beings, or, as the earliest Upanishads put it, their repeated death (punar-mrityu); (3) the doctrine of *karma and retribution, which seeks to explain the metaphysical effects of a person's actions; (4) the notion that the production of karma and future reincarnation can be prevented through spiritual practices, notably *renunciation and *meditation. In later periods, the practical way to *liberation became identical with the approach of Yoga, as is evidenced in the *Yoga-Upanishads. See also Samnyāsa-Upanishads; see also under individual Upanishads.

upasarga ("obstacle"). So long as one has not attained *enlightenment, or *liberation, one can always fall prey to a number of difficulties arising from the *ego. The yogic scriptures have detailed some of these problems, which are obstacles on the spiritual path. The *Maitrāyanīya-Upanishad (VII.8) mentions constant joking, traveling, begging, living by trickery, and wearing earrings or skulls out of spiritual hypocrisy as "obstacles to knowledge" (jnāna-upasarga). The *Mārkandeya-Purāna (XL.1ff.) also furnishes a long list of obstacles, ranging from desire-bound deeds to magic (māyā), to knowledge, to paranormal abilities. In order to overcome these obstructions, this *Purāna (XL.14) recommends that one should focus one's *attention on the *Absolute, wearing a "white mental blanket." The *Shiva-Purāna (VII.2.38.10) speaks of six obstacles: (1) *pratibhā ("flash of illumination"); (2) *shravana (auditory phenomenon); (3) *vārtā (superscent); (4) *darshana (visionary state); (5) *āsvāda (supertaste); (6) *vedanā (supersensation). The *Yoga-Sūtra (III.37) applies the term upasarga specifically to "flashes of illumination" (*pratibhā) in the five senses, which are obstacles to the enstatic (*samādhi) state. See also dosha, vighna.

upashama ("calmness") is sometimes regarded as one of the practices of moral observance (*yama).

upastha-nigraha ("genital control") is occasionally listed among the components of self-discipline (*niyama). It stands for one's mastery of the sexual drive. See also brahmacarya, ūrdhva-retas.

upavāsa ("fasting"), which is sometimes counted as one of the practices of self-discipline (*niyama), is also often considered to be a possible obstacle (*vighna) to spiritual progress. The *Gheranda-Samhitā (V.31) specifically mentions that fasting should be avoided in conjunction with the practice of breath control (*prānāyāma). Already the *Mahā-

bhārata (XII.214.4) deems prolonged fasting harmful and instead recommends abstention from eating between breakfast and the evening meal. The *Varāha-Upanishad* (II.39) explains that true fasting is the proximity between the individual self (*jīva-ātman*) and the transcendental Self (*parama-ātman*), and not the emaciation (*shoshana*) of the *body.

upāya ("means") is a technical term in northern (Kashmiri) *Shaivism. Thus, the *Shiva-Sūtra* distinguishes between three means of approach: (1) *shāmbhava-upāya* ("Shambhu's means") is alert passivity toward the *Divine; this is also known as "supportless Yoga" (*nirālamba-yoga*); (2) *shākta-upāya* ("means pertaining to *Shakti") involves the agency of the mind (*citta*), inquiring into its authentic nature (the true "I"); (3) *āṇava-upāya* ("individual means") is any of the many practices of Yoga, such as *breath control and *meditation.

ūrdhva-retas refers to the psychophysiological process by which the semen (*retas*) flows upward (*ūrdhva*), and to the *yogin in whom this process is alive. First mentioned in the *Maitrāyanīya-Upanishad* (II.3) as a practice of the *vālakhilyas* (a certain type of seer or *rishi), *ūrdhva-retas* has since ancient times been the esoteric reason for celibacy (*brahmacarya*). It is the process underlying sublimation, by which the semen is transmuted into vitality (*ojas*) that feeds the higher centers of the *body, notably the brain.

ushtra-āsana ("camel posture") is described in the *Gheranda-Samhitā* (II.41) as follows: Lying down, one should bend one's legs back and hold them with one's hands while energetically contracting the abdominal muscles and the mouth. A "camel seat" (*ushtra-nishadana*) is mentioned already in the *Yoga-Bhāshya* (II.46).

utkata-āsana ("raised posture") is described in the *Gheranda-Samhitā* (II.27) thus: Standing on one's toes with heels off the ground, one should place one's buttocks on the heels. This position is to be assumed particularly when doing the water enema (*jala-vasti*).

utsāha ("zest," "zeal") is, according to the *Hatha-Yoga-Pradīpikā* (I.16), one of six factors that promote Yoga. A positive, energetic attitude toward spiritual practice is an essential prerequisite on the path. Otherwise the *yogin cannot break his habit patterns and lay down new "tracks" that are conducive to wholeness and *liberation. See also *vīrya*.

uttāna-kūrma(ka)-āsana ("extended tortoise posture") is described in the *Gheranda-Samhitā* (II.33) as follows: One should assume the "cock posture" (*kukkuta-āsana*) and then hold the neck with one's hands, assuming the pose of a tortoise with its limbs extended. It is generally thought that this complicated posture is done while lying on one's back. This appears to be similar to the "womb posture" (*garbha-āsana*) mentioned in modern works, where one balances on one's but-

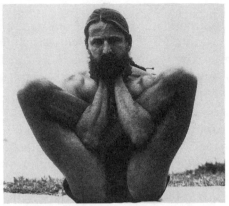

74. *Uttāna-kūrmaka-āsana.*

tocks. Some contemporary manuals of *hatha-yoga* contain a different description: Sitting on one's heels, one should arch backward until the head touches the ground. One's hands are kept on the thighs. Cf. *kūrma-āsana.*

uttāna-manduka-āsana ("extended frog posture") is described in the *Gheranda-Samhitā* (II.24) thus: Seated in the frog posture (*manduka-āsana*), one should hold one's head with the elbows and then stretch the body like a frog. Some contemporary manuals of *hatha-yoga* describe this differently: Sitting on one's heels, one should arch backward until the head touches the ground. One's arms are folded around the head in such a way that the forearms serve as a cushion.

utthāna ("levitation") is a phenomenon witnessed during the most advanced stage of breath control (*prānāyāma*). See also *lāghava.*

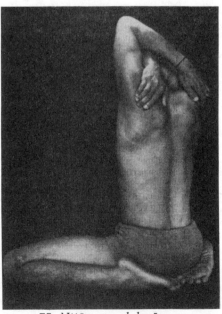

75. *Uttāna-manduka-āsana.*

utthāna-roma ("erect hair"). The *Laghu-Yoga-Vāsishtha* (V.6.158) mentions the bristling hair of the sage Uddālaka as a phenomenon accompanying his enstatic (*samādhi*) state.

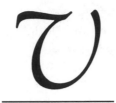

vāc ("speech") sometimes stands for *sound in general. According to the *Yoga-Kundaly-Upanishad (III.18ff.), there are four levels of sound—from the inaudible transcendental to the vocalized sound—which must be dissolved in reverse order until the supreme *Reality beyond all sound is realized. See also *shabda, vāk-siddhi*.

Vācaspati Mishra was a *Shiva-worshipping brahmin of Mithila who lived in the middle of the ninth century A.D. He was a distinguished scholar who commented on all major philosophical systems of *Hinduism, with the exception of the *Vaisheshika school, which he treated in conjunction with the *Nyāya system. His expositions are marked by their great learning and exemplary lucidity. Among his many works is a subcommentary on the *Yoga-Sūtra, entitled *Tattva-Vaishāradī.

vahni ("fire") is a synonym for *agni*.

vahni-sāra-dhauti ("cleansing by way of fire"), also known as *agni-sāra-dhauti*, is one of the techniques of "inner cleansing" (*antar-dhauti) employed in *hatha-yoga. It is described in the *Gheranda-Samhitā (I.20f.) thus: One should push the *navel back against the spine a hundred times. This is said to cure all *diseases of the stomach, to fan the fire in the belly (*jāthara-agni), and to yield a "divine body" (*divya-deha). This text also enjoins great *secrecy about this practice.

vahni-yoga ("fire Yoga"). See *agni-yoga*.

Vaikhānasa-Smārta-Sutra ("Aphoristic Lawbook for Forest Dwellers") is, as the title suggests, a work belonging to the *smriti* category that deals specificially with the duties of forest eremites, called *vaikhānasas*. It was composed some time in the fourth century A.D. and contains important references to *Yoga as practiced by certain ascetics (*tapasvin*). Thus, chapter VIII speaks of hermits who live with or without wives and mendicants (*bhikshu*) who dedicate their lives to the quest for *liberation. Greatest among the last-mentioned ascetics are the "supreme swans" (*parama-hamsa*). The same chapter also mentions three categories of yogic practitioners: (1) the *sāranga-* or "variegated" *yogins*, who comprise four kinds: those who do not practice *breath control but live with the conviction "I am *Vishnu"; those who practice *breath control and the other techniques of Yoga; those who follow an eightfold Yoga (*ashta-anga-yoga*) but begin with *breath control; and those who appear to practice an atheistic type of Yoga; (2) the *ekā-rishya-yogins*, who have a single *rishi* ("seer"), the meaning of which is not clear in this context; five types are distinguished on the basis of their spiritual accomplishment; and (3) the *visarga-yogins*, who adopt various questionable means of self-mortification, sometimes even rejecting the practice of *meditation, and who can attain "liberation only in a future life.

vairāgya ("dispassion"), also known as *virāga*, is sometimes counted as one of the components of self-discipline (*niyama*). It signifies the mood and practice of *renunciation, or the abandonment of passion (*rāga*). The *Yoga-Sūtra (I.15) defines it as the "awareness of mastery of him who is without thirst for seen (i.e., earthly) and revealed (i.e., heavenly) things." *Patanjali also speaks of a higher form of dispassion, consisting in one's nonthirsting for the primary constituents (*guna*) of *Nature, resulting from the "vision of the Self" (*purusha-khyāti*).

Vairāgya is one of the two fundamental aspects of spiritual life, the other being practical application (*abhyāsa*) of the various techniques, especially *meditation. Unless practice is accompanied by an attitude of dispassion, one runs the risk of inflating rather than transcending the *ego. Dispassion without practice, on the other hand, is like a blunt knife: The psychosomatic energies released through dispassion are not channeled appropriately and thus may lead to confusion and possibly *delusion instead of *liberation. Hence already the *Bhagavad-Gītā (VI.35) enjoins their simultaneous cultivation. The *Uddhāva-Gītā (IV.11) expresses the same conviction in the compound *vairāgya-abhyāsa-yoga*. See also Abandonment, Renunciation, *vīta-rāga*.

vaishāradya. See *nirvicāra-vaishāradya*.

Vaisheshika ("distinctionism") is one of the six philosophical systems (**darshana*) of *Hinduism. This school of thought, which was founded by Kanāda in the sixth century B.C., is concerned with the differences (*vishesha*) between things. The Vaisheshika system offers an approach to *liberation through rational understanding of the categories of existence. However, *Yoga is mentioned in the *Vaisheshika-Sūtra* (V.2.16), which is ascribed to the legendary Kanāda but was probably composed between 200 B.C. and A.D. 100. Here, Yoga is defined as "that which effects the cessation of suffering (**duhkha*)."

vaishnava ("pertaining to *Vishnu") is an adjective that is also employed as a noun to denote a follower of *Vaishnavism.

vaishnavī-mudrā ("seal pertaining to *Vishnu") is explained in the *Shāndilya-Upanishad* (I.7.14ff.) as one's external gaze (*bahir-drishti*) at an inner sign (**antar-lakshya*), while being unable to either shut or open the eyelids. The *Nāda-Bindu-Upanishad* (31) stipulates that this technique should be practiced for the manifestation of the inner sound (**nāda*). See also *shāmbhavī-mudrā*.

Vaishnavism is the religious culture centering on the *worship of God *Vishnu. Together with *Shaivism, this is one of the two great theistic traditions of *Hinduism. Originating in *Vedic times, the worship of Vishnu gained in popularity about the time of the *Buddha. The early phase of Vaishnavism is known as *Pāncarātra or the *Bhāgavata religion. The *Bhāgavad-Gītā*, a part of the *Mahābhārata* epic, is the oldest available scripture of this tradition. The *Gītā*, which styles itself a "textbook of Yoga" (*yoga-shāstra*), gives us an excellent glimpse into the yogic orientation of early Vaishnavism. Fragments of the Pāncarātra teachings have also been preserved in other sections of the epic. The early post-Christian era saw the rise of a vast *Vaishnava literature known as the *Samhitās ("Collections") of which over two hundred individual works are known to have existed. Only a few of these texts have been studied, one of them being the *Ahirbudhnya-Samhitā* (XII.31ff.), which mentions a *Yoga-Samhitā* by *Hiranyagarbha. Concurrently with the creation of this literature, South India celebrated its own Vaishnava poet-saints, the *Ālvārs. Vaishnavism blossomed around the turn of the first millennium A.D., receiving its greatest impetus through the teaching and missionary activities of *Rāmānuja and his numerous disciples. This is also the period in which the highly influential *Bhāgavata-Purāna* was composed. The Yoga characteristic of Vaishnavism, which is strongly theistic, is *bhakti-yoga*. This is tempered, however, by *karma-yoga*. See also Krishna.

vaishvānara ("pertaining to all men") is the "fire" situated in the center of the human *body, which is responsible for digestion. This is also known as the *jāthara-agni*.

vaitrishnya ("nonthirsting") is a synonym for *vitrishna*.

vajra ("thunderbolt" or "diamond") is a secret name for the penis (*linga*, *medhra*).

vajra-āsana ("adamantine posture") is described in the *Gheranda-Samhitā* (II.12) as follows: One should tighten the thighs like a thunderbolt and place one's legs under the anus. This is said to yield powers (*siddhi*). This practice is also called "adept's posture" (*siddha-āsana*) in some works. The *Yoga-Sūtra* (III.46) speaks of adamantine robustness (*vajra-samhananatva*) as one of the aspects of bodily perfection (*kāya-sampad*).

vajra-deha ("adamantine body") is the transubstantiated *body of an *adept of *hatha-yoga, which is as indestructible as a diamond. The *Mahābhārata* (XII.322.9) mentions a race of beings whose bones are like diamond (*vajra-asthi-kāya*), who were seen by the sage *Nārada when he ascended the sacred Mount *Meru. They are said to have a steady gaze, to live without eating, and to emit a beautiful scent. See also *divya-deha*, *dridha-deha*.

vajrā-nādī ("adamantine channel") is a conduit inside the central channel (*sushumnā-nādī*) of the *body. According to the *Shat-Cakra-Nirūpana* (1), it extends from the penis to the *head. See also *brahma-nādī*.

vajrolī-mudrā (*"vajrolī* seal"), also spelled **vajronī-mudrā,** is an important "seal" (*mudrā*) of *hatha-yoga. The *Gheranda-Samhitā* (III.45ff.) describes this technique as follows: One should place one's palms on the ground and raise one's legs without letting the head touch the ground. According to this manual, the *vajrolī-mudrā* is praised as the best of *Yoga practices, which awakens the "serpent power" (*kundalinī-shakti*), causes longevity, and leads to all kinds of powers (*siddhi*), notably control over the semen (*bindu-siddhi*). The *Hatha-

Yoga-Pradīpikā (III.85ff.) understands this practice differently: It is the sexual technique of sucking up the female ejaculate (*rajas) with the penis (*mehana*). In order to develop this ability, the *yogin is advised to blow into a tube which he has inserted into his penis. In his commentary on the *Yoga-Tattva-Upanishad* (126), *Upanishad Brahmayogin describes the following technique: Dipping the penis into cow's milk poured into a bronze vessel, the *yogin sucks up the liquid with his penile shaft "resembling a thunderbolt" and then releases it again. When he has acquired sufficient control, he should ejaculate his semen (*retas) into the vagina and then draw it up again together with the woman's ejaculate (*shonita). Reflecting the antinomian spirit of *Tantrism, the *Hatha-Yoga-Pradīpikā* (III.84) further observes that he who knows this technique may live as he pleases without detriment, and even disregard the practices of self-discipline (*niyama). Cf. *amarolī-mudrā, sahajolī-mudrā*.

vāk- or **vākya-siddhi** ("power of speech") is often mentioned as one of the paranormal abilities (*siddhi) acquired by the *yogin. See also *vāc*.

Vāmadeva is a *Shaiva *yogin whose teachings are recorded in the *Shiva-Purāna* (VI.18.7ff.). An *adept by the same name appears in the *Varāha-Upanishad* (IV.2.35) as a representative of "gradual liberation" (*krama-mukti).

vāma-krama ("left process") is one of the forms of *kapāla-bhāti. According to the *Gheranda-Samhitā* (I.56f.), it is practiced by repeated and unstrained inhalation through the left nostril and exhalation through the right nostril. This is stated to cure disorders of phlegm (*kapha).

vāma-mārga ("left path") is the left-hand approach in *Tantrism, which involves the literal enactment of the "five m's" (*panca-ma-kara). This is understood to be a dangerous orientation, which leads those who are impure to ruin. Cf. *dakshina-mārga*.

vamana-dhauti ("cleansing by vomiting") is one of the forms of "heart cleansing" (*hrid-dhauti). The *Gheranda-Samhitā* (I.39) explains this technique thus: After meals one should drink water filling up the stomach until it reaches the throat. Then one should direct one's *gaze upward for a short while and finally vomit the water out again. If practiced daily, this is said to cure disorders of phlegm (*kapha) and bile (*pitta). See also *gaja-karaṇī*.

vandana ("prostration") is one of the aspects of the *Yoga of devotion (*bhakti-yoga).

Varāha-Upanishad is one of the *Yoga-Upanishads. Presented as a dialogue between God *Vishnu and the sage *Ribhu, this work comprises five chapters with a total of 273 stanzas. It begins with a description of the categories (*tattva) of existence and then proceeds to elaborate the metaphysical principles of *Vedānta. The text (II.55) takes a critical stance toward what appears to be *Classical Yoga, which, it argues, is based on a misconception of the "Lord" (*īshvara). This *Upanishad (IV.2.39) is also critical of *hatha-yoga, though outlines that approach in the fifth chapter, which appears to be a later addition. Here *mantra-, *laya-, and *hatha-yoga are treated as stages of the eightfold path (*ashta-anga-yoga). It favors the practice called *samputa-yoga* ("Yoga of the bowl"), which is essentially *kundalinī-yoga. The designation *samputa* is not directly explained but can be understood as the intersection of the three principal pathways of the life force (*prana) in the *body—viz. *sushumnā-, *idā-, and *pingalā-nādī—and the *kuhū-nādī.

vāri-sāra-dhauti ("cleansing by means of water") is one of the techniques of "inner cleansing" (*antar-dhauti) employed in *hatha-yoga. The *Gheranda-Samhitā (I.17ff.) describes it as follows: One should fill the mouth completely with water and then swallow it slowly, move it into the stomach, and expel it through the rectum. This technique is said to be the foremost type of *dhauti, since it leads to a "divine body" (*divya-deha).

varna means both "coating" and "color." Its refers specifically to the four social estates of *Hinduism: the priestly estate (*brāhmana), the warrior estate (*kshatriya*), the merchant estate (*vaishya*), and the servile estate (*shūdra*).

In the sense of "color," *varna* refers to the frequency of *light that characterizes the psyche (*jīva). Thus, the *Mahābhārata epic (XII.271.33) mentions six colors: black, gray, blue, red, yellow, and white. These colors typify the *karma of a person, with black being the least favorable and white suggesting an advanced moral and spiritual level. "Clarity of color" (*varna-prasāda*) is mentioned in the *Shvetāshvatara-Upanishad (II.12) as one of the signs of progress (*pravritti) in *Yoga. Color also plays a role in the visionary experiences associated with *tāraka-yoga.

Finally, the word *varna* is also employed to denote "sound" and "letter" in *mantra-yoga.

vartamāna-karma ("present *karma*"). See *karma*.

varunā-nādī ("Varuna's channel"), also called **varunī-nādī,** is one of the principal "channels" (*nādī) through which the *life force (*prāna) circulates in the *body. Most texts locate it between the *yashasvinī- and the *kuhū-nādī. According to the *Yoga-Shikhā-Upanishad (II.26), it is situated below the *navel and is responsible for the function of urination.

vāsanā ("dwelling") stands for both "desire" and the subliminal trait left behind in the *mind by the exercise of desire. As the *Anna-Pūrna-Upanishad* (IV.78f.) declares: "So long as the *mind is not dissolved, so long the traits are not obliterated either. So long as the traits have not dwindled, so long the mind is not tranquil."

In *Classical Yoga, *vāsanā* is explained as a concatenation of "subliminal activators" (*samskāra). According to the *Yoga-Sūtra (IV.24), the mind (*citta) is speckled with countless *vāsanās*. They depend upon a person's stock of merit (*punya) and demerit (*apunya). The *Laghu-Yoga-Vāsishtha* (I.1.10) distinguishes between "pure" (*shuddha*) and "tainted" (*mālina*) *vāsanās*. The former are comparable to fried seed, which cannot sprout, the latter are the cause of reembodiment (*punar-janman). See also *āshaya, karma.

Vasishtha, or **Vashishtha,** is the name of several illustrious sages. In the *Vedic era, Vasishtha was a seer (*rishi*) who composed many of the hymns of the seventh book of the *Rig-Veda. In later times, a Vasishtha was a prominent sage in the *Rāmāyana and the *Mahābhārata epics, several *Purānas and *Upanishads, and not least in the *Yoga-Vāsishtha. According to legend, the *rishi Vasishtha's personal quarrel with sagely king Vishvāmitra escalated into a feud between their respective clans. However, the story of their abiding enmity is often taken as an expression of the clash of interest between the sacrificial ritualism of the priestly estate (*brāhmana) and the spiritual heritage of the warrior estate (*kshatriya).

vāshitva ("mastery") is one of the major paranormal powers (*siddhi) recognized in *Yoga. The *Mani-Prabhā (III.44), a commentary on the *Yoga-Sūtra, explains it as the "control over the elements" (bhūta-niyantritva).

vāso-dhauti ("cleansing [by means of a] cloth") is one of the forms of "heart cleansing" (*hrid-dhauti). The *Gheranda-Samhitā (I.40f.) describes it thus: One should slowly swallow a thick cloth four fingers wide and then draw it out again. This is said to cure abdominal diseases, fever, enlarged spleen, leprosy and skin diseases, as well as disorders of phlegm (*kapha) and bile (*pitta).

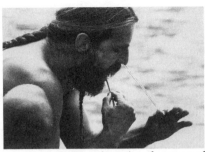

76. Vaso-dhauti: cleansing the stomach by means of a long piece of cloth.

The *Hatha-Yoga-Pradīpikā (II.24) calls this technique simply *dhauti. According to this scripture, the cloth is four digits broad and fifteen spans long.

vasti ("bladder") is one of the "six acts" (*shat-karma) of *hatha-yoga. According to the *Gheranda-Samhitā (I.45), it is of two types: *jala-vasti ("water enema") and *shushka-vasti ("dry enema"). The word is also sometimes rendered as "syringe," because the description given of this technique in the *Hatha-Yoga-Pradīpikā (II.26) involves the use of a tube inserted into the anus by which water is sucked up. The *Jyotsnā (II.26) mentions that the tube should be six fingers long and that two-thirds of it should be inserted.

vāta ("air, wind") is one of the five material elements (*bhūta) of the manifest *cosmos. Its symbol is the hexagon (shatkona), and it is associated with the color black, the "seed syllable" (*bīja-mantra) yam, and is thought of as ruling the area from the navel (*nābhi) to the middle of the eyebrows (*bhrū-madhya). The word vāta is also employed as a synonym for *prāna ("breath"). It also signifies one of the bodily humors (*dhātu) and has the qualities of dryness, coldness, and mobility. See also tattva, vāyu.

vāta-sāra-dhauti ("cleansing by means of air") is one of the four techniques of "inner cleansing" (*antar-dhauti) employed in *hatha-yoga. The *Gheranda-Samhitā (I.15f.) describes it thus: One should shape the mouth like the beak of a crow—in the manner of *kākī-mudrā—and slowly suck in the air, filling the belly with it and moving it around, and then slowly forcing it through the anus. This is stated to cure all *diseases and to increase the "abdominal fire" (*jāthara-agni).

vāyavī-dhāranā-mudrā ("aerial concentration seal") is one of the five *concentration techniques described in the *Gheranda-Samhitā (III.77ff.). This practice consists in focusing one's *attention and *life force, through *breath control, on the *wind element for 159 minutes. This is held to stimulate the life energy and to enable one to move through space (khe-gamana). See also dhāranā, mudrā, panca-dhāranā.

vāyu ("air," "wind") is a synonym for *vāta and *prāna. Expressing a universal yogic sentiment, the *Shāndilya-Upanishad (I.7.6) declares that the breath (vāyu) should be tamed as one tames a lion, an elephant, or a tiger—step by step lest it should kill one. Perfect mastery over the air element, known as vāyu-siddhi, culminates in the paranormal power of *levitation.

vāyu-sādhana ("discipline of the air") is a synonym for *prānāyāma, used in the *Shiva-Samhitā (III.68).

Veda ("Knowledge") refers to the oldest portion of the sacred canon of *Hinduism, the four hymnodies—*Rig-Veda, *Atharva-Veda, *Yajur-Veda, and *Sāma-Veda. The hymns (sūkta, *mantra) of these roughly three-thousand-year-old collections are traditionally said to have been "seen" by seers (*rishi), and are regarded as revelation (*shruti). See also Upanishads.

Vedānta ("Veda end") is a comprehensive term for the metaphysical speculations that originated with the *Upanishads, which are the eso-teric continuation of the *Vedic ritualism. Vedānta comprises a vast body of literature, both scholastic and popular. It is the dominant philosophy of *Hinduism, favoring a nondualist (advaita) interpretation of existence: There is only the one *Reality, which appears manifold to the unenlightened *mind but which reveals itself as singular (eka) and nondual (advaya). One of the six philosophical systems (*darshana) of Hinduism, Vedānta was systematized in the Brahma-Sūtra of Bad-ārāyana, who may have lived in the second century A.D. This concise treatment gave rise to a host of sometimes considerably divergent interpretations. The best known and most influential school is the Kevala-Advaita (absolute nondualism) of *Shankara (c. A.D. 788–820).

Its great historical rival is the *Vishishta-Advaita (qualified nondualism) of *Rāmānuja (A.D. 1017–1137). There is even a dualist school of Vedānta, the Dvaita of Mādhva (A.D. 1199–1270). *Yoga played a varyingly prominent role in these schools and was interpreted differently by their protagonists, though no systematic study of the yogic materials present in the Vedānta tradition has as yet been undertaken. See also Advaita-Vedānta, Ramakrishna, Vivekananda.

vedānta-shravana ("listening [to the teachings of] Vedānta") is, according to the *Tri-Shikhi-Brāhmana-Upanishad* (I.34), one of the ten practices of self-discipline (*niyama*). See also *shravana*.

Vedāntic is the anglicized adjective of *Vedānta.

vedāntin is a follower of the *Vedānta tradition.

Vedic is the anglicized adjective of the Sanskrit word *vaidika*, meaning "pertaining to the *Veda," that is, the ancient *Hindu canon. See also Veda.

Vedic Yoga is an analytical category referring to the proto-yogic elements in the *Vedas, especially the *Rig-Veda* and the *Atharva-Veda*, which were composed in the period 1500–1000 B.C.

Veneration. See *ācārya-upāsana*, *guru-bhakti*.

vibhūti ("manifestation"). In the *Bhagavad-Gītā* (X.16), the term is used to refer to the "far-flung powers" by which *Krishna pervades the universe. In *Classical Yoga, *vibhūti* is a synonym for "paranormal power" (*siddhi*). The word also signifies the ashes that the *Shaiva ascetics smear on their bodies to indicate their status as world renouncers (*samnyāsin*).

vicāra ("reflexion," "reflection") is one of the higher mental phenomena, or spontaneous thought processes, associated with a particular level of enstasy (*samādhi*), in which the object of *attention pertains to the "subtle" (*sūkshma*) dimension of *Nature. In *Vedānta and Vedānta-based schools of *Yoga, the word *vicāra* also stands for existential pondering. Thus, the *Laghu-Yoga-Vāsishtha* (II.1.69) explains it as consisting of asking searching questions such as "Who am I?" and "Whence this universe?" This kind of inquiry is said to be a panacea for the "chronic disease of worldliness" (*samsāra-roga*). See also *nirvicāra-samāpatti, savicāra-samāpatti*; cf. *vitarka*.

videha-mukti ("disembodied liberation") is generally understood to be *liberation that coincides with the shedding of the *body at *death. Those who enjoy this condition are traditionally thought to roam the invisible or "subtle" (*sūkshma*) dimensions of *Nature. However, Vidyāranya offers a different interpretation in his *Jīvan-Mukti-Viveka (II), arguing that the "disembodied" (*videha*) state refers to future embodiment only. Similarly, the *Tejo-Bindu-Upanishad (IV.33ff.) understands *videha-mukti* as the condition of perfect identity with the *Absolute to the point where all body consciousness has been lost. Cf. *jīvan-mukti*.

vidhi ("rule"). The *Shiva-Samhitā (V.4) lists the observance of rules and vows (*vrāta*) as a possible source of spiritual obstruction (*vighna*). This is meant to drive home the point that we benefit spiritually from what we do only if we are in right relationship to our *actions. So long as the *ego is involved, we are always in danger of mistaking the means (*upāya*) for the goal—that is, keeping a diet or practicing meditation (*dhyāna*) as if this was our ultimate concern.

vidyā ("knowledge," "wisdom") is the antithesis to *avidyā, or spiritual nescience. The ultimate condition of *Self-realization, or *enlightenment, is often characterized as one of gnosis, as opposed to the ignorance that marks the unillumined personality. As such, it is referred to as *bodha, prajñā*, and *vidyā*. However, this *wisdom transcends the dichotomy between subject (consciousness) and *object (world) that is an integral part of conventional *knowledge. It is not a content of consciousness (*citta*), but the very nature of pure Consciousness (*cit*).

In some contexts, the word *vidyā* stands for "technical knowledge," such as in the compound *khecarī-vidyā* or the technical knowledge regarding the "ether-walking seal" (*khecarī-mudrā*), an important technique of *hatha-yoga and *Tantrism.

Vidyāranya Tīrtha was a learned *Vedānta scholar who was probably born about A.D. 1314. He composed such fine works as the *Panca-Dashī* (or at least the first ten chapters of it) and the *Jīvan-Mukti-Viveka. He is often identified with Mādhava, the author of the *Sarva-Darshana-Samgraha* ("Compendium on All Systems"). He obviously had an intimate knowledge of Yoga, and appears to have followed the practical path of *ashta-anga-yoga.

vighna ("obstacle"). Spiritual life is uniformly characterized as being inherently difficult, because it is based not only on critical self-understanding but also on the radical transcendence of the self, or *ego. This involves the constant willingness to drop habit patterns and adaptations that are not in keeping with one's growing understanding of the nature of one's authentic identity as the *Self rather than the personality complex, or limited body-mind. Some of these emotional and mental patterns can prove very tenacious and then become veritable obstacles to change and maturation. The *Yoga scriptures mention many different obstacles, or obstructions. For instance, the *Yoga-Tattva-Upanishad (30f.) refers to the following obstacles that can occur at the outset of spiritual practice: (1) *ālasya ("sloth"); (2) katthāna ("boastfulness"); (3) dhūrta-goshthī ("fellowship with rogues"); (4) mantra-ādi-sādhana ("cultivation of *mantras and so forth"), that is, cultivation of such practices for the wrong reasons (e.g., to acquire magical *powers); (5) dhātu-strī-laulyaka ("longing for a physical woman" rather than the *Goddess). These, the text states, should be avoided through the accumulation of merit (*punya) and can be turned around through the practice of reciting the sacred *pranava (i.e., the syllable *om). Other works mention different remedies, but all imply that one should persist in one's spiritual efforts. In the *Yoga-Shāstra (101ff.) of *Dattatreya five obstacles are listed: *ālasya ("laziness"); prakatthāna ("gossiping"); mantra-sādhana ("cultivation of *mantras"); dhātu-vāda ("*alchemy"); khādya-vādaka ("dieting"). The last three are included because they are often employed for the wrong reasons, such as the acquisition of magical *powers.

The *Tejo-Bindu-Upanishad (I.40ff.) mentions the following nine obstacles: anusandhāna-rahitya ("lack of application"); *ālasya ("laziness"); bhoga-lālasa ("longing for enjoyment"); *laya ("inertia"); *tamas ("stupor"); *vikshepa ("distractedness"); *tejas ("overzealousness"); *sveda ("[excessive] sweating"); *shūnyatā ("voidness"), which probably stands for absent-mindedness. The *Yoga-Kundaly-Upanishad (I.56ff.) contains a similar catalogue of obstacles on the spiritual *path, which includes doubt (*samshaya) and sleep (*nidrā). A more extensive catalogue is furnished in the *Shiva-Samhitā (III.32f.), which includes undesirable types of *food, overeating (*atīva-bhojana), fasting (*upavāsa), misanthropy (jana-dvesha), cruelty toward animals (prāni-pīdana), female companionship (strī-sanga), and garrulousness (bahv-ālāpa). Elsewhere, this scripture (V.3ff.) notes that obstacles can arise not only from pleasure (*bhoga) but also from one's practice of virtue (*dharma) and from knowledge (*jnāna). Thus, it refers to ablutions (*snāna) and rules (*vidhi) as instances of the second group, and knowledge about the subtle channels (*nādī) of the *life force and the ability to stop one's *breath as instances of the third group. This text (III.47) emphasizes that even in the face of all these numerous difficulties, the *yogin should absolutely persist in his efforts.

Moreover, many scriptures state that the paranormal powers (*siddhi) are to be regarded as obstacles to the "great power" of *enlightenment. See also *antarāya, dosha, upasarga*.

vijnāna ("knowledge") usually stands for secular knowledge or intellectual understanding and as such is distinguished from wisdom (*jnāna). In some rare contexts, however, this word can also denote the ultimate liberating gnosis (*vidyā).

Vijnāna Bhikshu (A.D. 1525–1580) was a *Vedānta monk and scholar who, in addition to several shorter works, also composed authoritative commentaries on the *Brahma-Sūtra*, the *Sāmkhya-Sūtra*, and the *Yoga-Sūtra* (entitled *Yoga-Vārttika*). Vijnāna Bhikshu, an original thinker, promulgated a form of theistic Vedānta, which is close to the Sāmkhya-Vedānta orientation of the *Purānas and the *Bhagavad-Gītā*. In particular, he rejected *Shankara's more radical nondualist metaphysics and instead believed in the existence of a personal *God as the highest being, the multiplicity of souls (*purusha), and the reality of the world. Though not a follower of the *yoga-darshana himself, Vijnāna Bhikshu was obviously well acquainted with *Yoga theory and technology. In his exegesis, he tends to be more speculative than, for instance, *Vācaspati Mishra, another great Yoga savant, and often proposes interesting explanations where other commentators remain silent or merely reiterate previous opinions. His chief disciple was *Bhāva Ganesha.

vijnāna-maya-kosha ("sheath composed of knowledge") is the bodily "envelope" (*kosha) formed of higher understanding, or what in some schools is called *buddhi*.

vikalpa ("conceptualization"). In *Classical Yoga, this is one of the five categories of mental "fluctuation" (*vritti), and is defined in the *Yoga-Sūtra (I.9) as knowledge that is without perceivable object and that follows verbal distinctions. This term is often also understood in the sense of "imagination" or "fantasy."

vikāra ("modification") is an important *Sāmkhya term, which is also often employed in the commentaries on the *Yoga-Sūtra*. It signifies the transformations of the ground of Nature (*prakriti) into such distinct categories (*tattva) as the ten senses (*indriya), the five sense objects (*vishaya), and the lower mind (*manas). See also parināma.

vikshepa ("distraction"). In the *Yoga-Sūtra (I.30), this term is used as a synonym for *antarāya ("obstacle"). It suggests that obstacles such as *sickness, *laziness, and *doubt distract one's consciousness (*citta) from the task of focusing on the spiritual process. These distractions are accompanied, according to *Patanjali, by pain (*duhkha), depression (*daurmanasya), tremor of the limbs (angam-ejatva), as well as faulty inhalation (*shvāsa) and exhalation (*prashvāsa).

vipāka ("ripening" or "fruition") generally refers to the fructification of *karma, that is, the visible results (in the form of advantageous or disadvantegeous events) of former actions, whether they were committed in this lifetime or previous embodiments. Cf. phala.

viparīta-karanī-mudrā ("inverse action seal") is described in the *Gheranda-Samhitā (III.33ff.) as follows: One should place one's *head on the ground and, with one's hands spread out and legs raised, remain steady. This appears to be the original name for the headstand (*shīrsha-āsana). However, some modern manuals interpret it as the shoulder stand. The idea behind this potent practice is to achieve a reversal of the microcosmic "sun" (*sūrya) and "moon" (*candra). The "moon" oozes the precious ambrosia (*amrita), which trickles into the abdomen, where it is consumed by the "sun." Through this "seal" (*mudrā), the *yogin seeks to interrupt this process and save the nectar for higher purposes. Daily practice of this technique for up to three hours is said to greatly fan the "abdominal fire" (*jāthara-agni), which is why the practitioner should eat amply. This exercise is praised as a panacea for all ills and as a means of conquering *death itself.

viparyaya ("error") is one of the five categories of mental "fluctuation" (*vritti), and is defined in the *Yoga-Sūtra (I.8) as erroneous knowledge that is not based on the actual appearance of a thing. The *Yoga-Bhāshya (II.3) also treats viparyaya as a synonym for the term *avidyā ("nescience"), which is "five jointed." It is the arch error, as a result of which we misinterpret existence itself. Cf. pramāna.

vīra ("hero") is an important *Tantric category, referring to the spiritual practitioner who animates the "heroic" disposition (*bhāva), which is the only one suitable for the present "dark age" (*kāli-yuga). The *Kula-Arnava-Tantra (XVII.25) explains the term vīra as follows: "On account of being free from passion (*rāga*), intoxication (*mada*), affliction (*klesha*), anger (*kopa*), jealousy (*mātsarya*), and delusion (*moha*), and on account of being far removed from activity (*rajas*) and inertia (*tamas*), he is called a 'hero.' "

The above passage represents a fanciful etymological play on the words *vīra* ("hero"), *vīta* ("free"), and *vidhūra* ("far removed"), which contradicts other *Tantric scriptures that ascribe to the *vīra* a strong dynamic (*rajas*) quality. Often the *vīra* is understood to be the practitioner of the left-hand ritual involving the "five substances" (*pancatattva*), including sexual intercourse (*maithunā*). The implication is that the heroic practitioner risks everything in his or her struggle for *self-transcendence. See also *vīrya*.

vīra-āsana ("heroic posture"). Mentioned already in the *Mahābhārata* (XII.292.8), this posture (*āsana*) is described somewhat inadequately in the *Gheranda-Samhitā* (II.17): Placing one leg on the (opposite) thigh, one should turn the foot backward. Modern manuals often describe this posture differently: Kneeling down, one should sit between the thighs.

virāga ("nonattachment") is a synonym for *vairāgya*.

Virūpāksha is mentioned in the *Hatha-Yoga-Pradīpikā* (I.5) as a great *adept of *hatha-yoga*. No further information about him is given.

vīrya ("vitality, energy") is listed in the *Yoga-Sūtra* (I.20) as one of the requisites of the yogic *path leading to superconscious enstasy (*asamprajnāta-samādhi*). Elsewhere in this work (II.38), *vīrya* is stated to be acquired through the practice of chastity (*brahmacarya*). See also *vīra*.

vishāda ("despair"). When Prince *Arjuna faced his family, friends, and teachers on the battlefield, he fell into a mood of confusion and despair. Although he knew that he was fighting for a just cause, he could not conceive of slaying them. Seeing Arjuna's despondence, the God-man *Krishna, who served as the prince's charioteer, instructed him in the secrets of *karma-yoga*, the *path of self-transcending action. The eternal order (*dharma*), he taught in the *Bhagavad-Gītā*, must be maintained. It was the duty of a warrior to fight for justice, and despair was an unmanly thing. This has often been interpreted as an allegory of the human situation in general.

Vishāda is occasionally counted as one of the "defects" (*dosha*). The

Uddhāva-Gītā (XXIV.2) states that spiritual practitioners often tend to feel dejected either from exhaustion or because of their failure to control the *mind properly and recommends that they should then take refuge to the "lotus feet of the *Lord." The *Mārkandeya-Purāna* (XXXIX.16) soundly suggests the practice of breath control (*prānāyāma*) to overcome depression.

vishaya ("object") is the thing experienced through the senses (*indriya*). The *Yoga-Bhāshya* (IV.17) compares *objects to a magnet because they bind consciousness (*citta*) as if it had the properties of iron. Sensory awareness is the habitual condition of the *waking consciousness. In *Yoga, which typically endeavors to bring about the introversion *attention, sense objects are often regarded as the enemy. Thus, in his *Tattva-Vaishāradī* (II.55), the Yoga scholar *Vācaspati Mishra compares them to snake's venom (*āshi-visha*)—a sentiment that is echoed in numerous other works of different traditions. The *Bhagavad-Gītā* (II.59) speaks of the "eating" (*āhāra*) of objects, and this notion is also present in the Sanskrit term *bhoga*, meaning "experience" but being derived from the verbal root *bhuj* ("to eat, consume, enjoy").

In some contexts, *vishaya* stands for "worldliness," as in the *Yoga-Kundaly-Upanishad* (I.60), where it is named as one of the ten obstacles (*vighna*) and is contrasted with renunciation (*virati*). See also *artha*, *lakshya*.

vishesha ("special" or "particular"). In *Classical Yoga, *vishesha* represents the ontic level of the "particularized," which, according to the *Yoga-Bhāshya* (II.19), is composed of the five elements (*bhūta*), the ten senses (*indriya*), and the lower mind (*manas*). Cf. *avishesha*.

Vishishta-Advaita is the *Vedānta school of "Qualified Nondualism," for which *Rāmānuja was the most distinguished spokesman. In contrast to the radical nondualism of *Shankara, this school of thought defends the view that the ultimate *Reality is not merely an unqualified (*nirguna*), impersonal *Absolute but the suprapersonal *Being in which all qualities inhere. It appears that the early representatives of this school, such as *Nāthamuni and *Yamunācārya, practiced an eightfold *Yoga (*ashta-anga-yoga*) with a strong devotional (*bhakti*) orientation.

Vishnu was originally a minor *deity of the *Vedic pantheon but, possibly because mythology endowed him with a carefully delineated personality and history, grew quickly into one of the principal gods

of *Hinduism. His name means
"pervader" and refers to his omni-
presence. In the trinity of medieval India, Vishnu stands for the
principle of preservation, whereas
*Brahma represents that of crea-
tion and *Shiva that of destruction.

Vishnu is the supreme Godhead worshipped in *Vaishavism.
His benign qualities invite a devotional (*bhakti) response, and
*bhakti-yoga flourished in the reli-
gious culture of Vaishnavism.
Vishnu's most significant aspect
are his twenty-four "incarnations"
(*avatāra) in different world ages
(*yuga), among which the God-
man *Krishna is the most popular

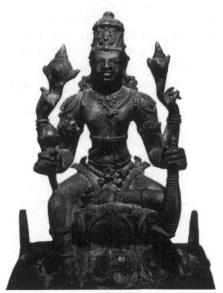

77. God Vishnu.

embodiment, *Rāma being a close second. The *Vaishnavas created
many remarkable works extolling Vishnu and pointing out a *path to
realizing unity or identity with that great God. Foremost among these
scriptures are the *Bhagavad-Gītā and the *Bhāgavata-Purāna. See also
deva.

vishnu-granthi ("Vishnu's knot") is the second of the "knots" (*granthi)
or blockages in the *body, preventing the free flow of the life force
(*prāna). It is located at the throat.

Vishnu-Purāna is one of the major works of the *Purāna genre. In its
earliest portions, it belongs to the pre-Christian era. It deals with *Yoga
in the sixth canticle and understands it as the *path of meditation
(*dhyāna).

vishuddha-cakra ("pure wheel") or **vishuddhi-cakra** ("wheel of purity") is the fifth psychoenergetic center (*cakra) in ascending order,
and is also known as jālandhara-pītha and "great doorway to *liberation"
(mahā-moksha-dvāra). It is located at the throat or, as the *Yoga-Shikhā-
Upanishad (I.174) puts it, at the "throat well" (kantha-kūpa). It is generally depicted as a sixteen-petaled lotus of a smoky purple hue. According to the *Shat-Cakra-Nirūpana (28), its pericarp is composed of
the "circle of space" (nabho-mandala), which resembles the

full moon. This center is connected with the "seed syllable" (*bīja-mantra) *ham*, the element ether (*ākāsha), and the Goddess Shākinī. The *Shiva-Samhitā (V.92) states that by contemplating this *cakra*, one acquires an instant comprehension of the *Vedas and all their mysteries.

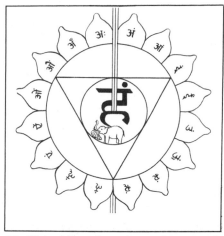

78. *Vishuddha-cakra, the psychoenergetic center at the throat.*

vishva ("world") is the *cosmos in its entirety, which *Hindu cosmology pictures as a vast, multidimensional, dynamic being arising in the infinity of the *Divine and governed by the law of *karma*. The ordinary, unenlightened psyche (*jīva) is entrapped in the processes of *Nature, and escapes this state of *bondage only through higher wisdom (*jñāna, *vidyā), that is, realization of the transcendental *Reality. *Yoga is one of the spiritual avenues elaborated in *Hinduism by which the world-bound psyche can awaken to its true identity as the Self (*ātman, *purusha) and recover its essential *freedom. On the way to *enlightenment, or *liberation, the *yogin may acquire all kinds of extraordinary insights and visions that reveal to him the immensity—in space and time—of the *cosmos. However, such privileged knowledge, especially of the "subtle" (*sūkshma) dimensions of the world, must ultimately be renounced as well, so that the universe as a whole can be transcended. For some but by no means all schools of Yoga, the world experienced by the unenlightened psyche is the great enemy of the spiritual process. They consequently regard transcendence of cosmic existence as the highest goal of human aspiration. This is the ideal of "disembodied liberation" (*videha-mukti). A more integrated viewpoint looks upon the world as a potential aid to *enlightenment. According to this second view, after one has awakened from the dream of separate existence as a worldly *ego (a subject confronting multiple objects), one enjoys the world as a manifestation, or play (*līlā) of the *Divine. This is the ideal of "living liberation" (*jīvan-mukti).

vishvāsa ("confidence," "trust") is mentioned in the *Shiva-Samhitā (III.18) as a precondition for successful spiritual practice. See also *āstikya*, *shraddhā*.

vishva-udarā-nādī ("world belly channel"), also spelled vishva-udarī-nādī ("world-swelling channel") is one of the principal conduits (*nādī) through which the life force (*prāna) circulates in the *body. It is generally thought to be located between the *hasti-jihvā- and the *kuhū-nādī. The *Yoga-Yājnavalkya (IV.44) places it in the middle of the belly (tunda), which would explain its curious name, since the *navel is the center of the *microcosm. This channel of the *life force is held to be responsible for the consumption of food.

Vitality. See vīrya.

Vital areas. See marman.

vīta-rāga ("free from passion") applies to both the condition and the person enjoying the state of freedom from attachment (*rāga). The Mundaka-Upanishad (III.2.5) sees this as a precondition for *Self-realization, while the *Bhagavad-Gītā (II.56) mentions it as a necessary qualification of the sage whose wisdom is firmly settled (*sthita-prajnā). The *Yoga-Sūtra (I.37) speaks of such an individual as a fit object for one's *meditation. See also vairāgya.

vitarka ("cogitation") Apart from its general application in the sense of "thought," this term has two basic meanings in *Classical Yoga. First, it stands for the spontaneous thought processes that occur in conscious enstasy (*samprajnāta-samādhi) in relation to a "gross" (*sthūla) object of *contemplation. Second, vitarka denotes the kind of unwholesome deliberations that can arise in the course of the day, such as the idea to take revenge or to lie. For their extirpation, the *Yoga-Sūtra (II.33) recommends that one should dwell on the opposite idea, such as to bless and to speak the truth regardless of one's emotional state. This practice is known as *pratipaksha-bhāvanā. See also nirvitarka-samādhi, savitarka-samādhi; cf. vicāra.

vitrishna, also called vaitrishnya ("nonthirsting"), is a synonym for *vairāgya ("dispassion").

Vivarana is a remarkable subcommentary on the *Yoga-Bhāshya of *Vyāsa, which is the oldest available commentary on the *Yoga-Sūtra, the textbook of *Classical Yoga. Its full title is Yoga-Bhāshya-Vivarana, and its author is *Shankara Bhagavatpāda, whom some Hindu authorities identify with the great teacher (*ācārya) of *Advaita-Vedānta. In importance, this work ranks with *Vācaspati Mishra's *Tattva-

Vaishāradī and *Vijnāna Bhikshu's *Yoga-Vārttika*. The *Vivarana* is noteworthy for its many original interpretations and metaphors, which show that the author must have been an intellectual giant.

viveka ("discernment") refers to the recognition of the distinction between the real and unreal, truth and fiction, and particularly the transcendental *Self and the "nonself" (*anātman*). This is an important notion in *Classical Yoga, which insists on the eternal separation between the Self (*purusha*) and Nature (*prakriti*). the (*Yoga-Shikhā-Upanishad* (IV.22), which is based on the nondualist metaphysics of *Vedānta, criticizes this view, stating that the *yogins distinction between Self and "nonself" springs from *ignorance. See also *viveka-khyāti, vivekin*.

Vivekananda, Swami. Among the many disciples of *Ramakrishna, Vivekananda is the best known. Born Narendranath ("Naren") Datta in 1863, he was educated at the Mission College in Calcutta, where he demonstrated a great talent for philosophy. He first met Ramakrishna at age eighteen, and joined his *āshrama* two years later. He became the favorite pupil of the unsophisticated but wise Ramakrishna, who assured the young man that he, Ramakrishna, had indeed "seen" *God as clearly as they were seeing each other. Shortly after the death of his *guru in 1886, Vivekananda renounced the world and, together with other close disciples, founded the

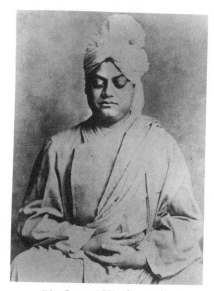

79. Swami Vivekananda.

Ramakrishna Order, which later developed into the Ramakrishna Mission. This organization has done much to disseminate *Hindu teachings in the Western hemisphere. Vivekananda gained world fame almost overnight by representing *Hinduism at the 1893 World Parliament of Religions in Chicago. He won the respect of such men as William James and Leo Tolstoy, and his teaching activity particularly attracted Aldous Huxley and Gerald Heard, who were instrumental in paving the way for *Vedānta in the West. Upon his return to India, he was celebrated as a national hero. Vivekananda has numerous books to his credit, consisting primarily of his talks to small groups. They include his widely read treatments of *rāja-yoga, *karma-yoga, *jnāna-yoga, and *bhakti-yoga. He interpreted *Yoga strictly from the viewpoint of the nondualist philosophy of *Vedānta. Vivekananda died in 1902.

viveka-khyāti ("vision of discernment"), also called "wisdom born of discernment" (viveka-ja-jnāna) and "vision of otherness" (*anyatā-khyāti), is a key concept of *Classical Yoga. According to the *Yoga-Sūtra (III.52), it is the direct means to *liberation and is said to be "omni-objective" (sarva-vishaya), "omni-temporal" (sarvathā-vishaya), and "nonsequential" (akrama). It is also referred to by *Patanjali as the "deliverer" (*tāraka), which should make it clear that this is not mere intellectual understanding. Rather, viveka-khyāti occurs at the highest level of conscious enstasy (*samprajnāta-samādhi).

Viveka-Mārtanda ("Sun-Bird of Discernment") is a short tract on *Yoga, consisting of only eight duplets, which were apparently composed for a certain Sultan Ghiyās-ud-dīn. The text is attributed to Rameshvara Bhatta, who lived in the fourteenth century A.D.

vivekin ("discerner") is, according to the *Yoga-Sūtra (II.15), the person who recognizes that sorrow (*duhka) lies hidden in everything, even in apparently pleasurable experiences. See also viveka.

vrāta ("vow") is sometimes mentioned among the constituent practices of self-discipline (*niyama). The *Yoga-Yājnavalkya (II.11) explains it as one's holding fast to the spiritual means (*upāya), in order to realize both virtue (*dharma) and the *Self. The *Shāndilya-Upanishad (I.2.11) defines it more conventionally as the steady performance of the regulations laid down in the *Vedas.

Vrātyas. The Vrātyas of ancient India were sacred migrant brotherhoods held together by vows (*vrāta). They were connected with the earliest *history of *Yoga, and may have invented the practice of breath control (*prānāyāma) in connection with the presentation of the songs and melodies (sāman) composed by them. The literature of *Hinduism contains many references to these enigmatic groups, but the most reliable information about them is given in the vrātya-khānda (Book XV) of the *Atharva-Veda. The Vrātyas, it appears, were among those many communities that did not belong to the orthodox kernel of *Vedic society but had their own customs. In the eyes of the brahmic custodians of the Vedic sacrificial religion, they were despicable outcastes, and may even have been the occasional victims of human sacrifices. The Vrātyas worshipped God *Rudra, the God of *wind (and *breath), who was later assimilated into *Shiva. The Vrātyas wandered primarily in the northeast of India, but in the course of time many converted to orthodox *Brāhmanism and became sedentary. Some of their members are said to have "quietened the penis" (*shamanica-medhra*), which suggests total celibacy (*brahmacarya*). Each group had a professional bard (known as *māgadha* or *sūta*) and a female called *pumshcalī* ("man mover"), who appears to have been a sacred prostitute. During the misummer ceremony, bard and prostitute enacted the creative, erotic play between God and Goddess—thus foreshadowing the *Tantric practice of ritual intercourse (*maithunā*).

vriksha-āsana ("tree posture"), a favorite posture (*āsana*) among contemporary practitioners of *hatha-yoga, is described in the *Gheranda-Samhitā* (II.25) thus: Standing straight like a tree on the ground, one should place the right foot on the left thigh. This is more than a balancing exercise, for it is thought to also stabilize the *mind.

vrisha-āsana ("bull posture") is described in the *Gheranda-Samhitā* (II.38) as follows: Placing one's buttocks on the right heel, one should place the left foot to the side of the right leg. See also *āsana*.

vritti ("whirl") can mean a number of things, including "activity," "mode of life," "livelihood," and "rule." In yogic contexts, the term stands specifically for the "fluctuations" of consciousness (*citta*). *Patanjali distinguishes five types of *vritti*: valid cognition (*pramāna*), misconception (*viparyaya*), conceptualization (*vikalpa*), sleep (*nidrā*), and memory (*smriti*). Obviously, these categories do not offer a comprehensive catalogue of psychomental states. However, they are all significant in the practice of *meditation and *enstasy. As the *Yoga-Sūtra* (I.2) states, "Yoga is the restriction of the fluctuations of consciousness" (*yogash citta-vritti-nirodhah*). According to aphorism II.11, the fluctuations are to be restricted by means of meditation (*dhyāna*). Their restriction (*nirodha*) leads over into the state of conscious enstasy (*samprajnāta-samādhi*). The reason the *yogin seeks to check these psychomental activities is that they obscure his true nature as the transcendental Self (*purusha*) and thus embroil him in inauthentic existence and suffering (*duhkha*), because they generate "subliminal activators" (*samskāra*), which then give rise to renewed psychomental activity.

vyādhi ("disease"). The *Yoga-Sūtra* (I.30) lists *vyādhi* among the obstacles (*antarāya*) on the spiritual *path. The *Yoga-Bhāshya* (I.30) explains the term as disorder of the bodily humors (*dhātu*), secretions (*rasa*), and organs (*kārana*). Since *body and *mind form a unity, it is easy enough to appreciate that illness (*roga*) may interfere with one's spiritual practice. It is difficult to concentrate and stay lucid when one has a fever or one's body is racked with *pain. It is therefore important that one should restore the body-mind to good *health, either through conventional means or, if possible, through yogic practices and the adoption of wholesome attitudes.

vyakta ("manifest") is a frequently used concept of *Epic Yoga. The *Mahābhārata* (III.211.12) has this instructive verse: "Whatsoever is 'created' by the senses (*indriya*) is called *vyakta*. That which is to be known as being beyond the senses and can be grasped [only] by symbols is the 'unmanifest' (*avyakta*)."

In the *Yoga-Sūtra* (IV.13) the term refers to the properties (*dharma*) of an *object existing in the present, in contrast to the properties pertaining to the past or the future, which are technically known as "subtle" (*sūkshma*). See also Cosmos, *parvan*; cf. *avyakta*.

vyakti ("manifestation") is the entire created *cosmos, which has evolved out of the transcendental ground (*pradhāna*) of Nature (*prakriti*).

vyāna is one of the five principal forms of the life force (*prāna*) circulating in the *body. Already in the *Maitrāyanīya-Upanishad* (II.6), it is said to support the activities of inhalation (*prāna*) and exhalation (*apāna*). It is widely held to be diffused throughout the body, though some texts mention specific areas, such as the eyes, ears, throat, and the joints, and is also often thought to make speech possible.

Vyāsa ("Gatherer") is the name of several legendary sages, and it is impossible to hold them apart. The *Vishnu-Purāna* (III.3) mentions that there have been twenty-eight Vyāsas, since the *Vedas have been arranged as many times. Generally, however, *Hindu tradition treats Vyāsa as a single individual, who is also called Krishna Dvaipāyana, son of the seer Parāshara and the beautiful fisher girl Satyavatī, who, after miraculously regaining her virginity, married King Shāntanu.

Vyāsa is said to have compiled the four *Vedas, the *Mahābhārata* epic, together with the *Bhagavad-Gītā*, the vast *Purāna literature, and a host of other works. He is also credited with the authorship of the oldest extant commentary on *Patanjali's *Yoga-Sūtra, the *Yoga-Bhāshya. The *Mahābhārata (XII.26.4) calls him the "foremost of *Yoga experts."

vyoma-cakra ("ether wheel") is a psychoenergetic center (*cakra) located, according to the *Hatha-Yoga-Pradīpikā (IV.45), at the "unsupported" (nirālambana) place between the *idā- and the *pingalā-nādī. The *Yoga-Rāja-Upanishad (17) speaks of it as the ninth center, having sixteen spokes and being the abode of the supreme *shakti that bestows great *bliss. See also ākāsha-cakra.

vyoman ("ether," "space") is a synonym for ākāsha.

vyutkrama ("inversion") is one of the three constituent practices of *kapāla-bhāti. According to the *Gheranda-Samhitā (I.58), it is practiced by slowly drawing water up through the nose and expelling it again through the mouth. This is said to cure disorders of phlegm (*kapha).

vyutthāna ("emergence"). See Waking consciousness.

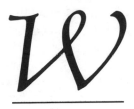

Waking consciousness is the predominant mode of awareness in which the ego-identity is either reinforced through habitual (*karmic) responses to life or gradually undermined through a spiritual reversal of one's values, attitudes, thoughts, and *actions. For this reason, it has special significance for the *yogin. However, the waking consciousness is by no means the only mode of awareness, and the *yogin* must learn to discipline himself progressively on all levels of possible experience. Thus, he must conquer his dreams (*svapna) and even deep sleep (*nidrā, *sushupti). This means that he must cultivate Self-awareness (the consciousness of the *witness) in all states of *consciousness. Even the higher stages of awareness, as realized in enstasy (*samādhi), are to be submitted to this discipline. See also *jagrat, jāgarita-sthāna*.

War, or conflict, characterizes much of ordinary human life. No comprehensive spiritual philosophy can afford to ignore this fact. Indeed, spirituality is often couched in terms of an endeavor to establish psychic equilibrium (*samatva). Such a state of inner balance is typically sought to be cultivated through withdrawal from life. The *Hindu tradition of abandonment (*tyāga) or renunciation (*samnyāsa) has generally taken this form. However, a different orientation has been espoused in the *Bhagavad-Gītā, a work composed in the pre-Christian era. Its teachings are set against the backdrop of one of the greatest wars fought on Indian soil. It seeks to resolve the tension between doing one's duty (*dharma) by fighting for what is true and good and striving for spiritual enlightenment (*bodha) or liberation (*moksha). In a crucial passage of the *Gītā* (II.18ff.), the God-man *Krishna offers his disciple Prince *Arjuna the following advice:

> Finite, it is said, are those *bodies of the eternal, indestructible, incommensurable embodied being (*sharīrin) [i.e., the *Self]. Hence fight, o son of Bharata.

> He who thinks of Him as slayer and he who thinks [that He can be] slain—they both do not know. He does not slay nor is He slain.

> Never is He born or dies. He did not come into being, nor shall He ever come to be. This primeval [Self] is unborn, eternal, everlasting. It is not slain when the *body is slain.

*Krishna's ethics seems to fly in the face of the fundamental moral rule of nonharming (*ahimsā). Hence his teachings about war have often been interpreted as being merely allegorical. However, Krishna does not condone war in general. Rather, the war in which he and *Arjuna were involved was to reestablish the moral order (*dharma) that had been lost through the egotism of the Kurus who had usurped Arjuna's kingdom. For only in a society whose moral order is intact are people free to devote themselves to the pursuit of the highest human aspiration—that of self-transcendence or liberation (*moksha). Krishna's nonpacifist ethics cannot be properly appreciated apart from his spiritual philosophy.

Water. See *ap, jala.*

Wisdom is knowledge that has sedimented in one's being to the degree that it transforms one's basic attitude to life and *death. It is a deep, lived understanding of the fact that individual human existence amounts to very little apart from the great *Being, or *Divine, in which it arises for a brief spell only to become dissolved again into That. Wisdom liberates one from the burden of the *ego consciousness and puts one in touch with the essential Identity that transcends the *body and the *mind. See also *jnāna, buddhi, manīshā, prajnā.*

Witness. Beyond the different states or levels of awareness lies the transcendental *Self, which is characterized as the witness (*sākshin) of all psychomental phenomena. This witness, also called the "Fourth" (*caturtha), is the single most far-reaching discovery of India's seers and sages, and undoubtedly their greatest contribution toward a universal psychology.

Work. See *karman*.

World. See Cosmos, *bhuvana*, *loka*, *samsāra*, *vishva*.

world ages. *Hindu chronology operates with vast time cycles. The manifest world is thought to depend for its existence on the life of the Creator-God, *Brahma. He is said to live for one hundred brahmic years corresponding to 311,040,000,000,000 human years. The universe is created concurrently with his birth, and upon his death it vanishes completely. After a period of latency, lasting a hundred brahmic years, a new Brahma springs forth from the *Divine and with him a new universe. Thus, the cycle of creation (*sarga*) and dissolution (*pralaya*) is repeated ad infinitum. There are also minor creations and dissolutions at the end of each brahmic day and night, corresponding to 8,640,000,000 human years. This period is known as a *kalpa*, which is composed of 1,000 *mahā-yuga* ("great aeons"). Each *mahā-yuga* is composed of 12,000 divine years, corresponding to 1,555,200,000 human years. The duration of each *mahā-yuga* is made up of four cyclic periods called *yuga*, which are marked by a progressive worsening of the moral order (*dharma*). These are the *krita-* or *satya-yuga* (lasting 4,000 divine years), the *tretā-yuga* (Lasting 3,000 divine years), the *dvāpara-yuga* (lasting 2,000 divine years), and the *kāli-yuga* (lasting 1,000 divine years). In between each of these four *yugas* is a period of latency lasting 800, 600, 400, and 200 divine years respectively. Present humanity is thought to live at the beginning of the *kāli-yuga*, the "dark age." With the collapse of the myth of progress. In the face of the far-reaching ecological crisis precipitated by technology and consumerism, this interpretation of contemporary history is believable enough.

Worship. See *arcanā*, *pūjā*.

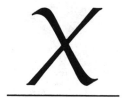

There are no entries under X.

Y

yajna ("sacrifice"). The notion of *sacrifice is one of the cornerstones of *Hinduism. Sacrificial rituals played an all-important role already in the *Vedic age. Through sacrifice, the ancient Indians sought to win and maintain the favor of the deities (*deva). As they saw it, the world itself is built on the principle of sacrifice: The primordial *Being, or *purusha, sacrificed itself to bring forth the *cosmos. Similarly, life perpetuates itself through the destruction of individual life forms.

Once this is understood, the only reasonable and mature response is to relate to existence as a continuous sacrifice. This idea was developed in the *Brāhmanas and earliest *Upanishads. For instance, the *Chāndogya-Upanishad (III.16.1) declares: "Verily, man (*purusha) is a sacrifice." This recognition led to the notion of the inner or spiritual sacrifice, that is, the dedication of one's life to a higher, cosmic purpose rather than the mere exoteric ritual offering of libations to the deities. Thus, *karma-yoga is essentially action performed in the spirit of sacrifice, or self-surrender. In the *Bhagavad-Gītā (III.10), the God-man *Krishna draws a parallel with the unselfish creation of the world by Prajāpati. In another passage of the same text (IV.25ff.), various forms of sacrificial action are mentioned—from offerings to the gods to the surrender of the senses (*indriya) into the fire of self-restraint (*samyama), or the restriction of one's *diet, or controlled *breathing, and so forth. In one stanza (IV.33), Krishna announces that the sacrifices of *wisdom (jnāna-yajna) is superior to material sacrifices (dravya-yajna), which captures the spirit of *Yoga in general. However, many yogic schools and *paths include material sacrifices in their daily exercitium. This is especially true of *bhakti-yoga.

Yājnavalkya is the name of several teachers who lived in different periods. The best known Yājnavalkya is the revered *adept of the *Brihad-Āranyaka-Upanishad, who lived with his two wives in a forest hermitage (*āshrama*). He was one of the first to teach the doctrine of rebirth (*punar-janman*) and *karma. Several centuries later, another Yājnavalkya authored the *Yājnavalkya-Smriti*, a work on law and ethics (*dharma*), probably written in the third century B.C. In one verse, this text (I.8) notes that the highest teaching (*dharma*) is that which leads to the vision of the *Self (*ātma-darshana*) by means of *Yoga. This Yājnavalkya has also been credited with the authorship of the *Yoga-Yājnavalkya-Samhitā*.

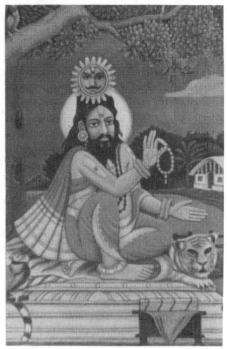

80. Yajnavalkya.

Yājnavalkya is also the name of a Yoga *adept who is frequently mentioned or quoted in the later *Upanishads, and who may have been the author of the *Yoga-Yājnavalkya-Samhitā*, among other works. There is also a *Yājnavalkya-Upanishad*, which belongs to the genre of *Samnyāsa-Upanishads and may have been composed around A.D. 1400.

Yajur-Veda ("Knowledge of Sacrifice") is the *Vedic collection (*samhitā*) that contains all the hymns relevant to the sacrificial rituals of the *brāhmanas. See also Veda.

Yāma ("Restrainer") is the *Hindu God of Death. In the *Katha-Upanishad* (I.1ff.), Yāma is introduced as the initiator of the young spiritual aspirant Naciketas. The story is a parable that makes the point that we must first face our own mortality before we can hope to transcend the fear of *death and to win *immortality.

yama ("restraint") is the first "limb" (*anga*) of the eightfold yogic *path taught by *Patanjali. It stands for the moral observances, which form the very foundation of spiritual discipline. According to the *Yoga-

Sūtra (II.30), there are five *yamas*. There are: nonharming (**ahimsā*), truthfulness (**satya*), nonstealing (**asteya*), chastity (**brahmacarya*), and greedlessness (*aparigraha*). These constitute the "great vow" (*mahā-vrāta*) of the **yogin* and are to be practiced on all levels, irrespective of time, place, or circumstance.

The **Tejo-Bindu-Upanishad* (I.17), which has *yama* as the first "limb" of its fifteenfold **Yoga* (**panca-dasha-anga-yoga*), defines it as the control of the **senses in the knowledge that "all is the Absolute (**brahman*)." The **Tri-Shikhi-Brāhmana-Upanishad* (II.28) explains it as dispassion (**vairāgya*) toward the **body and its **senses. The **Linga-Purāna* (I.8.10) interprets it as abstention (*uparāma*) in the form of asceticism (**tapas*). The **Kūrma-Purāna* (II.11.13) observes that the five disciplines of *yama* are conducive to the **purification of the mind (*citta-shuddhi*). Many works of **Post-Classical Yoga list ten practices under *yama*. Thus, the **Tri-Shikhi-Brāhmana-Upanishad* (II.32) mentions the following: non-harming, truthfulness, nonstealing, chastity, sympathy (**dayā*), recti-tude (**ārjava*), patience (**kshamā*), steadfastness (**dhriti*), moderate diet (**mita-āhāra*), and cleanliness (**shauca*). This series is repeated in several other **Yoga-Upanishads. However, the **Mandala-Brāhmana-Upanishad* (I.4) lists the following nine practices: devotion to the teacher (**guru-bhakti*), adherence to the **path of truth (*satya-mārga-anurakti*), enjoy-ment of the Real (*vastu*) as it is glimpsed in pleasurable experiences, contentment (**tushti*), nonattachment (**nihsangatā*), living in solitude (*ekānta-vāsa*), cessation of mental activity (*mano-nivritti*), nonattachment (*anabhilāsha*) to the fruit (**phala*) of one's **actions, and dispassion (**vairāgya*).

The **Siddha-Siddhānta-Paddhati* (II.32) speaks of calmness (*upashama*), mastery of the senses (**indriya-jaya*), mastery of diet (*āhāra-jaya*), mas-tery of sleep (*nidra-jaya*), and mastery of cold (*shīta-jaya*) as the con-stituent practices of *yama*, and makes the point that these have to be learned gradually. The **Yoga-Tattva-Upanishad* (28) treats scant diet (**laghv-āhāra*) as the single most important discipline.

yamin ("restrainer") is a synonym for **yogin*, the self-controlled spir-itual practitioner.

Yamunācārya, grandson of **Nāthamuni, was one of the great **Vaish-nava preceptors of the **Vishishtha-Advaita school of **Vedānta. He lived from A.D. 918–1038 and is said to have learned the eightfold **Yoga (**ashta-anga-yoga*) from the **adept Kurukanātha. He had nu-merous disciples, including **Rāmānuja. Yamunācārya wrote six works, the most important of which is his *Siddhi-Traya*.

yantra ("device") is a geometric representation of the levels and energies of the *cosmos and the human *body (as a microcosmic replica of the macrocosm). *Yantras* are widely used in *Tantric worship where they are treated as the "body" of one's chosen deity (*ishta-devatā*). They are drawn on paper, wood, and cloth, or inscribed on metal and other materials, or even constructed in three dimensions out of clay. They typically consist of a square surround, circles, lotus petals, triangles, and a central point known as the *bindu*, representing the creative matrix of the universe and gateway to the transcendental *Reality.

In the higher stages of the *Tantric ritual, the *yantra* must be completely internalized, that is, perfectly visualized. *Yantra-yoga* consists in the gradual dissolution of this inwardly constructed *yantra*, together with the dissolution of the individuated *consciousness. If successful, this exercise will catapult the practitioner (*sādhaka*) into pure *Consciousness, beyond the subject-object distinction. *Tantrism employs a large number of *yantras*, and the *Mantra-Mahodadhi* (XX) describes twenty-nine such geometric devices. The most famous *yantra* is the *shrī-yantra*. See also *mandala*.

yashasvinī-nādī ("splendid channel") is one of the principal channels (*nādī*) through which the life force (*prāna*) moves in the *body. Different scriptures mention different locations for this *nādī*. Some place it between the *pingalā- and the *pūshā-nādī, others between the *pūshā- and the *sarasvatī-nādī, and yet others between the *gāndhārā- and the *sarasvatī-nādī. It is widely thought to run from the "bulb" (*kanda*) to the left ear, though the *Shāndilya-Upanishad* (I.4.11) specifies the big toes as its termination point.

yati is any ascetic, including a practitioner of *Yoga.

yatna ("effort") or exertion is, according to the *Yoga-Sūtra* (I.13), the very essence of spiritual practice (*abhyāsa*): One cannot grow spiritually without applying oneself to the yogic disciplines. However, when spiritual striving becomes competitive it is counterproductive. See also Effort, *paurusha*, *prayatna*; cf. Grace.

yauga is sometimes used as a synonym for *yogin*, particularly in the *Nyāya and *Vaisheshika traditions.

Yoga is the name of a mythical sage mentioned in the *Mahābhārata* (XIII.150.45).

Yoga. The word *yoga* is derived from the verbal root (yuj, meaning "to yoke, harness." It has a wide range of applications in the Sanskrit language, from "union" to "team," to "sum," to "equipment," to "conjunction," and so forth. Early on, it came to also be applied to "spiritual endeavor," specifically the control of the mind (*manas*) and senses (*indriya*). This usage is first found in the *Taittirīya-Upanishad* (II.4.1), which dates back to the sixth or seventh century B.C.

By the time of the composition of the *Bhagavad-Gītā*—which can be assigned to the third or fourth century B.C.—the word *yoga* was widely used to denote the *Hindu tradition of spiritual discipline, comprising different approaches to *Self-realization, or *enlightenment. In that formative period, Yoga was still closely allied with *Sāmkhya. This fact is reflected in the *Mahābhārata epic, which frequently employs the compound *samkhya-yoga. In subsequent times, Yoga and Sāmkhya developed into separate philosophical schools, known as *Classical Yoga (*yoga-darshana) and Classical Sāmkhya respectively. The position of the former school was codified in the second century A.D. by *Patanjali in his *Yoga-Sūtra, while the latter's metaphysics was outlined one or two centuries later in the *Sāmkhya-Kārikā of *Īshvara Krishna.

If the schools of *Pre-Classical Yoga, as recorded in the *Bhagavad-Gītā, the *Moksha-Dharma, and other didactic portions of the *Mahābhārata epic, espoused a panentheistic philosophy, *Patanjali introduced, as far as one can tell, a dualistic metaphysics. He appears to have rejected the idea that the world is an aspect of the *Divine, and made a radical distinction between Nature (*prakriti) and the transcendental Self (*purusha). Hence *Bhoja, in his commentary (*Rāja-Mārtanda) (I.1), felt justified in characterizing *yoga* as *viyoga* ("separation").

However, even though *Patanjali's system came to be regarded as one of the six classical schools of *Hinduism, its dualism prevented it from assuming greater cultural significance. The dominant philosophical orientation within the fold of Hinduism has always been nondualist (*advaita*). Thus, the schools of *Post-Classical Yoga, as recorded in the *Yoga-Upanishads and the works of *Tantrism and *hatha-yoga, reaffirmed the panentheism of earlier times. This is also the essential position of the Integral Yoga (*pūrna-yoga) of Shri *Aurobindo. See also *ashta-anga-yoga, asparsha-yoga, bhakti-yoga, hatha-yoga, jnāna-yoga, karma-yoga, kriyā-yoga, kundalinī-yoga, lambikā-yoga, mantra-yoga, nāda-yoga, panca-dasha-anga-yoga, rāja-yoga, sapta-anga-yoga, shad-anga-yoga.*

yoga-agni ("fire of Yoga") is said in the *Yoga-Shikhā-Upanishad* (I.26) to "cook" the *body and bring it to sentience (*ajada*). This idea is fundamental to *hatha-yoga*, which seeks to transmute the body into a "divine" vehicle with great paranormal capacities (*siddhi*).

yoga-anga ("limb of Yoga"). See *anga*.

Yoga-Anushāsana-Sūtra-Vritti ("Commentary on the Aphorisms Expounding Yoga"), also called *Pradīpikā*, is a subcommentary by *Bhāva Ganesha Dīkshita, a pupil of *Vijnāna Bhikshu. It seeks to elucidate his teacher's commentary on the *Yoga-Sūtra*.

yoga-ārūdha ("Yoga ascended"). See *ārūdha*.

yoga-āsana ("Yoga posture") is described in the *Gheranda-Samhitā* (II.44f.) thus: Placing one's stretched (and crossed) feet on the knees with upturned palms on the ground, one should inhale and fix one's gaze at the tip of the nose (*nāsa-agra*).

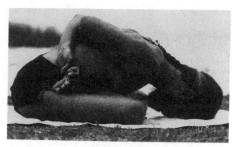

81. *Yoga-āsana.*

yoga-bala ("power of Yoga") is a phrase often used in the literature of *Pre-Classical Yoga. Thus, the *Bhagavad-Gītā* (VIII.10) observes that, at the time of *death, the *yogin* should employ the power of *Yoga and devotion (*bhakti*) in order to steady the *mind, so that he may reach the *Divine.

Yoga-Bhāshya ("Discussion on Yoga") is the oldest extant commentary on the *Yoga-Sūtra*. This work, which is attributed to *Vyāsa, was probably composed in the fifth century A.D. and is the basis for all subsequent exegetical efforts in *Classical Yoga. While Vyāsa shows great familiarity with *Yoga, he does not appear to have belonged to the direct lineage of *Patanjali, the author of the *Sūtra*. He seems, rather, to rely strongly on the ideas of the Sāmkhya teacher Vindhya-vāsin, who lived probably in the fourth century A.D. Some *Hindu authorities have expressed the belief that the *Bhāshya* was composed by Patanjali himself, but this does not seem to be very probable, because the interpretations and terminology of the *Bhāshya* are occasionally at variance with the *Yoga-Sūtra*.

Yoga-Bhāskara ("Illuminator of Yoga") is a no longer available work on *Yoga by Kavīndrācārya Sarasvatī (A.D. 1600–1675), who also authored a number of works on *Vedānta.

Yoga-Bīja ("Seed of Yoga") is a comparatively recent, short treatise of around ten printed pages on the rules of yogic practice, especially *breath control. It is ascribed to God *Shiva himself.

Yogācāra is the idealist school of Mahāyāna *Buddhism founded by Asanga in the fourth century A.D. This school is criticized by *Vācaspati Mishra in his *Tattva-Vaishāradī* (II.15) for its concept of *liberation. It is sometimes thought that *Patanjali's *Yoga-Sūtra* (IV.14–16) refers to Yogācāra as well, but the reference must be to an earlier Vijnānavāda tradition, such as the one represented by the *Lankā-Avatāra-Sūtra*.

Yoga-Cintāmani ("Thought-Gem of Yoga") is a work by Shivānanda Sarasvatī comprising around two hundred folios. It was probably authored in the late eighteenth or early nineteenth century A.D.

Yoga-Cūdāmany-Upanishad ("Secret Teaching on the Crest Jewel of Yoga") is one of the *Yoga-Upanishads and was probably composed some time in the fourteenth or fifteenth century A.D. consisting of 121 stanzas, it expounds *hatha-yoga* from a *Vedāntic point of view. The anonymous author of this work subscribes to the sixfold *path (*shad-anga-yoga*), paying particular attention to what he calls *prāna-samrodha* ("restraint of the breath"). The first seventy-one verses summarize the essential of *hatha-yoga* theory and practice. This is followed by an excursus on ontogenetic matters, which is probably an interpolation. The text concludes with a description of sense withdrawal (*pratyāhāra*), and appears to be incomplete. Indeed, it is presumably a fragment of the *Goraksha-Paddhati*.

yoga-darshana ("Yoga view") is a phrase first found in the *Mahābhārata* (XII.294.26), where it has a general meaning. Later, it came to refer specifically to the philosophical system formulated by *Patanjali and elaborated by his commentators. It is also known as *Classical Yoga.

yoga-griha ("Yoga house"). See *matha*.

yoga-kaksha ("yogic girdle"), as mentioned in the *Bhāgavata-Purāna* (IV.6.39), is a strap to secure the position of the knees while being seated in one of the postures (*āsana*).

Yoga-Kārikā is an original Sanskrit commentary on the *Yoga-Sūtra* largely based on the explanations of *Vyāsa and *Vācaspati Mishra. This work, which comprises 346 verses, was composed together with an autocommentary entitled *Saralā-Tīkā* by *Hariharānanda Āranya.

Yoga-Kārnikā ("Ear-Ornament of Yoga") of Aghorānanda was authored in the late eighteenth or early nineteenth century A.D. This compilation has thirteen chapters comprising over twelve hundred verses, and its value lies in the many quotations from other (including lost) works.

yoga-kritya ("Yoga praxis") is a synonym for *sādhana* and occurs in different passages of the *Mahābhārata* (e.g., XII.294.6).

Yoga-Kundaly-Upanishad is one of the *Yoga-Upanishads and probably belongs to the fourteenth or fifteenth century A.D. It consists of three chapters with a total of 171 stanzas. As the title suggests, this work deals with *kundalinī-yoga*, which is expounded from the perspective of the nondualist metaphysics of *Advaita-Vedānta. The first chapter outlines the spiritual *path; the second consists of a detailed exposition of the *khecarī-mudrā*; and the third describes the higher yogic processes and is interspersed with metaphysical speculations.

yoga-mārga ("yogic path"). The metaphor of spiritual life as a path or road (*mārga*) goes hand in hand with the image of the spiritual aspirant as an itinerant who progresses from one level of accomplishment to the next. The *Mahābhārata* (XII.289.53) observes that it is a great *sin to abandon the yogic way simply out of comfort (*kshema*). More radical schools of nondualism reject the path metaphor since it merely reinforces the illusion that there is a separate entity whereas, as they see it, only the one *Reality exists. Apart from such metaphysical objections, however, the path metaphor corresponds to psychological actualities and is useful to the degree that it does not serve goal-oriented striving.

Yoga-Mārtanda ("Sun-Bird of Yoga") is a work of 188 stanzas ascribed to *Goraksha and appears to be a fragment of the *Goraksha-Paddhati*.

yoga-mudrā ("seal of Yoga") is listed but not described in the *Hatha-Ratna-Āvali* (III.12) as one of the eighty-four postures (*āsana*). According to some contemporary works on *hatha-yoga*, this posture is executed by bending forward while seated cross-legged, with the arms behind one's back and the hands folded. *Upanishad Brahmayogin, in his commentary on the *Tri-Shikhi-Brāhmana-Upanishad (II.93), understands the *yoga-mudrā* as a hand gesture, equating it with the "seal of awareness" (*cin-mudrā*).

Yogananda, Paramahamsa (A.D. 1893–1952), was one of the early *Yoga masters to come to the West. Paramahamsa ("Supreme Swan") Yogananda, a pupil of Sri Yukteshwar (Sanskrit: Shrī Yukteshvara), founded the Self-Realization Fellowship in 1920 and achieved world fame through his book *Autobiography of a Yogi* (first published in 1946). He taught Kriya-Yoga (Sanskrit: *kriyā-yoga*), which is considered akin to *rāja-yoga*, and was eager to reconcile *Hinduism with Christianity.

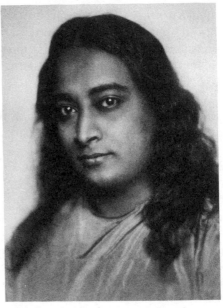

82. Paramahamsa Yogananda.

yoga-nidrā ("Yoga sleep") is an expression widely used in the literature of *Post-Classical Yoga to denote the highest state of *consciousness. In *Hindu mythology, *yoga-nidrā* is the state of God *Vishnu at the end of a world age (*yuga*), when the universe is temporarily dissolved until the great God reawakens.

Some contemporary *Yoga authorities employ the phrase *yoga-nidrā* to designate a state of deep relaxation. The term is also applied to a yogic posture (*āsana*), which is executed by interlacing the legs behind one's neck while resting on one's back with the hands clasped behind one's waist.

yoga-patta or **-pattaka** ("yogic table") is a contraption for resting the arms during meditation. It is mentioned in the *Tattva-Vaishāradī (II.46) and is also listed in the *Agni-Purāna (XC.10) as one of the paraphernalia of the newly initiated *disciple and in another passage (CCIV.11) as one of the utensils of a forest-dwelling ascetic (*vānaprastha*). *Yoga-patta* can also refer to a knee band, used during *meditation. In some contexts, furthermore, *yoga-patta* denotes a kind of ritual.

Yoga-Pradīpikā ("Light on Yoga") of Baladeva Mishra is one of the commentaries on the *Yoga-Sūtra*, composed in the twentieth century A.D.

Yoga-Rāja-Upanishad, which consists of only twenty-one stanzas, is one of the *Yoga-Upanishads. It speaks of *mantra-, *laya-, *rāja-, and *hatha-yoga, and deals particularly with the nine psychoenergetic centers (*cakra).

Yoga-Sāra-Samgraha ("Compendium of the Essence of Yoga"), also entitled *Jnāna-Pradīpā* ("Torch of Knowledge"), is a concise summary of *Classical Yoga by the renowned scholar *Vijnāna Bhikshu.

yoga-shāstra ("Yoga teaching/textbook"). See *shāstra*.

Yoga-Shāstra ("Textbook of Yoga") is a medieval work of 334 stanzas attributed to *Dattātreya, expounding the principles *hatha-yoga. This text has a *Tantric orientation, as is clear from its description of *vajrolī-mudrā, which involves sexual intercourse (*maithunā) in which both the male and female practitioner seek to absorb each other's "semen" (*bindu). Although the text knows of the tradition of 840,000 postures (*āsana), it only describes the lotus posture (*padma-āsana) and then proceeds to explain the more esoteric practices of the "seals" (*mudrā) and "locks" (*bandha).

Yoga-Shikhā-Upanishad ("Secret Doctrine of the Crest of Yoga") is one of the *Yoga-Upanishads. It comprises six chapters with a total of 390 stanzas. The last chapter was probably appended later. This *Upanishad is presented in the form of a didactic dialogue between *Shankara (here God *Shiva) and *Hiranyagarbha. On the basis of the nondualist metaphysics of *Vedānta, the anonymous author develops the outlines of a philosophy of the *body. The *yogin is asked to "energize" (*ranjayet*) his body (*deha) through the *fire of Yoga. The treatment that follows is a summary of *hatha-yoga lore, which ranges from brief instructions about rousing the *sarasvatī-nādī and the *kundalinī-shakti ("serpent power") to an original exposition of esoteric *anatomy. The fifth chapter repeats some of the information given in the first and also contains details about the psychoenergetic "channels" (*nādī). The concluding chapter deals specifically with the process of rousing the serpent power that lies dormant in the *body. Thus, the approach favored in this work is that of *kundalinī-yoga.

yoga-siddhi ("yogic perfection"). See *siddhi*.

Yoga-Siddhānta-Candrikā ("Moonlight on the Yoga System"), also entitled *Yoga-Sūtra-Gūdha-Artha-Dyotikā*, is work by Nārāyana Tīrtha, who also authored the *Sūtra-Artha-Bodhinī*.

Yoga-Sudhā-Ākāra ("Mine of Nectar on Yoga") is a work by Sadāshivendra Sarasvatī who lived in the eighteenth century A.D.

Yoga-Sūtra ("Aphorisms of Yoga") is the authoritative exposition of *Classical Yoga, which is ascribed to *Patanjali. This brief text was probably composed in the early post-Christian era, though some scholars place it into the second century B.C. Also known as *Pātanjala-Sūtra*, this work comprises four chapters (*pādā*) with a total of 195 aphorisms (some editions have one additional *sūtra*). Attempts to dissect this composition into independent textual units have failed to convince, and *Patanjali's work appears to be relatively homogeneous. There is some evidence, however, that the author incorporated a series of existing definitions dealing with the eight "limbs" (*anga*) of *Yoga—i.e., aphorisms II.28–III.3 (or III.8). If this conclusion is correct, *Patanjali's Yoga should be more appropriately called *kriyā-yoga* rather than *ashta-anga-yoga*.

The first chapter, entitled *samādhi-pāda* ("chapter on *enstasy"), outlines the principal processes involved in the systematic transformation of *consciousness. The second chapter, called *sādhana-pāda* ("chapter on the means"), introduces the basic concepts of *kriyā-yoga* practice. Then, at aphorism II.28 the discussion switches over to the eightfold path. The third chapter bears the title *vibhūti-pada*, as it deals with the paranormal manifestations of Yoga, which are known as *vibhūtis* or *siddhis*. However, this section also contains important information about the higher stages of yogic practice. The final chapter, styled *kaivalya-pāda* ("chapter on aloneness"), introduces important philosophical notions and also treats of the terminal stages of Yoga, including *liberation itself, which is called *kaivalya*.

Although *Patanjali understands his compilation merely as an "exposition" (*anushāsana*) of existing materials, his work nevertheless does not lack originality. In his endeavor to formalize the yogic tradition, he has introduced new concepts and terms that clearly evince the autonomy of *Classical Yoga as one of the leading schools or philosophical systems (*darshana*) of *Hinduism. In terminology, the *Yoga-Sūtra* is close to Mahāyāna *Buddhism, and the connection between *Classical Yoga and Buddhism has often been noted by scholars, though no detailed study has hitherto been undertaken. Particularly the parallels between the *Yoga-Sūtra* and the *Abhisamaya-Alankarā* deserve closer scrutiny.

Given the importance of the *Yoga-Sūtra*, it is not surprising that it has given rise to a large number of exegetical works. The oldest available commentary is the *Yoga-Bhāshya*, which furnishes the key to our understanding of *Patanjali's work. Other important commentaries are *Shankara's *Vivarana*, *Vācaspati Mishra's *Tattva-Vaishāradī*, and *Vijnāna Bhikshu's *Yoga-Vārttika*.

Yoga-Sūtra-Artha-Candrikā ("Moonlight on the Meaning of the Aphorisms of Yoga"), also entitled *Pāda-Candrikā*, is a commentary on the *Yoga-Sūtra*, authored by Ananta(-deva), who lived in the nineteenth century A.D.

Yoga-Sūtra-Bhāshya-Vivarana. See *Vivarana*.

Yoga-Sūtra-Gūdha-Artha-Dyotikā. See *Yoga-Siddhānta-Candrikā*.

Yoga-Taranga ("Wave of Yoga") is a treatise similar to the *Yoga-Sāra-Samgraha*. It was authored by Deva Tīrtha Svāmin, a disciple of *Vidyāranya Tīrtha.

Yoga-Tattva-Upanishad ("Secret Teaching on the Principles of Yoga") belongs to the genre of *Yoga-Upanishads. The anonymous author of this short tract of 142 stanzas seeks to integrate different forms of Yoga on the philosophical foundations of *Advaita-Vedānta. He emphasizes the interdependence of *Yoga and gnosis (*jnāna) and outlines the yogic *path, mentioning the four stages (*avasthā), the five obstacles (*vighna), the right environment (*desha) for the practice of *breath control, rules about *diet, the paranormal powers (*siddhi), the practice of concentration (*dhāranā), techniques of *hatha-yoga, and the condition of "living liberation" (*jīvan-mukti). This work decries intellectualism as well as ascetical torturing of the body (*kāya-klesha*).

Yoga-Upanishads are a group of twenty-one *Upanishads that were composed after the *Yoga-Sūtra* and that expound *Vedānta-based yogic teachings, particularly *hatha-yoga and *kundalinī-yoga. Many of these texts belong to the fourteenth and fifteenth centuries. The following are generally listed among this group: *Advaya-Tāraka-, *Amrita-Nāda-, *Amrita(-Nāda)-Bindu-, *Brahma-Vidyā-, *Darshana-, *Dhyāna-Bindu-, *Hamsa-, *Kshurikā-, *Mahā-Vākya-, *Mandala-Brāhmana-, *Nāda-Bindu-,

*Pāshupata-Brāhma-, *Shāndilya-, *Tejo-Bindu-, *Tri-Shikhi-Brāhmana-,
*Varāha-, *Yoga-Cūdāmany-, *Yoga-Kundaly-, *Yoga-Rāja-, *Yoga-Shikhā-,
and *Yoga-Tattva-Upanishad.

Yoga-Vārttika, also entitled *Pātanjala-Bhāshya-Vārttika,* is an extensive commentary on the *Yoga-Sūtra, composed by *Vijnāna Bhikshu.
It contains much original material and numerous quotations from
*Hindu philosophical and religious literature. Next to the *Yoga-Bhāshya
of *Vyāsa and the *Vivarana of *Shankara, this is the single most important commentary on *Patanjali's aphorisms.

Yoga-Vāsishtha-Rāmāyana, also called *Ārsha-Rāmāyana* or *Jnāna-
Vāsishtha,* is a didactic poetic work of around thirty thousand verses
written in elegant Sanskrit and attributed to Vālmīki, the composer of
the great *Rāmāyana epic. The *Yoga-Vāsishtha* is presented as a dialogue
between Prince *Rāma and his teacher *Vashishta. There has been
much scholarly speculation about the date of this work, and estimates
range from the ninth to the thirteenth century A.D. It is probable that
it was composed after the *Laghu-Yoga-Vāsishta, which can be assigned
to the early tenth century A.D. There are a number of abridgements
of this massive work, notably the *Yoga-Vāsishtha-Sāra-Samgraha.
   Be that as it may, the *Yoga-Vāsishtha* has inspired countless generations of spiritual aspirants. Its philosophical basis is *Advaita-
Vedānta: There is only the Single Consciousness (*eka-citta*), which is
formless, omnipresent, and omniscient. The multifarious objects of the
world are present in it like innumerable images carved in stone or, as
one passage (III.2.55) has it, like pictures in the artist's mind. The
world, which is perceived as a result of our congenital nescience
(*avidyā*), appears to the finite *mind as something external to itself. It
is described as a dream or a bubble arising in the *Absolute.
   However, this metaphysical truth is to be realized, through unmediated experience, rather than believed. The spiritual *path outlined
in the *Yoga-Vāsishtha* is that of *jnāna-yoga and has great similarity with
the *buddhi-yoga of the *Bhagavad-Gītā, which is founded in a harmonious blending of wisdom (*jnāna*) and action (*karma*). Since, according
to this work, the *mind creates its own *bondage and *liberation, there
is no need to renounce the world physically once the truth of the single
*Consciousness has been experienced. This is called the path of "men-
tal liberation" (*cetya-muktatā*).
   *Yoga is variously defined as "restraint of the fluctuations of *con-
sciousness," "freedom from sensation," and "separation from the effects of the poison of passion." Sage *Vashishta, who acts as a

spokesman for this Yoga, teaches a discipline comprising seven stages (*bhūmi*), terminating in the *yogin's "abiding in the *Fourth" (*turya-ga*).

Yoga-Vāsishtha-Sāra-Samgraha ("Compendium of the Essence of the *Yoga-Vāsishtha*) is a digest of the teachings of the *Yoga-Vāsishtha-Rāmāyana*, compiled by *Vidyāranya.

yoga-vid ("Yoga knower") is, according to the *Yoga-Cūḍāmany-Upanishad* (64), one who knows about the harmonious identity (*samarasa-aikyatva*) of the two forms of the human semen (*bindu*). This is a common esoteric explanation in the *hatha-yoga* tradition. Elsewhere, the term is often simply used as a synonym for *yogin.

Yoga-Vishaya ("Object of Yoga") is a short work of thirty-three stanzas ascribed to *Matsyendra, though belonging to a later date. It covers such basic topics as the nine psychoenergetic centers (*cakra*), the three "knots" (*granthi*), and the nine "gates" (*dvāra*).

Yoga-Yājnavalkya(-Samhitā), whose full title is ***Yoga-Yājnavalkya-Gītā*** (or ***-Gītā-Upanishad***), is a work on *hatha-yoga*, consisting of 506 stanzas. It is written in the form of a dialogue between *Yājnavalkya and his wife Gargi. P. C. Divanji (1954), the editor of this Sanskrit text, has placed it in the second century A.D. This assignment is based on the identification of the author of the *Yoga-Yājnavalkya* with his namesake who composed the *Yājnavalkya-Smriti* and who in one stanza (III.110) recommends the study of "the Yoga teachings (*yoga-shāstra*) promulgated by me." However, an analysis of the contents and terminology of the *Yoga-Yājnavalkya* suggests a much later date, perhaps the thirteenth or fourteenth century A.D. There are many parallels between this work and the *Yoga-Upanishads, notably the *Shāndilya-Upanishad*. Cf. *Brihad-Yogi-Yājnavalkya*.

yoga-yuj ("Yoga joined") sometimes stands for the spiritual novice, as in the *Vishnu-Purāna* (VI.7), where he is enjoined to first contemplate the "gross" (*sthūla*) form of existence before proceeding to the more "subtle" (*sūkshma*) aspects.

yoga-yukta ("Yoga yoked") is a synonym for *yogin, used particularly widely in the literature of *Pre-Classical Yoga. It denotes the practitioner who has brought his *senses and *mind under control by means of the techniques of *Yoga.

yogi-deha ("*yogin's* body") is the transubstantiated *body of the *adept of *hatha-yoga. According to the *Yoga-Shikhā-Upanishad (I.41), this body is invisible even to the *deities. It is free from change and *bondage and is endowed with a variety of paranormal powers (*siddhi). It is described as resembling the ether (*ākāsha). See also *divya-deha*.

yogin is a male practitioner of *Yoga. The *Shiva-Samhitā (II.5) defines the *yogin* as someone who knows that the entire universe is situated within his own *body. Similarly, the *Siddha-Siddhānta-Paddhati (II.31) states that he is called a *yogin* who fully knows the nine psychoenergetic centers (*cakra), the three "signs" (*lakshya), the fivefold ether (*ākāsha), and the "ambrosial shower" (*dhāra*) issuing from the *kāla in the *head.

There are different categories of *yogins*, depending on the type and rigor of their yogic disciplines, as well as their spiritual attainment. The *Yoga-Shikhā-Upanishad (I.75f.) distinguishes two kinds of *yogins*: those who pierce through the "sun" (*sūrya) by means of the yogic techniques and those who break down the door of the central conduit (*sushumnā-nādī) and drink the nectar from the cranial bowl. *Upanishad Brahmayogin explains the former type as *samnyāsa-yogins* (renouncers) and the latter as *kevala-yogins* (radical practitioners). The *Shiva-Purāna (VII.2.38.25ff.) groups *yogins* according to their different paranormal abilities (*siddhi). The *Yoga-Bhāshya (III.51) offers the following fourfold classification: the *prathama-kalpika (neophyte); the *mādhu-bhūmika (who has reached the "honeyed level"); the *prajnā-jyotis (the advanced practitioner enjoying the light of gnosis); and the *atikrānta-bhāvanīya (transcender).

yoginī is a female practitioner of *Yoga. According to the *Hatha-Yoga-Pradīpikā (III.99), a *yoginī* is more specifically a *woman initiate who can preserve her own genital ejaculate (*rajas) and suck up the male semen (*bindu) through the practice of the *vajrolī-mudrā. In *Tantric contexts, the term *yoginī* can also refer to the group of eight, sixteen, sixty-four or more female divinities, which are forms of the Goddess *Durgā. The cultic worship of these *yoginīs* emerged in the ninth century A.D. and is related to the tradition of *Shaktism.

yogi-pratyaksha ("yogic perception") is another term for "direct apprehension" (*sākshāt-kārana), which involves the *yogin's conscious identification with an object. This is the basis of the practice of "coincidence" (*samāpatti) through which various paranormal powers (*siddhi) can be acquired.

yogi-rāj ("ruler of *yogins*"), also sometimes called *yoga-rāj* ("ruler of Yoga") is an honorific title granted to a spiritual master.

yogyatā ("fitness") is a technical term of *Classical Yoga, which was introduced by *Vācaspati Mishra in his *Tattva-Vaishāradī* (I.4) to explain the special correlation (*samyoga*) between the transcendental *Self and the finite *consciousness or *mind, which is not spatiotemporal but a kind of "preestablished harmony." *Yogyatā* denotes a dual capacity (*shakti*), namely *Nature's capacity to be experienced (*bhogya-shakti*) and the *Self's capacity for experiencing (*bhoktri-shakti*). See also *pratibimba, samnidhi*.

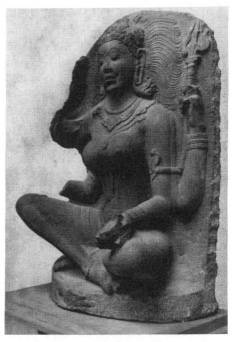

84. A yoginī.

yoni is derived from the verbal root *yu* ("to fasten, join") and means literally "holder." This word has a wide spectrum of applications—ranging from "source" to "home" to "vulva." In yogic contexts, it principally stands for the perineum or the vagina. Some texts describe it as being situated in the pericarp of the lotus at the base of the spine, known as the *mūlādhāra-cakra*. This area is also called *yoni-sthāna* ("perineal place") and *kāma-rūpa* ("desire formed") and in the *Dhyāna-Bindu-Upanishad* (45) is

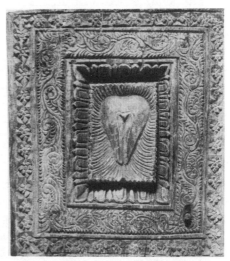

85. The vulva (yoni) is a symbolic representation of the Goddess and is used in ritual worship.

said to be "adored by all *yogins*." It is thought to contain an inward-facing "phallus" (*linga*), which is a symbol of creativity.

yoni-bandha ("perineal lock") is a technique of *hatha-yoga, which is described in the *Yoga-Tattva-Upanishad (120f.) as follows: Pressing the heels firmly against the perineum (*yoni), one should force the *apāna life force upward.

yoni-mudrā ("perineal seal") is occasionally used synonymously with *yoni-bandha. Some authorities identify this practice with the *shāmbhavī-mudrā, which they explain as the means for finding the "source" (*yoni) within oneself. It is referred to but not described in the *Hatha-Yoga-Pradīpikā (III.43). However, Brahmānanda in his *Jyotsnā commentary explains it as the "contraction of the penis" (medhra-ākuncana), equating this technique with the *vajrolī-mudrā. The *Shiva-Samhitā (IV.1ff.) states that one should concentrate on the "prop" (ādhāra), that is, the lowest psychoenergetic center of the *body at the base of the spine, and contract the perineum while inhaling. The *Gheranda-Samhitā (III.38) further specifies that inhalation should be done by means of the *kākī-mudrā. The yoni-mudrā is widely praised in the scriptures of *hatha-yoga and *Tantrism for enabling the *yogin to arrest ejaculation, even after the semen (*bindu) has begun to flow already. See also mudrā, shakti-cālana-mudrā; cf. ashvinī-mudrā.

yuga ("aeon"). See World ages.

yukta ("yoked") is often found in combination with other words, such as yukta-svapna ("controlled dreaming"). It is derived from the same verbal root—yuj—as the word *yogin. See also yoga-yukta.

yukta-ātman ("yoked self") is a common synonym in the scriptures of *Pre-Classical Yoga for the self-controlled *yogin, who, as the *Bhagavad-Gītā (VI.29) puts it, regards everything with the same calm indifference, or *sama-darshana. The *Uddhāva-Gītā (II.45) compares him to fire, for he has become bright through his *asceticism.

yukti ("means"). The *Laghu-Yoga-Vāsishtha (V.10.128f.) mentions the following four means of controlling the *mind: the acquisition of Self-knowledge (adhyātma-vidyā-adhigama), mixing with holy men (sādhu-samgama), abandonment of desire (vāsanā-samparityāga), and restraint of the motion of the breath (prāna-spanda-nirodhana). Elsewhere (VI.1.58), it speaks of two principal means: Self-knowledge (*ātma-jnāna) and *breath control (prāna-samyama).

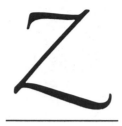

Zen. The Japanese word *zen* is derived from its Chinese equivalent *ch'an*, meaning "meditation," which is a direct translation of the Sanskrit term **dhyāna* (in Pali, the language of the Buddha: *jhāna*). Zen is Japan's form of **Yoga and is close in spirit to the spontaneous (**sahaja*) approach characteristic of certain schools of medieval **Tantrism. Through meditative sitting (Japanese: *za-zen*) and the use of attention-focusing devices known in Japanese as *koans*, the Zen practitioner endeavors to break through to the pure "Buddha mind" in sudden illumination (Japanese: *satori*). The state of *satori* is to be distinguished from the average yogic **samādhi*. Whereas the former occurs on the basis of the **waking consciousness, the latter is a mental transmutation that is preceded by sensory inhibition (**pratyāhāra*) in deep **meditation. Rather, the fleeting *satori* illumination is similar in nature to the permanent condition of **sahaja-samādhi*. Both reveal reality "as it is" (*yathā-bhūta*), free from all mental distortions.

Zest. See *utsāha, vīrya.*

BIBLIOGRAPHY

1. References

Aurobindo, Sri. *The Life Divine*. 2 vols. Pondicherry, India: Sri Aurobindo Ashram, 1977. First publ. 1955.

⸺. *The Synthesis of Yoga*. Pondicherry, India: Sri Aurobindo Ashram, 1976. First publ. 1948.

⸺. *Essays on the Gita*. Pondicherry, India: Sri Aurobindo Ashram, 1949.

Bharati, Agehananda. *The Tantric Tradition*. London: Rider, 1965.

Divanji, P. C. "The Yogayājñavalkya." *Journal of the Bombay Branch of the Royal Asiatic Society*, new series, vol. 28 (1953), pp. 99–158, 215–268; vol. 29 (1954), pp. 96–128.

Eliade, Mircea. *Yoga: Immortality and Freedom*. Princeton, N.J.: Princeton University Press, 1969.

Hacker, Paul. "Śankara der Yogin und Śankara der Advaitin: Einige Beobachtungen." *Beiträge zur Geistesgeschichte Indiens: Festschrift für E. Frauwallner*. Vienna, 1968. pp. 119–148.

Jung, Carl Gustav. *Psychology and the East*. Princeton, N.J.: Princeton University Press, 1978.

Krishna, Gopi. *Kundalini: The Evolutionary Energy in Man*. London: Robinson & Watkins, 1971.

Linquist, Sigurd. *Die Methoden des Yoga*. Lund, Sweden: 1935.

Nowotny, Fausta. *Eine durch Miniaturen erläuterte Doctrina Mystica aus Srinagar*. The Hague, Netherlands: Mouton & Co., 1958.

Radhakrishnan, Sarvepalli. *The Bhagavadgītā*. London: Routledge & Kegan Paul, 1960. First publ. 1948.

Singh, Mohan. *Gorakhnath and Mediaeval Hindu Mysticism*. Lahore, India: Mohan Singh, 1937.

van Buitenen, J. A. B. "Studies in Sāṃkhya." *Journal of the American Oriental Society*, vol. 76 (1957), pp. 15–25, 88–107.

Wilber, Ken. "Are Chakras Real?" in John White, ed., *Kundalini, Evolution, and Enlightenment*. Garden City, N.Y.: Anchor Books, 1979. pp. 120–131.

Woods, James Haughton. *The Yoga-System of Patañjali*. Delhi, India: Motilal Banarsidass, 1966.

Yogananda, Paramahamsa. *Autobiography of a Yogi*. Los Angeles, Calif.: Self-Realization Fellowship, 1987. First publ. 1946.

Zvelebil, Kamil V. *The Poets of the Powers*. London: Rider, 1973.

2. Recommended Reading

Alyar, K. Nārāyanasvāmi. *Thirty Minor Upanishads*. El Reno, Okla.: Santarasa Publications, 1980. First publ. 1914. This volume contains renderings of a fair number of minor Upanishads, including some of the Yoga-Upanishads. The translations are not always accurate but are still useful.

Avalon, Arthur (alias Sir John Woodroffe). *The Serpent Power*. New York: Dover Publications, 1958. First publ. 1919. A classic study of the esotericism and complex symbolism of *hatha-yoga*. It contains renderings of the *Shat-Cakra-Nirūpana* ("Specification of the Six Centers") and the *Pādukā-Pancaka* ("Five [Verses] on the Footstool").

Basham, A. L. *The Wonder That Was India: A Survey of the History and Culture of the Indian Sub-Continent Before the Coming of the Muslims*. New York: Grove Press, 1954. The best general introduction to India's pluralistic culture.

Da Free, John. *The Enlightenment of the Whole Body*. Middletown, Calif.: Dawn Horse Press, 1978. An excellent account of esoteric anatomy, founded in the author's personal experience and examined from the viewpoint of enlightenment.

Daniélou, Alain. *The Gods of India: Hindu Polytheism*. New York: Inner Traditions International, 1985. First publ. 1964. A systematic, illustrated presentation of Hindu mythology, which is helpful to a proper understanding of Yoga.

Deussen, Paul. *Sixty Upanishads of the Veda*. 2 vols. Transl. from the German by V. M. Bedekar and G. B. Palsule. Delhi, India: Motilal Banarsidass, 1980. First publ. 1897. This is the English translation of Deussen's path-making renderings of no fewer than sixty Upanishads, including many of the Yoga-Upanishads. Although the translations can now be improved upon, this compilation is still the most comprehensive attempt of its kind.

Eliade, Mircea. *Patanjali and Yoga*. New York: Schocken Books, 1975. A short illustrated account of Yoga theory and practice, culled from the author's classic study *Yoga: Freedom and Immortality*.

Feuerstein, Georg. *Yoga: The Technology of Ecstasy* (Los Angeles, Calif.: J. P. Tarcher, 1989). An in-depth survey of the history, literature, and branches of Yoga, with numerous quotations from the Sanskrit scriptures, written for the lay reader and also useful to the professional.

————. *The Yoga-Sūtra of Patañjali: A New Translation and Commentary*. Rochester, Vt.: Inner Traditions, 1990. A word-by-word translation of the *Yoga-Sūtra*, the textbook of Classical Yoga, together with a succinct commentary, based on the author's extensive philological and philosophical research on Classical Yoga.

————. *Introduction to the Bhagavad-Gītā: Its Philosophy and Cultural Setting*. Wheaton, Ill.: Quest Books, 1983. One of the few books to present the *Bhagavad-Gītā* in its historical and cultural context, without which the teachings in this important Yoga text are rather difficult to appreciate in full.

————. *Holy Madness: The Outer Limits of Religion and Morality*. New York: Paragon House Publishers, 1991. An examination of antinomian behavior among spiritual adepts, particularly as manifested in the *guru*-disciple relationship.

Goswami, Syundar Shyam. *Layayoga: An Advanced Method of Concentration*. London: Routledge & Kegan Paul, 1980. A wide-ranging treatment of esoteric anatomy and *kundalinī-yoga*, based on the original Sanskrit scriptures of Yoga and Vedānta and featuring numerous quotations from the native Indian texts.

Iyengar, B. K. S. *Light on Yoga: Yoga Dīpikā*. New York: Schocken Books, 1966. One of the most comprehensive and widely read presentations of *hatha-yoga* by a master of this branch of Yoga.

Larson, Gerald James, and Ram Shankar Bhattacharya, eds. *Sāmkhya: A Dualist Tradition in Indian Philosophy*. Princeton, N.J.: Princeton University Press, 1987. The single most comprehensive study of the Sāmkhya tradition with numerous renderings from, or summaries of, the Sanskrit sources.

Panikkar, Raimundo. *The Vedic Experience—Mantramañjarī: An Anthology of the Vedas for Modern Man and Contemporary Celebration*. London: Darton, Longman & Todd, 1977. A penetrating, detailed study of the religiophilosophical ideas in the Vedas, the most ancient part of the canonical scriptures of Hinduism.

Sannella, Lee. *The Kundalini Experience: Psychosis or Transcendence?* Lower Lake, Calif.: Integral Publishing, 1987. A simple introduction to the *kundalinī* phenomenon, based on clinical case studies of subjects who experienced spontaneous *kundalinī* awakenings. This book should be read in conjunction with the autobiographical account by Gopi Krishna (see under References).

Walker, Benjamin. *Tantrism: Its Secret Principles and Practices.* Wellingborough, England: Aquarian Press, 1982. A simple, short introduction to Tantrism.

For further references, the reader is referred to the notes and bibliography in Georg Feuerstein's *Yoga: The Technology of Ecstasy*, the extensive bibliography in Mircea Eliade's *Yoga: Freedom and Immortality*, and the *International Yoga Bibliography* compiled by Howard R. Jarrell and published in 1981 by Scarecrow Press (Metuchen, N.J.). These works also contain references to editions of the Sanskrit texts cited or referred to in this encyclopedic dictionary.